The Herbs of Life

The Herbs of Life
Health & Healing Using
Western & Chinese Techniques

■ Lesley Tierra, L. Ac., Herbalist ■

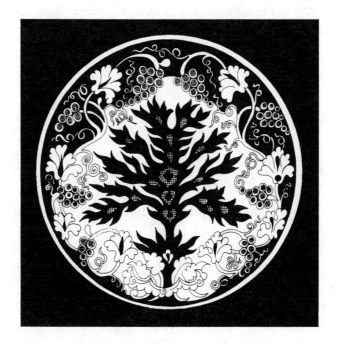

 The Crossing Press ■ Freedom, CA 95019

Copyright © 1992 by Lesley Gunsaulus Tierra

Cover art and design by AnneMarie Arnold
Interior design by Sheryl Karas
Illustrations, pages 25-34 by Amy Sibiga
All other illustrations by Candis Cantin

Printed in the U.S.A.

Library of Congress Cataloguing-in-Publication Data

Tierra, Lesley.
    The herbs of life : health & healing using Western & Chinese techniques / by Lesley Tierra
        p. cm.
    Includes bibliographical references and index
    ISBN 0-89594-499-5 — ISBN 0-89594-498-7 (pbk.)
    1. Herbs—Therapeutic use. 2. Medicine, Chinese. I. Title.
RM666.H33T5
615'.321—dc20   91-38511
                                                           CIP

For

*my husband, Michael, and
our son, Chetan,
my greatest teachers, loving support
and encouragement.*

In Thanks...

Many people have helped me bring this book into greater clarity and purpose.
To them I give my thanks and appreciation:

Michael Tierra, my first and greatest herb teacher, from whom I am always learning more;
Shasta Tierra, for her tremendous enthusiasm and wonderful insights; Steve Blake, for his wonderful ideas and clarity; Mariah Wentworth, Candis Cantin, Savarna (Diana McCabe), Darlena LaOrange-Theocradies and Janet Davis, for their encouragement and support; John Gill, for his openness and belief in me for writing this book; Baba Hari Dass, the Hanuman Fellowship and the Sri Ram Foundation, for their unending inspiration; Senta Tierra, for her unflagging support with the household; Chetan Tierra, for sharing his mom with the computer and for the title of this book; and my parents, Bonnie and Gus Gunsaulus, who taught me that I could accomplish anything I desired.

CONTENTS

CONTENTS

FOREWORD BY MICHAEL TIERRA, L.AC., O.M.D.

The practice of herbalism can be defined as the systematic use and application of herbs and related materials for the purpose of healing. We find evidence of various systems and approaches to the use of herbs throughout ancient and native cultures of the world. *The Herbs of Life* shows the way by which we in the West are able to benefit from the great herbal traditions of China and India which, as it turns out, are not so unlike the way our own once were, previous to the 18th century and the advent of so-called scientific rationalistic thought.

By offering a practical approach to the classification of the therapeutic properties of herbs and foods, this book provides a good introduction to the important process of integrating Eastern and Western approaches into a kind of Planetary Herbalism. Through a renewed appreciation of traditional "energetic" systems especially Chinese herbal medicine, this should allow one to go beyond the overly simplistic "this for that" approach so characteristic of many popular herbals written by non-herbalists.

It is at this point that one might ask what is meant by an energetic approach to healing and classifying herbs for medicine, and how or to what degree does it differ from the predominant Western medical model? To begin with, the Western medical model, which is often imitated by inexperienced herbal practitioners in a kind of "allopathic" herbalism, focuses almost exclusively on relieving the primary symptom of the patient. The traditional wholistic herbalist treats not only the primary symptom, but the underlying causes which precipitate it. *The Herbs of Life* takes this second approach—recommending herbs and other foods which tend to strengthen underlying deficiencies as well as clear the body of toxic wastes. By following the simple guidance which this book provides, the reader can discover the true healing power of herbs and foods with absolutely no risk of the insidious long-term side effects of many, if not most, Western drugs.

Implied in the pages of this work is the belief that the essential principles and methods of traditional herbal medicine are capable of being understood and utilized not only by the professional health practitioner but also by the lay public. This book provides a simple and practical guide to aid in a first attempt at shopping for herbs. It then details the traditional principles of "simpling," or making various effective herbal preparations in a kitchen with only basic kitchen utensils.

Herbalism has been sometimes called "the simpler's art." This is to identify its common bond with folk practice based upon empirical evidence of "what works." This is in contrast to scientific medical knowledge which is primarily derived from research and laboratory experiments. With the present crisis in medicine and health care in the orthodox professions, its increasing exclusivity in terms of cost and availability, the side effects and risks of medical drugs and procedures, most of which are more serious than the disease they are intended to cure, it is no wonder that natural medicine, especially herbal medicine, is on the rise.

There are many unique aspects about this book which place it as a worthy addition to the noble tradition of self-help herbals. It clearly sets forth the way an herbalist thinks about herbs, foods and disease and unites them with various methods that, while presently used as part of the practice of acupuncture, were once and still continue in many places of the world to be the domain of the folk healer. These include such techniques as cupping, moxibustion, meditation and breathing practices along with other simple home remedies that are bound to support one's quest for greater health and wellness.

In terms of nutrition and diet, the book presents a system of energetic classification of foods based on their heating and cooling energies and the principle of "empty and full." This chapter should prove most interesting and of great practical value especially for those who are attempting to find a broader, more universal approach to nutrition based on traditional Chinese energetic principles.

Finally, the book invites the reader to share the experience of an herbalist and healer in the process of furthering the integration of the ancient healing wisdom of the East with the West as we evolve towards a more global awareness. Through this process, it is hoped that the reader will feel empowered to further continue to explore on his or her own the beautiful world of herbalism.

Introduction

I felt invulnerable to disease as a teenager and in my early twenties. I experienced illness, like a cold or flu, as a normal life experience from which I quickly healed. However, in my mid-twenties I began experiencing problems which medical tests couldn't discover or define. I was one of those "doomed" to have recurring bouts of illness with no known cure.

Eventually I discovered the use of herbs and their tremendous healing effects. Attending Heartwood College in Santa Cruz, California, I studied herbs and herbal energetics, Shiatsu massage, dietary therapy, beginning acupuncture theory and wholistic healing. There, I learned how to look at my illness in a different way, and I determined the appropriate diet for healing my condition. With this new perspective, a cure was possible. All together, these factors not only helped me heal my "incurable" problem, but have strengthened me so that ten years later, they have not recurred.

At that point in my life, I had spent five years in managerial work with a large company and then two years doing freelance photography. When I first learned about herbs, it appeared as a vast complicated field in which only well-studied "experts" knew enough to use them for healing. In my first tentative explorations, I discovered this is not so.

Learning to use herbs can be as simple as picking raspberry leaves in your backyard or getting roasted dandelion root from the local herb store. It can also extend to in-depth study of one of several traditional herbal systems still in use by other cultures around the world. The study of herbs is accessible to everyone.

In my own search for healing, I have found five factors to be essential: 1) breathing exercises and contemplation, 2) physical exercise, 3) proper diet, 4) appropriate lifestyle habits, and 5) natural medicines. I have seen over and over with hundreds of patients that these same five factors make all the difference in the quality of their health and lives.

Looking at ourselves as integrated beings, we see how these five aspects interrelate in promoting our health. Sometimes one category needs emphasis over the others. Yet, usually all need to be taken into account to regain and maintain health. Therefore, I have written this book to focus on these five categories, with an emphasis on the fifth, using herbal medicines.

Breathing exercises may at first seem strange to many of us in the West. Yet, when we look deeper at the role of oxygen in our health, we recognize breathing exercise as essential. Oxygen is carried by the blood to every cell of our bodies. With a lack of oxygen, a myriad of problems results—tiredness, poor memory, impaired mental function, heart and lung problems, blood-related conditions and the growth of cancer, viruses and bacteria. Exercising the breath sends oxygen throughout the entire body, cleansing the cells, vitalizing the system, feeding the body with important nutrients, and purifying and relaxing the nervous system and mind.

Contemplation, be it an inward silence, prayer or meditation, is invaluable for creating peace and calmness and relaxing nervous tension, a major contributing factor in modern diseases. Because contemplation is such an individual matter and many books are available on various approaches, only breathing practices are covered in this book. Several specific ones are given in the chapter entitled *Home Therapies*.

Much has been written about the importance of exercise. Therefore, I do not cover it except to say that whichever method you choose should be enjoyable and fun. Otherwise, it creates a poor mental state which defeats the health benefits of the exercise. Stretching, movement and aerobics in some form or another are essential three times a week for good health. Many people need more and should incorporate it as needed.

Proper dietary habits is an old and controversial topic. We are told we "should" follow everything from the five basic food groups to the latest fad. However, every one of us has a unique body based on a different constitution with its own needs. Thus, each of us requires an individualized dietary program; there is no such thing as one diet which is good for every one of us.

When food is looked at in terms of its energy, it is possible, however, to give basic food guidelines which help heal or promote balance for each of us . Further, every type of food can be viewed as a healing agent or a disease culprit. Which it is for you depends on your constitution and individual needs. This way of looking at and using food is covered in the chapter *The Energy of Food*, with further details in *Living With the Seasons*.

Lifestyle habits is a broad category, encompassing our daily patterns, mental attitudes, emotional health and spiritual well-being. While not usually considered a part of health in the West, they are intimately connected with healing and health by traditional Chinese and East Indian Ayurvedic medicines. Our sleeping, eating, working, living and socializing habits all contribute to our health and well being, or to our diseased state.

Just as appropriate diet varies for each of us, so do lifestyle habits vary according to each of our constitutions and health needs. Several of the effects of various lifestyle habits are considered in the chapters *The Process of Health and Healing* and *Living With the Seasons*.

Herbs have formed the basis of most healing methods throughout the world for thousands of years. There is a rich heritage of wisdom and experience to draw upon in using herbs as our natural medicines.

In this book we learn about the many aspects which give herbs their healing potential and how to use them, including their various therapies, remedies and preparations. Herbal healing is included in all chapters of the book, yet Part I specifically introduces and teaches the beginning basics of herbal medicine.

The Herbs of Life is organized to encompass the five factors involved in health and healing in the following way:

Part I encompasses the various aspects of herbs and how they are used for healing. This includes their heating or cooling energies, tastes, properties, chemical constituents, families, formulas and individual information on each herb with projects, preparation recommendations, doses and cautions. It also covers how disease manifests in the body and how to choose herbs accordingly.

Part II covers the various aspects involved in the process of regaining and maintaining health and gives many valuable tools for both healing and preventing sickness. These include learning about the effects of food, the various factors which affect the health and healing process, specific home remedies made with foods, spices and herbs and valuable home therapies as adjunct healing agents.

Part III contains information on how to obtain and make your own healing tools. It has directions for creating herbal medicines and gives information on how to harvest, prepare and store your herbs. Step-by-step instructions on each type of herbal preparation, a guide to shopping for herbs, and herbal medicine kit instructions and contents are provided as well.

This book may be used in several ways. You may choose to read it from cover to cover starting at the beginning. You may also start by just exploring the herbs, remedies, therapies and preparations, leaving the energy of herbs for later in-depth study. Or, you may choose to learn first about the energy of healing, including the energy of herbs, illness and foods. The herbs given may be studied in total, or better yet, you may get to know a few very well before starting to learn them all.

What is important is to take your time: experiment, let it become a part of you, go slowly with areas you don't understand. This is a new way of thinking to most people in western cultures. It takes time and patience to absorb it.

Getting to know herbs is like gaining new friends. It is very rewarding to recognize in the mountains or woods, or even in a local vacant lot, a plant which has helped you or someone you know heal some physical problem. Then the plant is your ally. Every spring I watch for the comfrey to unfold in my yard. It has been a tremendous friend, healing my spider bites and my son's broken arm. I have used it in salves for my son's wounds and the family's summer mosquito bites. This is just one example; many more exist and are waiting to unfold for your use and delight.

Plants are so integrated into our lives that we may not even be aware of how many of the things we use come from them: straw, popcorn, pasta, bread, perfumes, cork, rubber, wood, paper, rope, cotton, beverages, dyes and many chemical drugs are just a few. Many people throughout the world still use tree twigs to clean their teeth. In India people use Neem tree twigs, and the Pueblo people in New Mexico use red willow twigs. The Shikakai tree bark is used to make shampoo in India, while jojoba and soaproot in North America are used for shampoo and soap respectively.

In addition to providing most of our food, plants are the source of our air: in breathing we inhale oxygen and exhale carbon dioxide while plants do just the opposite. This symbiotic relationship between people and plants keeps our atmosphere balanced with the proper amount of elements for the health of both. Further, when plants die, they compost the earth, which provides fertile soil from which new plants can emerge to keep this cycle going. The current deforestation of much of our planet should evoke deep concern from each of us. Without sufficient plants, our own health and the health of the entire planet is severely jeopardized.

It has been written in one of the world's most ancient books, the *Rig Veda*, that the sun is part of the Creator, plants are part of the sun and we are part of plants. This saying poetically demonstrates our intimate connection with plants. They are the gifts of Nature for our healing and well being.

As I have learned to use and cherish herbs and natural healing for my health and that of many others, so do I desire to pass this knowledge on for your betterment and good health, also. I invite you on a journey of looking at your environment as a mystery, where you learn step by step about the exciting world of herbs and what might be at your very fingertips for many of your needs. May you find tremendous benefits and joy in learning about herbs and their myriad applications in promoting health and healing, both for yourself and in serving others!

I.
How to Use Herbs for Health & Healing

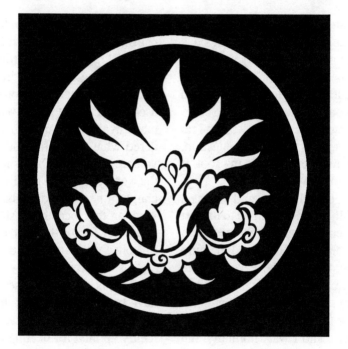

The Nature of Herbal Healing

One night my husband and I were at a family party. We were dancing and enjoying ourselves out on a deck crowded with other people. I had my shoes off. As the night wore on, the dance floor became even more crowded and, suddenly, my foot was impaled by a spike heel from a woman dancing a bit too close to me. The pain was excruciating. Not only could I no longer dance, but walking was out of the question. There was a perfect square indentation on my foot. It began bleeding, bruising and swelling.

My husband quickly looked around and, noting a tree that the deck was built around, climbed to its first branches and picked several leaves. He chewed them up into a pulp and spit them out. He placed the pulp on my wound, creating a poultice of the leaves. Within ten minutes the pain decreased by 50%, and in a half hour I could walk by myself. We replaced the poultice with another, one or two more times that night, and by morning not only could I walk normally, but there was hardly a sign of the wound left!

This experience is one of many I've had proving over and over the powerful and practical healing ability of plants. In this case, leaves from an oak tree healed my wound. Oak leaves are high in tannins which relieve pain and promote wound healing. Yet, many other plants would have also worked. The chlorophyll (making the greenness) in their leaves is extremely healing for the type of wound I had.

Combining the simple knowledge of making a poultice with the awareness of the healing abilities of green leaves, we were able to heal my wound immediately, right there on the dance floor. There was no need to wait until getting home to find something to heal it or to suffer through the next several days of pain and debilitation before it slowly healed on its own, risking a possible infection.

Knowing this basic information has helped me tremendously and many other people as well. It is this useful practical wisdom which I wish to pass on and make available to more people. Have you ever wondered what the plants and "weeds" growing around you are good for? Or has it ever occurred to you that the very thing you need to help you sleep, clear a cough or heal a cold might be right in your very own yard or the local herb shop? There is a veritable pharmacy for most of our ailments right at our fingertips once we learn how to use them.

Using herbs externally, like the poultice that healed my foot, is only one of the many uses of herbs. Herbs have been employed for thousands of years all over the world in a myriad of ways. They are still predominantly applied for healing by several major cultures, such as the Chinese, East Indian and Tibetan. Yet, over the last one hundred years in the West, herbs have been relegated to the status of spices or quaint "folk medicines" with little or no healing value. There are two main reasons for this: 1) the loss of a systematic method for using herbs, and 2) the advent of science with technological industries and their resulting chemical medicines.

Mechanistic Healing

Originally, herbs were used in the West according to a systematic approach called the Humour system.

Promoted by Hippocrates in Greece, this system categorized each person as one of several physiological types. It likewise classified herbs and applied them for healing in a corresponding fashion. In this system, like all traditional healing systems with a theoretical foundation, the individual was evaluated, taking into account any strengths and weaknesses causing the disease. Then the effect the herbal medicine had on the organs, the person and the disease was considered. It was next matched with the cause of the individual's condition.

With the advent of materialistic thinking in the 17th and 18th centuries due largely to Newtonian physics, a mechanistic view of nature has occurred. This proclaims that only what can be substantiated materially is reality. Extending to the human body, this way of thought views the body as a machine governed by mechanical laws and comprised of chemical constituents. As a result, modern medicine has come to view and treat disease separately from the person who experiences it. The disease is identified and then the common treatment for it given. Thus, everyone who receives the same diagnosis gets the same cure.

Likewise, Western herbology has turned from applying herbs according to the Humour system to using them mechanistically. Herbs are applied to treat diseases solely according to their therapeutic properties and chemical constituents. The disease is separated from the individual, and a plant's components are separated from the whole plant to treat the disease.

Such an approach is based on the fallacy of isolation. It sees that one aspect of a person can be isolated and treated separately regardless of the other aspects of the person, or that an herb's part can be used in isolation irrespective of the rest of the plant's components. It results in our simplified approach of asking, "What is in this herb and what is it good for?" and, "What herb can I use for my headache?" This simplistic method of using herbs isolates the disease from the person and the chemical aspects of an herb from its overall individual therapeutic effect.

This view of modern medicine and Western herbology was fully launched when substantial financial support was given only to allopathic medical schools committed to scientific research and high technological needs in the early twentieth century. This was done after a survey of medical schools was completed at the turn of the century to determine which ones were most interested in promoting "scientific medicine," or the newly developing drug and hospital industries.[1]

As a result, 80% of the current schools, including naturopathy, homeopathy and herbology, were closed and ultimately relegated to the status of interesting but ineffective folk medicine. These same schools were the ones which promoted a wholistic and systematic way of viewing individuals, their disease and herbs to heal them.

This shift from traditional medicine to modern medicine has taught us to think that science knows more about us than we could ever understand about ourselves. Yet, as we gain further experience with chemical medicine, we are learning that perhaps Nature knows more about us and healing than we can ever assume with the modern medicine approach.

We are finding that: chemical drugs often create worse problems than the ones they are solving; chemical drugs frequently only maintain a person's condition without ever healing it; sometimes the condition is healed but the person develops other problems later on; and, this method ignores other important and essential factors involved in true healing, such as a person's emotions, family life, work, lifestyle practices, dietary habits and personal needs and satisfaction. It is only when we take these last factors into account that we are effecting a wholistic healing approach.

Symptomatic Versus Energetic Herbology

Thus, a new model for healing is needed. In our search for this new healing model we are experiencing a resurgence of interest in the West in herbs and their healing effects. In exploring this herbal renaissance, it is important to renew our use of herbs according to a wholistic model, one which evaluates every element involved in an individual's condition, takes into account all aspects of an herb's energy and then matches the herbs to the condition accordingly.

Current Western herbology doesn't do this.[2] Instead, it applies herbs *symptomatically*. With this approach, the disease is isolated from the person and herbs are given to treat the disease symptoms, just like modern medicine. For example, if we get a headache, we take willow bark. Sometimes we combine several herbs into a formula for this ailment, yet our approach is always the same: willow bark is good for headaches; therefore, if you have a headache, take willow bark. While this frequently works, it doesn't always. Not every headache is relieved by the same herb. Thus, it is a "hit or miss" approach—something is missing.

Traditional cultures which use herbs according to a theoretical system use herbs *energetically*. Chinese, East Indian Ayurvedic, Tibetan, Middle Eastern Unani and Native American Cherokee medicines are all founded on an energetic basis, although each system is different. To use herbs energetically, we look beyond the symptoms of the disease to alleviating the underlying imbalance which caused the disease. This cause varies according to each individual because all aspects of a person are taken into account, not just the disease itself.

Likewise, each herb is evaluated energetically according to all of its aspects, such as its hot or cold effects, tastes, properties, colors, growing conditions, chemical constituents and so on. The appropriate herbs are then selected which alleviate the underlying cause of the disease. The herb's energies are matched with that of the person, the disease and its cause.

Thus, rather than making the headache the main treatment focus, we look at the person to see what is occurring in the body to cause the headache. The cause for it is then treated instead of just the headache itself. In eliminating the cause, the headache goes, too.

Some causes of a headache may be: 1) liver congestion, 2) stomach upset, 3) tension or 4) weakness in the body. Which cause it is varies according to each person's body and whatever health imbalances exist. Dandelion and feverfew help headaches due to liver congestion; catnip can relieve headaches due to stomach upset; valerian often eases tension headaches; and cinnamon can eliminate headaches due to weakness in the body. Each of these herbs is different, yet each relieves a headache in its own way. This is quite a different approach as opposed to simply giving willow bark for any one of these types of headache.

What is missing in the symptomatic method of giving herbs, therefore, is that only the headache is looked at while the person who has the headache is completely ignored! We assume that every headache is the same and forget that because every one of us is different, each headache is due to a different cause. Thus, the symptomatic way of using herbs is to treat the disease, while the energetic method is to treat the person who has the disease.

A New View of Healing

This book, therefore, is not a typical western herbal where herbs are described symptomatically: "this herb is good for that." Rather, it teaches us how to herbally treat the whole person and the underlying imbalance. It is also geared toward the beginner, both for those who know little, if anything, about herbs and their uses, and also for those who already use herbs but want to move beyond using them symptomatically to applying them energetically.

Because we are going to look at herbs and the process of healing differently in this book, it is important to put all your preconceptions about herbs, health and healing aside for awhile before reading further. Since the principles we are going to learn are quite new to our Western way of thought, they may not fit in with our preconceived notions of health. We are going to build a concept of health based upon ancient principles used by many other cultures around the world.

In the West we have little understanding of how to maintain health and prevent sickness. We have more understanding of how to deal with disease, except those which have multiple causes, such as cancer, arthritis, AIDS and chronic fatigue syndrome. The energetic concept of medicine is important, therefore, because it provides a method for understanding and treating the cause of these complex conditions.

It also takes into account all aspects a person is experiencing. Some of us think we have a disease, like candida or chronic fatigue syndrome, but when we look deeper at the cause of the problem we learn we really don't have that disease. Further, many of us experience problems which can't be identified as a known disease. Instead, we are told to go home because there is nothing wrong with us, or else to seek psychiatric help. That is why it is important to treat the person, not the condition. In treating the person the imbalance can be discovered and corrected. When treating the condition, often a "cure" doesn't exist or our condition doesn't exist!

There are definite strengths of modern medicine, including its ability to heal mechanical injuries, such as broken bones, to perform necessary surgery and to probe the micro-universe. Interestingly, it is through this last means that science is now corroborating the energetics of herbs. Biochemical components are being discovered that have specific properties, tastes and so forth which account for the previously known energetic effects of plants. In most cases they are validating what the common knowledge of that herb has been. This deepens our appreciation of traditional plant wisdom.

For example, herbs which cause a sweat are found to contain volatile oils which open the surface of the body and are known to be antibiotic and antiviral in action. Also certain flavors are caused by specific biochemical agents in the herbs. Sweet indicates there is sugar in the herb, sour indicates the presence of an acid, bitter means it possibly contains an alkaloid, and salty indicates sodium or mineral salts are present. Each of these are used in drugs but are found in herbs in a more balanced way.

While modern medicine is being adopted by many traditional cultures around the world, some countries are extracting its advantages and integrating them with their traditional medicines. For example, many hospitals in China integrate the practice of both modern and traditional medicine. Modern medicine is used for surgery, yet it is often combined with Chinese acupuncture for anesthesia and herbs for recovery. Such a synthesis would be valuable to us in the West.

To learn how to use herbs for healing according to an energetic system, many factors are involved. We first learn how to determine an herb's energy, taking into account all of its various aspects. Then we determine the underlying factors causing the illness. Next, we match the appropriate herbs to the determined condition.

However, this is not all, for other considerations are involved in order to regain and maintain health. It is not always enough just to give the right herbs. Dietary factors may also be involved. If someone is eating foods which contribute to their problem, even when herbs are taken the problem will persist. Therefore, disease-causing foods for that person need to be determined and eliminated, and health-promoting foods substituted. Likewise, lifesyle habits contributing to the illness need to be identified and changed.

How the herbs are going to be used is another element. There are many different applications for the internal and external use of herbs, such as teas, fomentations, poultices, tinctures and pills. Each one has a different purpose and effect. Obtaining the herbs, making your own remedies or knowing how to purchase them is also important to learn.

Extent of Herbal Healing

Before beginning, a basic understanding of the extent and limitation of herbal therapy is important. First, there are three different categories of herbs: mild, strong and toxic. Herbalists mainly use mild herbs because they have nutritive, energetic and therapeutic value without causing reactions or toxic effects.

This is one of the values of using herbs instead of chemical medicines. While mild herbs don't compete with the strong effects of drugs, their food-like nature and complex biochemical processes are more able to affect the entire body and mind. Likewise, they don't throw off any one aspect of the body and cause a reaction or another disease. Therefore, when you find the right herb, you can use less of it and affect more areas of the body than with chemical drugs.

Secondly, wholistic herbal therapy is appropriate to use in almost all conditions, either by itself or as an adjunct to other methods. Because mild herbs do not interfere with chemical drugs, they can be taken to assist modern medical procedures, from surgery and hospitalization to the intake of daily medicines. Herbal therapy can thus be used in complex, serious conditions or in more simple situations.

When using herbal therapy to heal an illness, however, it is important to know when it is not working and other help is needed. For acute ailments, if no improvement is noted within three days, then it may be wise to consider other approaches. For chronic ailments, if no improvement is noted within a month, then another course of treatment might be considered.

Quite often, treating ourselves is difficult since we cannot always see ourselves clearly. Going to an experienced professional, such as an acupuncturist, naturopath or homeopath, can then be invaluable for obtaining an evaluation and an herbal healing program. Further, mechanical injuries are best treated initially with modern medical techniques.

Learning to use herbs can be simple. It can also be a joyous life-long pursuit when all of its complex and various aspects are delved into. On whatever level you choose to encompass herbs within your life, I am sure you will feel enriched and rewarded. We can begin now to reclaim the ancient knowledge of regaining and maintaining health through wholistic herbal healing.

---

[1] This survey was subsidized by the Carnegie and Rockefeller foundations and resulted in the Flexner Report issued by the American Medical Association in 1910.

[2] In England herbs are used more systematically and wholistically today. Yet, it is still based on pathology, not energy.

The Energy of Herbs

In the West, we use herbs symptomatically. We give an herb to treat the symptoms of the illness according to its known use, such as giving willow bark for a headache. This method does not treat the cause of the illness, nor does it take into account all the effects an herb has, most especially its energy. As a result, sometimes the herb is effective, while other times it isn't.

Traditional cultures throughout the world apply herbs according to their energetic effects on the body. The traditional Chinese, East Indian Ayurvedic and Tibetan healing systems, the ancient Greeks and Romans, herbalists throughout Europe until the 17th century and many Native American tribes, most especially the Cherokee, all evolved energetic healing systems which are still in use today.

In the West, we again need to start using an energetic system of healing. By doing so we use herbs efficiently and effectively. Further, we avoid using them improperly, possibly either resulting in no effect, or creating an opposite and undesired effect. Learning the components which comprise the energy of an herb enables us to apply these principles to herbs we aren't familiar with in our own area or in other places we visit while traveling.

Traditional Oriental Medicine offers a useful system because it is practical and simple and has a tradition of 5000 years experience and application. In this system, the energy of an herb has several different aspects which work together to give the herb a unique personality and use. They also determine the conditions for which the herb is effective or ineffective. These aspects are:

- heating or cooling energy
- the five tastes
- the four directions
- other energies and special properties

The first and most important aspect of an herb's energy is it's heating or cooling quality. The effects of tastes, directions and other energies all contribute to this basic heating-cooling category. All together, these components comprise an overall energetic effect. This is then termed the energy of the herb. Each herb has a different effect on the body according to these various parts which comprise its energy.

Heating-Cooling Energy

Energy is defined by Webster's dictionary as "vitality of expressing" and "the capacity of acting." The energy of an herb, therefore, has the capacity to act on the body in a certain way. Specifically, this is its heating or cooling effect, or the capacity to warm the body up or cool the body down.

Imagine how you feel lying down in an open meadow on a bright summer day. Next imagine how you feel sitting by a bubbling stream in the woods. In the sun and meadow you feel warm, while by the stream in the shade of the woods you feel cool.

The same warm or cool energy can occur in us through the use of herbs. Every herb has a heating or cooling energy which is a natural part of that herb. When we use the herb, that energy causes warmth or coolness in the body.

Another way of looking at it is the effect an herb has on the body's metabolism. When it causes the metabolism in the body to speed up, it is heating. When it causes the metabolism to slow down, it is cooling. In the first case we feel warmer; in the second, cooler.

If there is already heat in the body, then taking a warm-natured herb will create further heat. However, taking an herb with a cool energy will clear the heat, creating balance. Likewise, if there is coldness in the body, taking a cool-natured herb will create more coldness. Taking a warm-natured herb will warm that coldness and create balance. This concept is simplified, but it demonstrates how the warming and cooling energies of herbs can affect the body and how we feel.

The energy of an herb is an inherent part of the herb. It can never be changed because it was created this way, just as a dog can't become a cat, or a flower a rock because their inner natures are to be what they are. Yet, it can sometimes be slightly altered to be less cool or less warm through external applications, such as warming it up in the oven, or cooling it down in the refrigerator, although its inner nature still remains warm or cool.

Warming and cooling energies are on a continuum, as in this diagram:

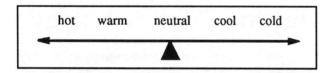

Some herbs are hot, some slightly warm, others cool, some very cold and others neutral. Each herb varies in energy, yet overall it is stated that the herb is either hot, warm, neutral, cool or cold. There are very few hot or cold herbs, and so warming or cooling energies are the most common seen.

Let's use an example. Peppermint is an herb that has a cooling energy. It will cool the body either by causing a sweat or cooling the metabolism. Now, drinking hot peppermint tea may make you feel warm at first since it is heated up; however, the peppermint will eventually cool the body since its energy is cooling. Drinking cold peppermint tea will cool you off since the peppermint is cooling and the tea is also cold from the refrigerator. Either way, if the outside temperature of peppermint is changed, it still doesn't alter its inner cooling energy.

Now let's try an experiment to test the warming or cooling energy of herbs. First, eat a few fresh mint leaves. Now, take a big breath in and out through your mouth. Does it feel cool or warm from the mint? Mint usually causes coolness in the mouth, and it has this same cooling effect inside the body. Next, sprinkle a little cinnamon powder on your index finger and taste it. Notice how this makes your mouth feel after you eat it. Does it feel cool and numb, or tingly and warm? Cinnamon tastes spicy and warm, and its warm energy stimulates metabolism in the body.

It is easy to feel the energy of mint or cinnamon right away, but with most herbs it takes time to feel their warming or cooling energies in our bodies. Therefore, we want to learn what the energy of each herb is before we take it so we know which effect it will have and if this is the effect we want to happen.

There are some herbs which have a neutral inner nature. This means that they are neither warm nor cool but balanced and so will not change the energy of your body when you take them. Licorice is an example. If you chew on a slice of licorice root, it will feel neither warm nor cool. This means it has a neutral energy and will not warm or cool the body.

Therefore, one of the best ways to tell the inner nature of an herb is to see how you feel after eating it. If you eat mint you feel cool, and if you eat cinnamon you feel warm. Another way is to look at its color. As a general rule red, yellow, orange and pink herbs have a warm energy, and white, blue, purple and other dark-colored plants have a cool energy.

A further key to learning the energy of an herb is how our bodies react from it. Herbs which give us more energy and strength and activate our blood circulation generally have a warm energy. Herbs which cause us to go to the bathroom, sweat or feel calm usually have a cool energy.

The Five Tastes

The taste of an herb helps determine its heating or cooling energy. It also gives the herb other qualities and effects which are helpful in learning more uses of the herb. In the West there are four tastes recognized, but in the Orient there are five: sweet, bitter, spicy, salty and sour. Sometimes astringent is placed in a sixth category, but essentially it belongs to the sour taste.

Pungent

The pungent taste is also called acrid or spicy, and it is *warm to hot* in energy.[1] It stimulates the circulation of blood, energy, lymphatic fluid and nerve energy. It counteracts poor digestion and circulation, feelings of coldness and mucus production. It moves energy from the inside to the outside of the body, opening the pores and allowing a sweat to occur. Thus, it is especially useful for surface ailments such as colds, flu and mucus congestion. It also stimulates the circulation of fluid, secretions and saliva. The spicy taste has a direct effect on the Lungs and Colon.[2]

Since pungent herbs are dispersing, in excess they can exhaust energy reserves, cause the finger and toe nails to wither and tighten the tendons, thus decreasing flexibility. Therefore, they should be used only as needed. Examples include *ginger*, *prickly ash*, *cayenne*, and *aconite*.

Salty

The salty taste is *cold* in energy. It stabilizes and regulates fluid balance. It also has a softening effect and so is good for hardened lymph nodes, tight muscles, constipation, hard lumps and cysts. The salty taste has a direct effect on the Kidneys, Adrenals and Bladder. In fact, a craving for salt is often indicative of adrenal exhaustion. Some systems, like Macrobiotics, say salt is heating in energy, which is probably referring to its ultimate effect on the body in excess, when it can be irritating.

In excess, salt can cause water retention and high blood pressure and injure the blood. Herbs high in mineral salts will not create the complications of excess salt in the body. All seaweeds are salty, and herbs such as *plantain* and *nettles*, while classified as bitter, are high in mineral salts.

Sour

The sour taste is *cooling*, drying, astringent and refreshing. It dries up mucus and tightens the tissues and muscles, thus toning them. It helps stop excessive perspiration, loss of fluids and excess secretions of mucus and bleeding. It also stimulates digestion and metabolism and aids in breaking down fats through its stimulation of bile, thus aiding their absorption. The sour taste has a direct effect on the Liver and Gallbladder as it drains and expels any excess in those organs.

In excess, however, the sour taste can actually harm digestion, as it can coat the mucus linings of the stomach and intestines, thus causing poor digestion and absorption. It can also toughen the flesh. Example herbs are *raspberries*, *blackberries*, *schisandra*, *orange peel* and *lemons*.

Bitter

The bitter taste is *cooling*, drying, detoxifying and anti-inflammatory. It stimulates the secretion of bile, which in turn sparks the digestive fires and stimulates normal bowel elimination. It also helps protect the body against parasites and clears the blood of cholesterol. As such, this taste strengthens the Heart and Small Intestines and cleanses the blood. Sweet cravings can be alleviated through ingestion of something bitter. It also dries dampness and secretions in the body, such as diarrhea, leucorrhea and skin abscesses.

Bitter in excess can be too drying and eliminating. It can also cause the skin to wither and body hair to fall out. Example bitter herbs include *dandelion*, *gentian* and *golden seal*.

Sweet

Perhaps the most well known taste, sweet can actually be separated into two types: *empty sweet* and *full sweet*. Empty sweet includes simple sugars like honey, juices and sugar. Full sweet includes complex carbohydrates and herbs which build, tonify, harmonize and nourish. The *empty sweet* taste varies in energy according to the sugar. Essentially, it is *cooling* and eliminating in effect, although very small amounts of honey and raw sugar can help strengthen. (This is a case showing how a little bit of something can strengthen whereas a lot can be depleting.)

The *full sweet* taste is *warming* and strengthening. Herbs with the full sweet taste build those with weakness and lack of energy and blood. Because they also satisfy the body's true craving for sweet, they have a direct effect on the Spleen and Stomach. However, in excess sweet can cause congestion and lethargy and sedate the digestive fires. It can also cause the bones and joints to ache and hair to fall out. Examples of the sweet taste are *ginseng*, *red dates* and *cinnamo*n.

Most herbs have two or more tastes in combination which give them multiple uses, although usually one taste predominates. These tastes can also be used to alter the energy of an herb or herbal combination through their external application.

For example, herbs stir-fried in vinegar have a greater effect on the liver and are better absorbed. Stir-frying herbs in a little honey adds the sweet quality so that they are more strengthening to the digestive organs. Adding salt to an herb tea helps take its energy to the kidneys and bladder. A small amount of a spicy herb added to a formula helps stimulate its circulation throughout the body, more quickly moving the herbs to their destination.

The following diagram gives a representation of herbal energies on a continuum from warm to cool energies:

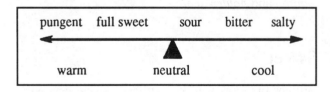

The Four Directions

All herbs have a tendency to move in one of four directions in the body: *rising* or upward, *sinking* or downward, *floating* or outward, and *descending* or inward. The rising energy helps remove obstructions and promotes circulation, as stimulating herbs do. Examples include *prickly ash* and *motherwort*. The floating energy disperses colds and flus, for example, to the outside of the body and eliminates toxins through the pores of the skin. Herbs with volatile oils have this energy. Examples are *ginger*, *peppermint* and *yarrow*.

The sinking energy causes elimination through the bowels or urine, activates menses and lowers fevers. Example herbs include *yellow dock*, *uva ursi*, *angelica* and *scullcap*. The descending energy strengthens the inner organs and treats the deep-level functions of the body. Examples include *ginseng*, *licorice* and *fenugreek*.

Overall, lighter herbs, like leaves and flowers, tend to float and rise, making them effective for more acute and surface conditions like colds, flus and inflammations. Heavier herbs, such as roots, barks and seeds, tend to move inward, being more useful for treating deep and chronic conditions.

The way herbs are prepared and taken also influence their directional energy. Herbs made into a tincture with wine or alcohol have a rising tendency since alcohol has a rising energy. Herbs mixed with ginger juice move outward to the extremities since ginger is spicy and dispersing. Herbs taken in vinegar sink downwards since vinegar is heavy in energy.

Further, by adding herbs with a spicy rising energy to a combination of herbs, the formula's actions can be made to ascend more to treat the upper part of the body. Likewise, by adding herbs with downward moving energies to a combination of herbs, the formula's actions can be made to descend more to treat the lower part of the body. Thus, the method of preparing herbs has an effect upon where they are directed in the body.

When treating ailments, herbs are used which have a similar movement tendency to that of the disease. For instance, if a disease is superficial and located in the upper part of the lungs, it would be best to use rising and floating herbs that cause sweating and expectoration of mucus. For a disease that is in the intestinal or urinary tracts, sinking herbs with laxative or diuretic properties would be appropriate. Inward moving herbs with strengthening properties would be useful for weakness in an internally operating organ system resulting in, for instance, poor digestion associated with lowered appetite, bloating and gas.

Other Energies

There are other qualities which affect the application of herbs. In Traditional Chinese Medicine, all universal phenomena are delineated as Yin or Yang. These are broad terms which encompass specific characteristics, and they include hot and cold energies. In terms of herbs, Yang is defined as warm, energizing and circulating; Yin is defined as cool and moistening. An herb which is warming, gives energy and/or circulates, is Yang. An herb which is cooling and moistens any body fluids is Yin.

The Yin-Yang system encompasses other qualities besides hot-cold energies. It includes the actions of the herb, its density, size, part and environmental aspects. These are summarized in the following chart:

Yin	Yang
cooling	warming
relaxing	energizing
moistening	circulating
grows quickly	grows slowly
expansive	compact
larger	smaller
soft	hard
fast-growing roots, leaves, flowers, fruits	slow-growing roots, root bark, tree barks

Plants possess both Yin and Yang qualities in them. Thus, with the Yin-Yang paradigm we look beyond hot-cold energies to the greater effects herbs have on the body. For example, a warming herb with a spicy or sweet taste has a hot or warm energy but may not be considered a Yang herb because of other qualities it has.

For instance, cayenne is a hot, spicy herb but is fast-growing, light and dispersing to the energy. When taken in larger quantities, it is extremely weakening to the body. In this way it can eliminate heat and energy and so is not a Yang herb as such. In small amounts, however, it can generate warmth and stimulate circulation. Then it has a Yang effect.

As another example, ginseng is sweet and slightly bitter whereas cinnamon is spicy and sweet. Ginseng is a dense and slow-growing root which warms and strengthens the energy while cinnamon is a bark which warms and stimulates circulation. In terms of energy, cinnamon is hot and ginseng warm, yet in terms of Yin and Yang, ginseng is more Yang than cinnamon. This is because it strengthens and doesn't over-stimulate as too much cinnamon can.

The parts of an herb usually vary according to Yang and Yin. Twigs, branches, barks and long roots which take time to grow and mature are generally Yang. Fruits, flowers, leaves, herbs with copious volatile oils (and so are strong-smelling) and fast growing roots are generally Yin in nature. Seeds are usually neutral in energy.

The following diagram gives a representation of herbal parts on a continuum from Yang to Yin energies:

Yin and Yang helps us see the additional qualities of an herb. These can be valuable in determining the effects herbs can have on the body. However, rather than learning herbs as either Yin or Yang, look at their hot-cold energies and their effects on the body. These are the most important determining factors.

Special Properties

Each herb has properties which make it useful for particular organs or physiological systems in the body, such as the heart or urinary system. This is determined by its predominant properties or actions, described in the chapter *Herbal Properties, Constituents, Families and Formulas*. The properties of an herb are derived from its biochemical constituents and the physiological effect these then have on the body. Some herbs even have a special ability to strengthen the body and its immune system and help adapt to stress and external influences. Called adaptogenic, this special quality is an inherent part of that herb. *Ginseng* and *astragalus* are good examples.

Altering Energies

The energy of an herb can be altered somewhat by where it grows, how and when it is picked, and by external applications. These do not change the herb's inherent warm or cool energy but can alter it slightly so that it is warmer or less warm, cooler or less cool than normal. For instance, herbs that grow in cold, northern climates, such as long roots or the barks of trees, tend to be more warming and building in energy. Herbs which grow in warm, southern climates, such as many fruits and flowers, tend to be more cooling and eliminating in energy.

This makes sense when you think about it, as people living in colder climates and using what grows locally need herbs and foods that are heartier and warmer. Thus, the herbs that grow there tend to have a warmer energy to help warm the body in cold weather. Likewise, those living in hotter climates need herbs and foods that are more cooling and eliminating in nature. The herbs that grow in hot climates tend to have a cooler energy to help cool the body in hot weather.

Herbs that grow in higher and more mountainous regions also tend to be warmer, while those growing in flat lowlands near water are more cooling. These locations can make some difference in the energy of one herb, also. For instance, dandelion has a slightly less cold energy when grown in northern climates than when grown in southern climates.

Herbs picked in late morning after the sun rises, at noon or at middle afternoon become more warming in energy. When herbs are dried in the sun (this is done quickly and with much turning of the herbs to prevent their being burned) their warming energy is

also enhanced. Similarly, herbs picked in the early evening, at night or before dawn are more cooling. Herbs exposed to the cooling rays of the moon also have their cooling energies increased.

The energy of an herb can also be altered somewhat by external applications. To make an herb warmer in energy (or less cool): 1) add heat or cook; 2) cook a long time; 3) use pressure (pressure cook or use weights, as for making pickles); 4) roast; or 5) use dry. To make an herb cooler in energy (or less warm): 1) add liquid or make soupy; 2) prepare with vinegar; 3) add simple sweets such as sugar, fruit or fruit juice; 4) cook quickly; 5) use cool; or 6) use raw.

Putting it together, we can look at the overall qualities which give an herb its warming or cooling energy and other effects. In general, warming herbs have a spicy or complex sweet taste (made up of complex carbohydrates), with more minerals and protein. Examples include *fennel, elecampane, angelica, prickly ash, cinnamon, ginseng* and *astragalus*. Overall, cooling herbs have a sour, bitter or salty taste. They are more eliminating in effect. Examples include *dandelion, golden seal, red clover* and *peppermint.*

Yang herbs are warming, energizing and circulating. They include hard leaves, twigs, branches, seeds, barks and roots which take a long time to grow and mature. They have little or no volatile oils. Yin herbs are cooling and moistening. They include leaves, flowers, juicy fruits, fast growing roots and tubers. They contain an abundance of volatile oils. They tend to grow and mature quickly and have a detoxifying effect in the body.

All of these aspects of the energy of herbs are summarized in the following chart. Once we can determine the energy of the physical ailment in the body, then we can properly choose an herb with an energy that matches it appropriately. This is what we will learn in the next chapter.

---

[1] As with everything in Nature, there are exceptions to the rule. Although the pungent taste is warm in energy, there are some herbs which are pungent with a cool energy, such as peppermint and lemon balm. Similarly, though the bitter taste is cooling in energy, there are some bitter herbs with a warm energy, like angelica and ginseng.

It is necessary to not be dogmatic with herbal energies. The most definite aspect of an herb which determines its energy is the final effect it has on the body. The two most important criteria for this are tastes and actions (properties), and each serves only as one determining factor. This is important to keep in mind as we discuss the tastes.

[2] Throughout the book all capitalized organs, like Lungs and Colon here, refer to the Chinese concept of organ systems. This concept does not refer to the organs themselves as we know them in Western medicine, but to a group of functions represented by those organ names. Thus, they are capitalized to differentiate them. Refer to the Bibliography for books with further information on this.

THE ENERGY OF HERBS

Qualities:	
Energy	← hot warm neutral cool cold →
Taste (*example herbs*)	pungent mildy sweet bland sour bitter salty *angelica* *licorice* *slippery elm* *lemon balm* *goldenseal* *seaweed, nettles*
Directions (*example herbs*)	descending rising warm-floating cool-floating sinking (inward) (upward) (outward) (outward) (downward) *ginseng* *prickly ash* *ginger* *peppermint* *yellow dock*
To Make Less Warm or Less Cool	add water, vinegar, salt add heat, pressure, time (age) cook quickly or use raw or cool cook longer or use cooked or dry (to make less warm) (to make less cool)
Yin/Yang	← yang neutral yin →
Herb Parts (*example herbs*)	slow-growing roots root & tree barks seeds faster-growing roots leaves flowers fruits *ginseng* *cinnamon & bayberry* *fennel* *burdock* *comfrey* *honeysuckle*
Other	dense grows slowly small hard mild large soft watery/juicy grows quickly
	picked late morning, noon, or mid-afternoon picked early evening, at night, before dawn grown in cold climate, mountain regions grown in warm climate, flatlands or near water sun-dried moon-dried

Note: This is a very general overview of warming-cooling and Yin-Yang qualities of herbs. There are exceptions! The inherent energy and taste of the herb are its primary energy indicators.

The Energy of Illness

In the first chapter we talked about the difference between using herbs symptomatically and energetically. When herbs are given symptomatically, the known use of an herb is matched with the symptoms of the illness. When herbs are applied energetically, the individual characteristics of the herb are matched with the qualities causing the illness and with the various traits of the person experiencing the illness. This energetic method is an approach of treating the person who has the disease rather than treating the disease itself.

When we experience illness, we are used to defining our condition in terms of its symptoms. For example, we define a cold as a stuffy nose, sneezing, possible cough, head congestion and low energy; a bladder infection as frequent and burning urination, possible blood in the urine and a sense of bloatedness; and bronchitis as inflamed bronchioles in the lungs with mucus congestion and cough. Our treatment approach for each of these is to directly eliminate the symptoms with medications in order to "get rid of" the illness.

This symptomatic treatment approach is used by both modern medicine and western herbalism. It gives decongestants or expectorants for colds, antibiotics and diuretics for bladder infections and antibiotics or anti-inflammatories for bronchitis. In many cases this works, but in others it doesn't, making it a rather hit-or-miss approach. When it doesn't work, it can cause a prolonged healing process, a weakening of the body and/or a suppression of the true cause of the illness.

The reason the symptomatic treatment approach doesn't always work is because not every cold, blad-der infection or bronchitis is the same. Further, not every body they are manifesting in is the same. A cold you have can be totally different from a friend's cold because both of you are different. Therefore, one overall treatment approach does not heal each type of cold, bladder infection or bronchitis inflammation. Rather, each illness manifests with a different energy that varies according to the energy in each person's body.

Let's look at an example a little more deeply. If you say that you have a throat infection, it does not tell very much about either the particular nature of the infection or your overall condition. Using the symptomatic treatment method, a laboratory analysis is made to determine the specific type of bacteria causing the infection. Then the indicated antibiotic is prescribed. This approach only alleviates the symptoms of the throat infection. It does not eliminate the deeper cause of the infection.

When using the energetic method, we look at the various factors causing the throat infection. It may be due to a type of heat in the throat arising out of a lack of cool fluids in the body. Or, it may be caused from a true excess of heat and toxicity in the body. The treatment is different in each case. With the energetic method we do not have to know the nature of the particular bacteria in the throat infection. This is because we are looking at the cause of the infection, not the infection itself.

Thus, to learn an energetic model for healing with herbs, we are first going to look at how we determine the cause and symptoms of an illness, often called the root and branch of a disease. Next we look at how to determine the warm-cool energy of our constitutions and its effect on the state of illness. Then we consider the various qualities which comprise an illness: its hot-cold energy, location, strength and damp/dry aspects. All these qualities combine together to give specific information on the illness and the resulting treatment approach.

Root and Branch of Disease

In treating illness it is important to realize that it has two aspects: a root and a branch. The root is the underlying cause while the branch is its symptoms. In the example above, the throat infection is the symptom, or branch of a disease. Its underlying cause is the root. As another example, a bladder infection is the branch of a disease. Its underlying cause, or root, can be from too much heat in the bladder or from a cold and weakened body. Each of these causes is different, so each should be approached differently.

In treating disease, if you only relieve the superficial branch, either the symptoms recur or other problems eventually develop because the root has not been eliminated. It is like weeding a garden. If only the leaves and stem are pulled, the weed grows back because the root remains. In order to eliminate the weed entirely, the root needs to be fully dug up.

Determining the root and branch, or cause and symptoms, of an illness automatically indicates the appropriate treatment approach. Thus, the energetic method of diagnosis is closely integrated with the cure. For instance, once we determine that the bladder infection is from too much heat in the bladder, then we know to use cooling and eliminating herbs which clear the heat and toxins from the bladder (herbal alteratives, antibiotics and diuretics). Likewise, when we determine that the sore throat is from a type of heat in the throat arising out of a lack of cool fluids in the body, then we know to treat it by giving a combination of both cooling (herbal alteratives and antibiotics) and fluid-strengthening herbs ("fluid" tonics) and diet.

The protocol for treating illness then, is to treat the root along with the branches. To do this, first look

at the branch, or all the symptoms occurring. Then look at what commonalities these symptoms have. From the commonalities we can determine the root cause of the symptoms. In acute conditions it is important to treat the branch of a disease first. This is because acute conditions are critical and so need to be healed quickly. Then the root, or original cause, of the condition can be treated. In chronic conditions the branch and the root can be treated simultaneously.

Energetic Treatment Approach

To determine the root of a disease we look at the commonalities of the symptoms to determine its cause. The cause of a disease has energetic qualities. Further, the person the disease is manifesting in has energetic qualities. However, the qualities of the disease and the person are interrelated. The energy of a disease develops out of the energy occurring within the person. Thus, there is a direct relationship.

Just as herbs and foods have warm and cool energies, so do illnesses manifest as warm or cool conditions. Colds, bladder infections and bronchitis, therefore, can be conditions of either heat or coldness. Which it is will determine which treatment will heal them. The warm or cool energy of the illness varies for each person. It is analyzed according to various signs. Once it is determined if the illness is from heat or coldness, one can choose the appropriate herbs and foods to heal it.

If the energy of the illness is not determined before it is treated, then the problem can get worse or reappear at a later date. In either case, the energetic cause of the illness still remains. As an example, one female patient I worked with had a bladder infection. She first treated herself by drinking cranberry juice copiously and taking goldenseal until the infection was gone. This worked for several days, yet in another few weeks the infection returned. After she continued her treatment, the infection again cleared, yet re-manifested in another month. She then tried antibiotic drugs which didn't work either. This woman also felt continuously cold and ate a lot of salads and fruit in her vegetarian diet.

This chronic recurrence of her bladder infection continued because her overall condition was one of coldness and she was giving it further cold treatment with cranberry juice, goldenseal (a cold herb) and antibiotics. Because an infection itself is hot, the condition would be temporarily cured. Yet, overall, such treatment only contributed more coldness to her already cold body and metabolism. Thus, her body continued to manifest the bladder infection.

When I saw her for treatment I first gave her a warmer diet to eat. This was essential because the continued intake of cold food would only negate the herbal treatment I was suggesting. Also, her body needed the warmth and strength of this type of food. I then gave her warm herbs to build and heat up her body along with more energetically balanced herbal antibiotics and anti-inflammatories. In time, not only did her bladder infections clear up, but the repetitive recurrences stopped.

Not applying herbs energetically to an illness like this is often the reason that herbs seemingly "don't work." Yet, the herbs are not impotent or useless. Improper application gives poor results.

The energy of an illness arises out of the individual qualities and traits of the person. The aspects that define or frame this are the person's constitution and the energy, location, strength and damp/dry qualities of the illness. Let's look at these in detail.

Constitution

When determining the energy of an illness, it is helpful to first look at the energy of the person's body, that is, the constitution, because this affects how the illness develops in that body. The constitution develops from birth, yet it can be altered over time according to the foods eaten, drugs taken, lifestyle habits adopted and mental attitudes maintained. Therefore, when determining a person's constitution, figure the attributes in the person's overall life, especially the last several years, and not just what imbalance is currently occurring.

Every person's constitution is unique. Yet, its energy may be seen on a continuum of hot to cold according to various attributes in the body. These are outlined in the following chart:

INDIVIDUAL'S CONSTITUTION

Attribute	Hot	Warm	Neutral	Cool	Cold
Spirit	aggressive	outgoing	joyful	sad	depressed
Body Type	large & robust or thin & wiry	muscular	normal build	thin	emaciated or fat
Posture	erect	stiff	relaxed	hunched over	limp
Activity	overactive	animated	normally active	little movement	still
Respiration	heavy & loud	loud sighing & stretching	normal	shallow & light	soft sighs
Voice	loud & rough	strong	regular & moderate	soft	almost inaudible
Skin	very red	reddish	normal	pale	very light or white
Lips	very red	reddish	normal	pale	very light
Moistness of Lips	cracked	dry	moist	wet	overly wet
Mucus	red or yellow & thick	yellow, green, or white & thick	white, slight	thin & white	clear & copious
All Body Odors	strong	somewhat strong	mild	somewhat faint	faint
Urine Color	red or dark yellow	dark yellow	golden	light	clear
Stool	dark, hard	slightly dark & hard	medium	slightly light & loose	light, loose

Because we are dynamic beings, we experience variations in each of these attributes. Yet, if we put a check by each attribute on the continuum where appropriate, add up each column and then look at the overall picture, we will usually see that we have more attributes on one side or the other of the balance point. This determines whether our constitution is either warm or cool in energy.

Constitutions closer to the balance point usually experience less illness than those close to the extremes where imbalance occurs more easily. Those with hot or cold constitutions, therefore, tend toward disease more frequently and more easily than those with just warm or cool ones. Altering the foods we eat, herbs we take and lifestyle habits we keep will, over time, help to adjust our current imbalance closer to the neutral zone.

Energy of Disease

Illnesses manifest according to the hot-cold continuum. A person who has a hot constitution tends toward experiencing illnesses of heat. Likewise, a person with a cold constitution tends toward experiencing illnesses of coldness. Yet, it is possible for a hot constitution to experience an illness of coldness and vice versa. The best way to determine which is occurring, therefore, is to look at the illness and determine its energy independently first and then include the information found on the person's constitution. This will help give a better overall picture of what is going on.

The energy of an illness refers to its hot-cold state. Conditions not as extreme are classified as warm or cool and most illnesses fall under this. Illnesses of heat are characterized by heat signs and illnesses of cold are characterized by cold signs. To determine if an illness is one of heat or coldness, at least three or more signs of its category will occur.

Heat

Heat causes extreme activity in the body with a tendency to rise up and out, like the heat from a fire. When it does this, it often moves other things with it, like blood (high blood pressure or blood in the mucus, stool and so forth) or the tongue (being loud and talkative).

SIGNS OF INTERNAL HEAT

- constipation
- thirst
- dark yellow/red urine
- craving for cold
- bloody nose, stools, urine
- yellow mucus, stools, urine
- blood in any discharges
- red tongue body
- burning digestion
- infections, inflammations
- dryness internally or externally
- red face, eyes
- aversion to heat
- dark, scanty urination
- hemorrhaging
- irritability
- fast pulse
- sweats easily
- yellow-coated tongue
- strong appetite
- fever
- sticky, thick and hot-feeling excretions

Extreme heat causes a more severe condition which includes several of the heat signs above plus:

- delirium
- shortness of breath
- restlessness
- depletion of fluids
- sudden high fever
- coma
- heat stroke
- disturbed mind
- exhaustion
- profuse sweating

Coldness

Coldness tends to congeal and contract, like ice. It causes a person to hunch over or curl up in order to minimize body surface and maintain inner warmth. With lack of heat, activity in all forms slows down. Usually there is tiredness, lack of energy or weakness.

SIGNS OF INTERNAL COLDNESS

- feelings of coldness
- diarrhea or loose stools
- aversion to cold
- craves warmth
- pale moist tongue
- slow or deep pulse
- lack of circulation
- low blood pressure
- poor appetite
- clear discharges, urine, nasal, mucus, etc.
- no thirst
- no sweating
- slowness
- sleeps a lot
- white tongue coat
- pale, frigid appearance
- achy pain in joints, flesh
- cold extremities
- poor digestion
- tendency toward stagnation and contraction

Look carefully at the chart below for a clear delineation of each of these symptoms. Remember that this represents a continuum, so that a person with a little coldness, for instance, will show only a few of the cold signs, and these will not be very pronounced or only occur occasionally. The same is true for someone with just a little heat.

Sometimes there are mixed signs of both hot and cold, such as a hot disease manifesting in a cold body and vice versa. To determine which it truly is and how to treat it, combine the information on the constitution with that of the illness.

For instance, the bladder infection example cited earlier is a condition of a hot disease manifesting in a cold body. The infection itself is hot with burning, scanty and yellow or bloody urine. Yet, the body was cold with feelings of cold, lowered immunity, little energy and strength. In this case there are signs of both heat and coldness. To treat this, the heat of the infection needs to be cleared directly and gently, while the coldness of the body needs to be warmed.

This can be done by using warming herbs, such as ginger, parsley and buchu, with a slightly cool antibiotic herb such as echinacea given with a little cold goldenseal. Ginger fomentations over the bladder can be added to heat the cold bladder surrounding the infection.

An example of a cold disease manifesting in a hot body is chronic asthma with clear to white phlegm, yet the body and breathing are strong, the person feels warm and perhaps the face is red. In this case, the cold mucus needs to be cleared with warming expectorants while the excess heat in the body needs to be eliminated with cooling alteratives.

False Heat and False Cold

Further conditions of hot and cold may occur which are less common. These are termed *false heat* and *false cold* conditions.

SYMPTOMS	
Hot	**Cold**
• hard, dry, solid stool, usually constipated; strong-smelling	• watery stool, frequent, or diarrhea; little odor
• yellow and thick urine; interrupted or stopped urine	• clear or white urine, usually frequent and copious
• appears very excited	• appears very depressed
• strong, stout, muscular, restless, active, irritable	• weak, tired, thin, quiet
• warm skin temperature, hands and feet; five senses are strong	• cold skin temperature, hands and feet; five senses are weak
• stretching posture in sleep; likes to stretch	• curled lying posture
• loud voice, talkative	• soft voice, silent
• heavy coarse breathing	• soft and shallow breathing
• thirst, dry mouth; prefers cold drinks & food, good appetite	• wet mouth, poor taste and appetite; prefers warm food and drinks
• dislikes pressure, massage	• prefers deep massage
• red, solid tongue; cracks, yellow thick coat	• fat, pale, wet tongue; no or white coat

To determine if it is a false heat or cold condition rather than a true one, it is necessary to take into account the entire person's constitution and condition rather than look at one or two symptoms.

In a *false heat* situation, there are heat signs but the signs or the person does not have strength as is seen in an excess condition. The face may be flushed, but it is superficial. The voice may be loud, but it comes in spurts and there is no strength behind it, only nervous energy. Hot flashes can occur or even night sweating, but the person doesn't feel hot all the time. Usually these people are thin, even emaciated, possibly being periodically talkative, restless and/or having insomnia.

In this situation, rather than an excess of heat, there is a lack of moisture in the body resulting in apparent heat signs, although there is not a true over-abundance of heat. These cases often occur from burn-out: over-working, -thinking, or -doing which depletes the essential fluids of the body. In this case, the heat needs to be gently cleared, but the substance of the body also needs to be nourished and moistened. Herbs to strengthen the substance of the body, cool the deficient heat and moisten and build the substance and fluids are used such as demulcents, emollients and heat-clearing herbs.

In a *false cold* condition, there are cold signs but the person does not have weakness as is seen in a true cold condition. The face may be pale, voice soft, hands and feet cold, or a lack of sweat or appetite occur, but overall the person is strong, buoyant and active.

In this situation usually the heat or fluids of the body aren't circulating properly and so they stagnate, resulting in various cold signs throughout the body. Yet overall, the person isn't hot and his/her action and constitution are of a heated person. In these cases the coldness needs to be gently warmed by giving circulating and stagnation-dispelling herbs, such as stimulants and warming diaphoretics and diuretics. Look at the chart below for a clear differentiation between true and false heat and coldness.

SYMPTOMS

True Heat	False Heat
high fever	low grade, even chronic fever
red face	superficially flushed face
can't go to sleep at all	falls asleep, but wakes frequently and perhaps can't go back to sleep
consistently loud voice	usually a soft voice with loud spurts that lose energy fast
sweats easily, copiously	night sweats only

True Cold	False Cold
fear of cold	no fear of cold
whole body is cold	just hands and feet are cold
lethargy, little movement	usually still active
low energy	normal energy to sometimes weak
hunched over	erect posture
diarrhea or loose stools	possibly the same as true cold
clear discharges	possibly the same as true cold
poor appetite, digestion	normal appetite, digestion
	could have lowered immunity

Location of Illness

Whether a disease is *internal* (in the body) or *external* (more on the surface of the body) defines the depth of the disease. Internal conditions affect the internal organs and bodily systems. Herbs whose energy is inward and downward and some with an upward energy are used, such as tonics, diuretics, laxatives, emmenagogues and some stimulants.

External conditions affect the skin, nose, throat and outer parts of the body. This includes chills, fever, sore throat, body aches, sinus conditions and skin eruptions. Herbs with an outward and upward energy are used, such as diaphoretics, expectorants and some stimulants and alteratives. Knowing the proper location of the illness then helps determine which herbal approach to use.

Internal hot and cold symptoms were given under the previous section on the energy of disease. External hot and cold symptoms include signs of internal hot or cold along with several of the following:

EXTERNAL HEAT SIGNS

- sudden onset of illness
- high fever
- great thirst
- carbuncles
- red skin eruptions
- fear of heat, throws covers/clothes off
- craves cool food and drinks
- profuse sweating
- headaches
- boils
- slight chills
- sore, swollen and possible red throat

EXTERNAL COLD SIGNS

- sudden onset of illness
- mild fever
- needs lots of covers
- craves warm foods and drinks
- no thirst
- fear of cold
- strong chills
- little sweating
- body aches

Strength of Illness

The strength of the disease in relation to the strength of the patient defines whether the illness is one of *deficiency* or *excess*. An excess condition occurs when there is too much of something, such as too much heat or dampness. A deficient condition occurs when there is a lack of something, such as a lack of blood (anemia), energy, heat, or fluids.

To determine which it is, we look at the root cause, not just the symptoms, and gauge that according to the capacity of the individual to maintain a continued resistance to the onslaught of disease. This is taken in a general sense and denotes the overall condition of the patient and/or the disease.

Excess states are characterized by the person having strength in either the acute or chronic condition and buoyancy of spirits, and the condition itself is extreme in its manifestation. In these instances there is an abundance of whatever is occurring, be it fever, phlegm, weight, heat, coldness, dampness and so forth. Herbs which have an eliminating or dispersing quality are used, such as purgatives, alteratives, diuretics, expectorants or diaphoretics. The idea here is to eliminate the excess.

It is not unusual for Western people, whose diets are high in meat protein, to experience excess diseases more frequently. Taken to extreme, they result in congestion and deficient states where the immunity of the body is so taxed that it can no longer deal with the excessive conditions created. In other words, all states eventually lead to deficiency when left untended over time.

Deficient states are those which hang on, take a long time to develop and have a tendency to recur. There is weakness, lack of blood, fluids, energy or heat, or lingering symptoms which don't go away, such as a constant low grade fever. This is a situation of chronic conditions and usually is accompanied by weakness and tiredness. Often there is not enough energy to throw off the disease.

Deficient states are an incapacity to find or produce what is necessary for the body to maintain its immunity to disease. It often takes a longer time to reach a deficient state, and so treatment to restore the body can take longer, too. Here herbal tonics for the blood, energy, fluids, or heat of the body are given.

If we look at the body as a container which holds its energy, heat, blood and fluids, we can view excess and deficient conditions in a different way. In an excess condition, the container is over-packed and bulging. There is no room, so the energy, blood or fluids tend to stop moving and stagnate. Heat can increase until steam needs to be released, like a pressure cooker. If the excess continues, it eventually blows holes in the sides and weakness results. Thus, the excess needs to be eliminated to create a healthy container with its contents flowing easily and smoothly.

In a deficient condition, the container is porous. It allows the energy, heat, blood or fluids to leak out. Thus, a person with this type of container is weak in any of these qualities. This person is overly sensitive to everything. Strong nourishment is needed to plug the holes and build a strong container. See the diagram below.

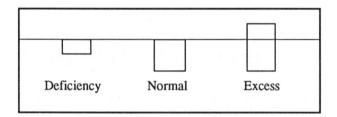

The following chart gives characteristics of excess and deficient states:

STRENGTH OF ILLNESS	
Excess	**Deficiency**
strong	weak
talkative	silent
strong smells	odorless
buoyancy of spirits	depressed
heavy sweating, breathing, and discharges	light sweating, breathing, and discharges
too much dampness or heat	lack of blood, energy, fluids
congestion & stagnation	flaccidity
high fever	low grade, even chronic fever

In treating excess conditions, especially acute ones, one should never tonify as this will only feed the disease rather than the body's normal energy. Elimination first needs to occur, even if there is a weakness. After the first stages of elimination are complete, some tonifying therapy can be given concurrently if appropriate.

In treating deficient conditions, it may be necessary to combine both tonifying and eliminative treatment. This needs to be done to build the person's strength to aid the deficiency while giving eliminative treatment to cure the particular symptoms. Applying both may be done in a single herbal formula.

False heat and false cold conditions definitely come into play here, too. If someone has cold symptoms, for example, it may be due to an excess of coldness or a deficiency of heat. Or if someone has heat symptoms, it may be due to an excess of heat or a deficiency of coldness. To see which it is, refer back to the chart under the section on the energy of disease which differentiates the true from the false heat and cold signs.

Damp/Dry Quality of Illness

Another quality of illness has to do with the moisture of the body. When excess fluid collects in the body, damp conditions result, such as edema, bloatedness and excessive mucus. When there is a deficiency or lack of fluids in the body, dryness results, such as chapped hands and lips and extreme thirst.

Dampness

In the body dampness is like rain—wet, heavy, congesting and stagnating. It can occur with either cold or heat signs. Dampness is treated by either eliminating the dampness or circulating the excess moisture in the body. Diuretics, expectorants, laxatives, energy tonics and bitter herbs all help do this. If there is accompanying coldness, then herbs in these categories with a warm energy are used. If there is also heat, then herbs in these categories with cool energy are used.

INTERNAL DAMPNESS SIGNS

- nausea
- watery stool
- no desire to drink, even if there is thirst
- tendency toward heaviness and turbidity
- distention or soreness in chest, head, flank or abdomen
- copious, turbid, cloudy or sticky excretions and secretions
- leukorrhea
- lassitude
- feeling of fullness
- lack of appetite and sensation of taste
- heavy, stiff or sore joints
- heavy diarrhea or vaginal discharge
- has a tendency toward thickness and stagnation

EXTERNAL DAMPNESS SIGNS

Includes any of the above signs plus:

- acute onset
- oozing ulcers and abscesses
- low fever
- skin eruptions containing fluids

Dryness

Dryness is a lack of moisture and fluids, like a dessert. Dryness can occur from an excess of heat which, over time, dries up the body's moisture. In this case there is also high energy. However, sometimes dryness occurs when the body's fluids and reserves are depleted. This person tends to burn the candle at both ends, overworking or being overactive for that person's needs. Thus, there is also a lack of energy.

Dryness is treated by moistening, lubricating and aiding the body to absorb the moisture it already contains. Demulcents, emollients and certain diuretics do this. It is also important to eliminate heating foods and herbs from the diet and include more moistening, cooling ones.

DRY SIGNS

- dehydration
- dry, rough, chapped or cracked
- dry cough
- dry stools
- dry skin
- dry tongue
- unusually thirsty

Dampness or dryness in the body can also result from fluids being out of place. In some cases, there may be a sign of dampness which is not due to an excess of moisture in the body. Instead, it may be caused by the existing fluids congealing and robbing fluids from somewhere else in the body.

For instance, some people may experience a runny nose along with a dry mouth, such as cottonmouth. In this case, both the dampness and dryness need to be regulated. If herbs are only given to moisten the throat, the body may take the moisture and create an even runnier nose. Of if herbs are given to only dry the nose, the dry mouth may become even dryer. Thus, damp and dry signs need to be worked with together.

Therapeutic Principles

Combinations of these conditions can also occur, and most mixed symptoms come under this. They include half external-half internal, half excess-half deficient, half cold-half hot symptoms. These kinds of conditions are treated with harmonization therapy. This therapy is one of using integrated approaches such as varied combinations of detoxification and tonification, cooling and warming, internal and external applied simultaneously as seems appropriate.

Overall, these qualities of illness often appear together in various ways. Which way they combine determines the treatment approach. First, we determine the root and the branches of the illness. Next, we look at the person's constitution to see where it lies on the hot-cold continuum. Then we consider the qualities causing the illness including its hot or cold energy, its location, its strength and any damp/dry aspects. Finally, we combine all the resulting information to determine the appropriate treatment approach and match the proper herbal energies for healing.

At the end of the chapter are several diagrams displaying various combinations with examples of their signs and symptoms and possible appropriate treatments. There is also a simple test to help you determine your current condition according to these principles. This test may be copied and used for others, too.

Determining the cause and nature of illness can be complicated. It can also involve more principles than those discussed here, such as stagnant blood and energy and energy moving in the wrong direction. Yet, what has been given can definitely help the identification of many illness conditions and indicate the proper treatment direction. Knowing this and the energy of herbs and foods can help one look for the appropriate herbal and therapeutic dietary approaches for correcting the condition found.

---

[1] For all herbal properties mentioned, such as expectorants, diuretics, demulcents, emollients, diaphoretics and so forth, refer to Chapter 4 for their definitions.

Self Test

The following is a simple test to help you determine your current state of imbalance. Check each item which seems to describe you. For the category which has the most checks, follow the corresponding description and instructions given on the reverse side of this page. If you have three or more checks in another category, that means you have a combination of causes. In that case include the other category's instructions also. (For more in-depth information on pulse and tongue diagnosis, see *The Web that Has No Weaver* by Ted Kaptchuk.)

One

- [ ] 1. Hypersensitive to cold in climate, food and drinks.
- [ ] 2. Slow movements and mannerisms.
- [ ] 3. Catches colds easily.
- [ ] 4. Pale complexion.
- [ ] 5. Frequently feels cold. Doesn't sweat. No thirst.
- [ ] 6. The tongue looks pale with a whitish coat.
- [ ] 7. The pulse feels deep and slow (less than 60 beats per minute).

Three

- [ ] 1. Feels heavy; hard to move.
- [ ] 2. Tends to be overweight.
- [ ] 3. Easily develops phlegm or mucus.
- [ ] 4. May have tendency to diarrhea, edema or mucus discharges from lungs, vagina or anus.
- [ ] 5. May feel warm or cool. May sweat easily. Possible thirst, but no desire to drink.
- [ ] 6. The tongue looks swollen and greasy.
- [ ] 7. The pulse feels fluidic, slippery and full.

Two

- [ ] 1. Hypermetabolic; easily flushed and irritated.
- [ ] 2. Moves quickly; very active.
- [ ] 3. Is prone to inflammatory diseases and conditions.
- [ ] 4. Red face and/or neck.
- [ ] 5. Frequently feels warm or hot. Wears light summer clothes in early spring. Sweats easily. Thirst.
- [ ] 6. The tongue looks red with a thick white or yellow coat.
- [ ] 7. The pulse feels fast and on the surface of the skin (80 or more beats per minute).

Four

- [ ] 1. Intolerance to extremes of either cold or heat.
- [ ] 2. Feels tired; lacks energy.
- [ ] 3. Prone to sickness, including colds, flus and fevers.
- [ ] 4. Pale complexion; anemic.
- [ ] 5. Doesn't want to move; hard to complete things.
- [ ] 6. The tongue looks pale with a thin coat.
- [ ] 7. The pulse feels thin and thready.

Five

☐ 1. Chest, palms and soles feel hot. Night sweats.
☐ 2. Feels tired easily; lacks energy or has energy in spurts.
☐ 3. Prone to sickness; lowered immunity.
☐ 4. Pale or superficially red nose and cheeks; anemic.
☐ 5. Restless, irritable; poor sleep or insomnia. Dryness.
☐ 6. The tongue looks thin, reddish and shiny with no coat.
☐ 7. The pulse feels thin and thready.

One

In this condition there is too much coldness in the body. Subsequently, the immunity is weakened and the metabolism is slowed. These people benefit from spicy, dry, warm and tonifying foods and herbs. They should avoid bitter, sour, cold and eliminating foods and herbs.

Two

This is a condition of excess heat in the body. These people should avoid spicy, sweet, dry, warm and building foods and herbs. Bitter, sour, salty and eliminating foods and herbs are beneficial for these people.

Three

This is a condition of excess dampness in the body. The tendency towards overweight is caused by food and fluid stagnation. Use bland, diuretic herbs, especially teas made from mushrooms. Include foods and herbs that are bland and bitter. Avoid dairy products and excessive intake of fluids. For those who also feel hot, include sour, cooling herbs and foods and avoid spicy ones. For those who also feel cold, include spicy, warming herbs and foods and avoid sour ones.

Four

This is a condition of having a deficiency of body energy and blood. Thus, both energy and blood in the body need to be tonified. Use mildly sweet and some spicy foods and herbs. Include energy and blood tonics. Cook herbs with food and make sure food is strengthening and nourishing. Avoid excessively spicy, dry, salty or sour foods and herbs.

Five

This is a condition of a lack of fluids and substance in the body, often called dryness. In this case, there is a low tolerance for dryness, especially in autumn. Daily warm sesame oil massage is very good for these people to strengthen their nervous systems. They benefit from mild, sweet, moistening and cooling foods and herbs. They should avoid spicy, dry, sour and bitter foods and herbs.

EXTERNAL EXCESS
Heat and/or Damp Condition

Overall: Acute condition, comes on quickly; usually good spirits, has strength and healthy immunity; has energy, strong odors; restless, irritable; hot: throws covers off; aversion to heat, wind and possibly dampness; with dampness feels heavy, labored

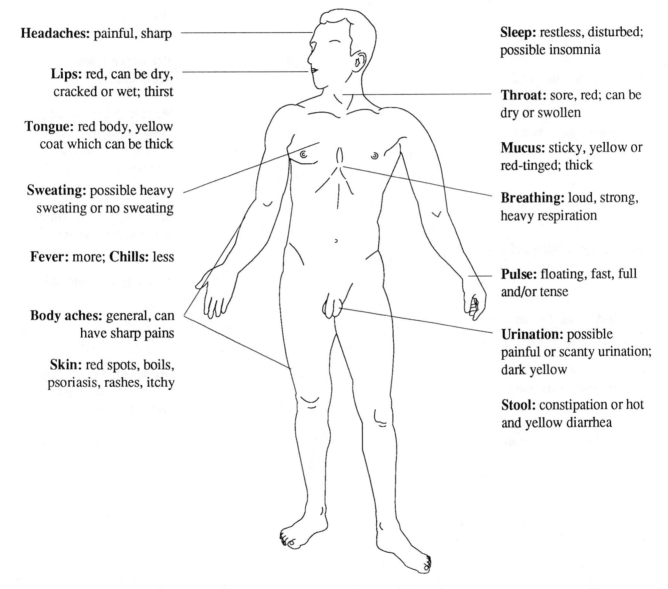

Headaches: painful, sharp

Lips: red, can be dry, cracked or wet; thirst

Tongue: red body, yellow coat which can be thick

Sweating: possible heavy sweating or no sweating

Fever: more; **Chills:** less

Body aches: general, can have sharp pains

Skin: red spots, boils, psoriasis, rashes, itchy

Sleep: restless, disturbed; possible insomnia

Throat: sore, red; can be dry or swollen

Mucus: sticky, yellow or red-tinged; thick

Breathing: loud, strong, heavy respiration

Pulse: floating, fast, full and/or tense

Urination: possible painful or scanty urination; dark yellow

Stool: constipation or hot and yellow diarrhea

Treatment Principle: Clear the External Heat, eliminate toxins, dry upper and lower Damp Heat

Herbal Energy to Use: cool, cold

Herbal Properties to Use: cooling diaphoretics, antispasmodics, diuretics, nervines, expectorants, antipyretics, alteratives, febrifuges, laxatives, astringents

EXTERNAL EXCESS
Cold and/or Damp Condition

Overall: Acute condition, comes on quickly; usually good spirits, has strength; can be overweight, edemic, swollen appearing; energy ok, though somewhat slow; normal to no odors; lowered immunity; cold: needs covers and clothes; aversion to coldness, wind and dampness; with dampness feels heavy, labored

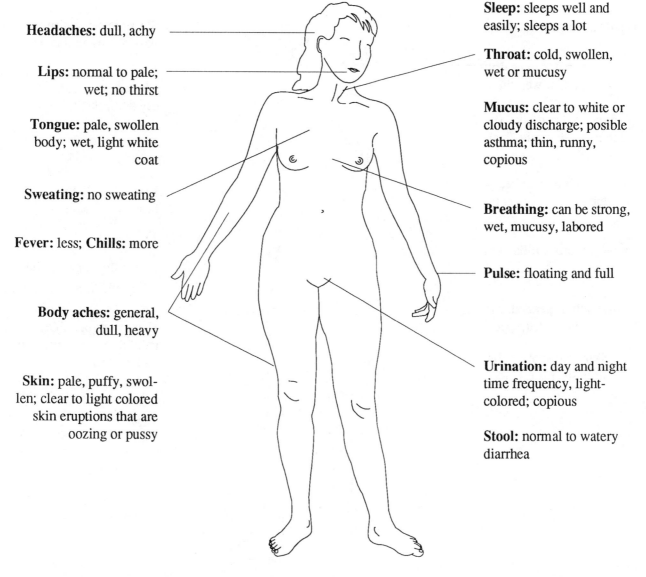

Headaches: dull, achy

Lips: normal to pale; wet; no thirst

Tongue: pale, swollen body; wet, light white coat

Sweating: no sweating

Fever: less; **Chills:** more

Body aches: general, dull, heavy

Skin: pale, puffy, swollen; clear to light colored skin eruptions that are oozing or pussy

Sleep: sleeps well and easily; sleeps a lot

Throat: cold, swollen, wet or mucusy

Mucus: clear to white or cloudy discharge; posible asthma; thin, runny, copious

Breathing: can be strong, wet, mucusy, labored

Pulse: floating and full

Urination: day and night time frequency, light-colored; copious

Stool: normal to watery diarrhea

Treatment Principle: clear External Cold, dry damp

Herbal Energy to Use: warm, some hot; drying

Herbal Properties to Use: warming diaphoretics, antispasmodics, diuretics, nervines, expectorants, carminatives, stimulants, astringents

EXTERNAL DEFICIENT
Heat Condition

Overall: Acute condition, comes on quickly; spirits change from good to poor; no strength, weak though restless; possibly thin and emaciated; some odors; lowered immunity; periodic hot flashes: covers and clothes go on and off; aversion to heat and wind

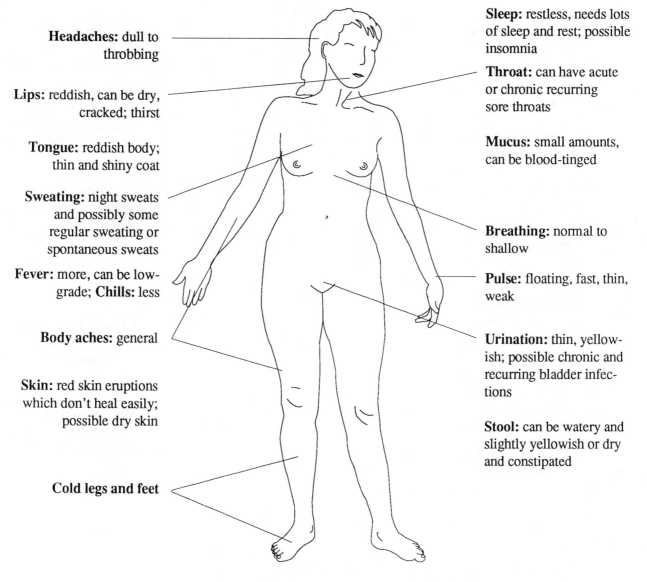

Headaches: dull to throbbing

Lips: reddish, can be dry, cracked; thirst

Tongue: reddish body; thin and shiny coat

Sweating: night sweats and possibly some regular sweating or spontaneous sweats

Fever: more, can be low-grade; **Chills:** less

Body aches: general

Skin: red skin eruptions which don't heal easily; possible dry skin

Cold legs and feet

Sleep: restless, needs lots of sleep and rest; possible insomnia

Throat: can have acute or chronic recurring sore throats

Mucus: small amounts, can be blood-tinged

Breathing: normal to shallow

Pulse: floating, fast, thin, weak

Urination: thin, yellow-ish; possible chronic and recurring bladder infec-tions

Stool: can be watery and slightly yellowish or dry and constipated

Treatment Principle: clear External Heat, strengthen immunity; moisten

Herbal Energy to Use: cool and building

Herbal Properties to Use: cooling diaphoretics and alteratives, with demulcents, emollients and energy tonics

EXTERNAL DEFICIENT
Cold Condition

Overall: Acute condition, comes on quickly; low spirits, depressed, sad, insecure; no strength, weak; exhausted; lowered immunity; no body odors; thin, pale, anemic; recurring colds and flus; cold: needs a lot of clothes and covers; aversion to cold, wind and damp

Sleep: sleeps a lot and a long time

Throat: can feel wet, cold, swollen, mucusy

Mucus: thin, clear colored and copious

Sweating: no sweating or spontaneous sweating

Fever: mild or sub-normal; **Chills:** more

Body aches: general

Skin: infections that don't come to a head; watery skin conditions; pale, puffy, edemic skin

Cold hands and feet, legs and arms

Pale face; anemic

Lips: pale, wet; no thirst

Tongue: pale, wet, swollen and flabby body; wet, thin, white or clear coat

Breathing: shallow, weak, soft, light; possible mucus, cough

Pulse: floating, slow, weak

Urination: clear, frequent, copious; night-time urination

Stool: diarrhea or frequent, light colored, watery, runny

Edema

Treatment Principle: clear External Cold; warm the internal body; strengthen energy and immunity

Herbal Energy to Use: warm, hot and building

Herbal Properties to Use: warming diaphoretics, diuretics and astringents; heat and energy tonics

INTERNAL EXCESS
Heat Condition

Overall: Strong spirits; bouyant; can be overweight or thin; active, energetic; can have blood in stools, urine, vomit, mucus or nose; strong body odors; hot: wears few clothes; can be irritable, aggressive, impatient, excitable, angry; aversion to heat

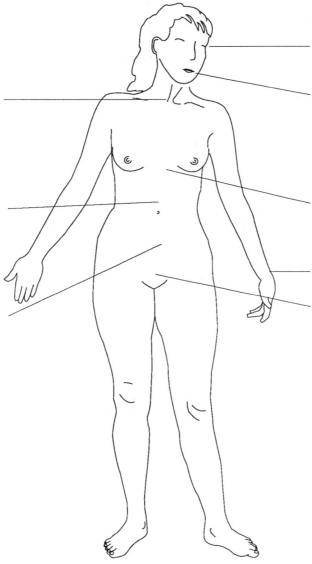

Sleep: restless, insomnia–can't go to sleep at all

Voice: loud, sharp, strong, commanding; talkative

Mucus: yellow, red-tinged, green, sticky with odor

Digestion: good appetite and digestion; can be burning or heartburn; prefers cool food and drinks

Abdomen: hard; obstructions

Infections and inflammations: acute, extreme; sharp or stabbing pain, burning

Skin: red, especially face; possibly yellowish

Sex: strong sexual drive; fertile

Eyes: red, yellow or bloodshot

Lips: red, maybe dry and cracked; thirst

Tongue: red body; full; yellow, sticky coat

Breathing: heavy, coarse, strong, raspy; possible shortness of breath

Pulse: fast, full

Urination: dark yellow, scanty or stopped; acute bladder infections; blood in urine

Stool: hard, solid, dry; constipation; hot yellow diarrhea; bloody

Menses: strong, heavy, painful; can come early; lasts long

Treatment Principle: clear the Internal Heat; eliminate toxins; cool blood

Herbal Energy to Use: cool and cold; detoxifying

Herbal Properties to Use: cooling alteratives, antipyretics, diuretics, demulcents, emollients, antispasmodics, nervines, purgatives, laxatives, refrigerants

INTERNAL EXCESS
Cold Condition

Overall: Usually good spirits; solid, strong; pale; possibly overweight or edemic, swollen appearing, flaccid; energetic and consistent, but may be slow; normal to light body odors; cold or warm: cheerful and joyful to sad, depressed, melancholic but there is energy; possible aversion to coldness

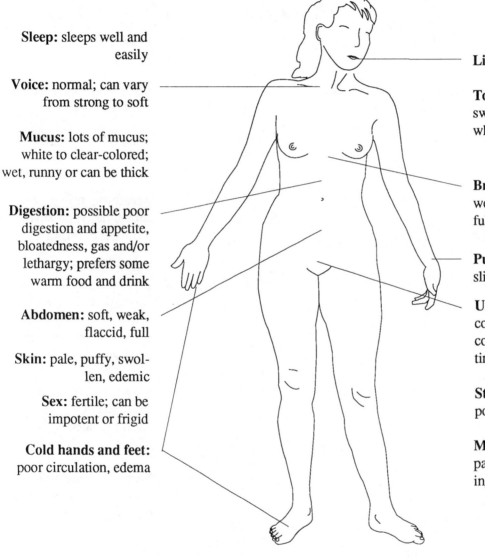

Sleep: sleeps well and easily

Voice: normal; can vary from strong to soft

Mucus: lots of mucus; white to clear-colored; wet, runny or can be thick

Digestion: possible poor digestion and appetite, bloatedness, gas and/or lethargy; prefers some warm food and drink

Abdomen: soft, weak, flaccid, full

Skin: pale, puffy, swollen, edemic

Sex: fertile; can be impotent or frigid

Cold hands and feet: poor circulation, edema

Lips: pale, wet; no thirst

Tongue: pale, flabby, swollen body; wet, thick white coat

Breathing: strong; can be wet or mucusy; chest fullness, asthma

Pulse: slow, deep, full, slippery

Urination: frequent and copious; clear to light-colored; possible night-time urination

Stool: normal to watery; possible diarrhea

Menses: can have dull pain; heavy; slow bleeding; can come early

Treatment Principle: warm the Interior Cold; eliminate Cold Damp; circulate blood and energy

Herbal Energy to Use: warm; stimulating, drying

Herbal Properties to Use: stimulants; warming expectorants, carminatives, diuretics, astringents, emmenagogues, antispasmodics, nervines; heat tonics

INTERNAL DEFICIENT
Heat Condition

Overall: Spirits appear good but can change to depression; thin or emaciated; tired; usually overactive or in "burn-out"; overwhelmed, restless with no underlying strength; weak, lowered immunity, chronic conditions that never seem to completely go away; can be anemic; can have low-grade recurring fever; can have low blood pressure; hot flashes: yet can feel cold; irritable, impatient but lacks strength and energy; possible aversion to heat, cold and/or wind

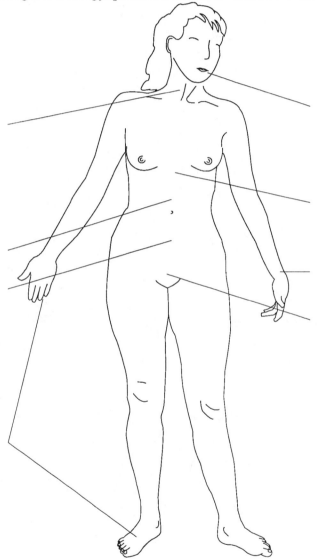

Sleep: restless; insomnia—goes to sleep fine but wakes frequently and can't go back to sleep

Voice: periodically sharp, but doesn't hold out; can be talkative in spurts

Mucus: none to thin, dry; can be blood-tinged

Digestion: possibly good or slow; can be burning

Abdomen: weak and lax

Infections and inflammations: chronic; low-grade

Skin: dry, superficially red cheeks and/or nose; dry hair

Hands and feet: burning sensation in palms and soles

Sex: sexual drive in spurts and not long-lasting; some fertility

Night sweats

Lips: dry, cracked; thirst

Tongue: red, thin body; no coat, shiny in appearance

Breathing: normal to shallow

Pulse: rapid and thin; weak

Urination: normal to scanty; possible recurring bladder infections with blood at times

Stool: possible constipation from dryness or lack of energy

Menses: light periods to heavy but short; can have some pain; irregular

Treatment Principle: clear the Deficient Heat; moisten and strengthen fluids

Herbal Energy to Use: cool and strengthening

Herbal Properties to Use: cooling demulcents, emollients, alteratives, antispasmodics, nervines, laxatives, hemostatics; fluid tonics with some neutral-energied energy tonics

INTERNAL DEFICIENT
Cold Condition

Overall: Low spirits; depressed; tired, exhausted, doesn't want to move, no energy; pale, anemic; possible swollen or puffy; lowered immunity; can be thin or overweight; cold: always wears lots of clothes; fearful, insecure, sad; aversion to coldness

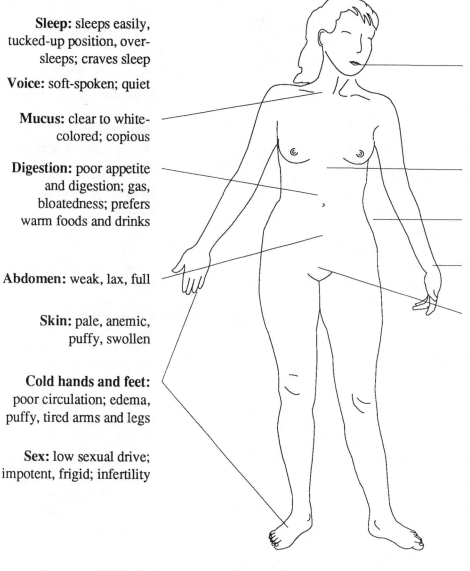

Sleep: sleeps easily, tucked-up position, over-sleeps; craves sleep

Voice: soft-spoken; quiet

Mucus: clear to white-colored; copious

Digestion: poor appetite and digestion; gas, bloatedness; prefers warm foods and drinks

Abdomen: weak, lax, full

Skin: pale, anemic, puffy, swollen

Cold hands and feet: poor circulation; edema, puffy, tired arms and legs

Sex: low sexual drive; impotent, frigid; infertility

Lips: pale, moist; no thirst

Tongue: pale, swollen, wet body; thin, white or clear coat

Breathing: slow, shallow, light, soft; sighs a lot

Lower back pain and achy joint pain

Pulse: slow, deep, thin, soft

Urination: clear, copious, frequent; night-time urination

Stool: light, watery, even diarrhea—clear and runny and frequently undigested food in stool

Menses: pale blood, very light; slow, late or irregular; there can be dull pain

Treatment Principle: warm the Internal Cold; tonify energy and build strength and resistance

Herbal Energy to Use: warm and hot

Herbal Properties to Use: warming antispasmodics, expectorants, nervines, emmenagogue, diuretics, astringents, stimulants, carminatives; heat and energy tonics

INTERNAL DAMP
Heat Condition

Overall: Good spirits; buoyant, strong; good energy though feels heavy; strong body odors; outgoing, active; possible high blood pressure and tendency to bleeding; good immunity; warm: but heavy, slow, labored; irritable, impatient; possible aversion to heat and dampness

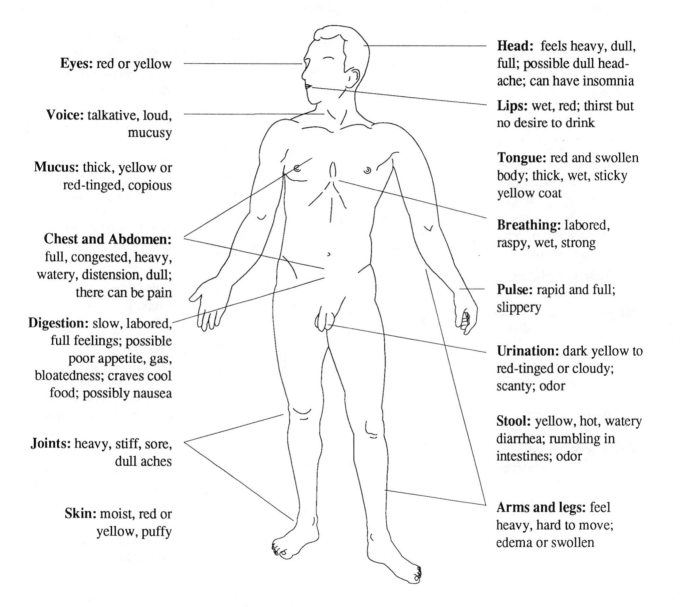

Eyes: red or yellow

Voice: talkative, loud, mucusy

Mucus: thick, yellow or red-tinged, copious

Chest and Abdomen: full, congested, heavy, watery, distension, dull; there can be pain

Digestion: slow, labored, full feelings; possible poor appetite, gas, bloatedness; craves cool food; possibly nausea

Joints: heavy, stiff, sore, dull aches

Skin: moist, red or yellow, puffy

Head: feels heavy, dull, full; possible dull headache; can have insomnia

Lips: wet, red; thirst but no desire to drink

Tongue: red and swollen body; thick, wet, sticky yellow coat

Breathing: labored, raspy, wet, strong

Pulse: rapid and full; slippery

Urination: dark yellow to red-tinged or cloudy; scanty; odor

Stool: yellow, hot, watery diarrhea; rumbling in intestines; odor

Arms and legs: feel heavy, hard to move; edema or swollen

Treatment Principle: clear Dampness and Heat

Herbal Energy to Use: cool, cold; drying

Herbal Properties to Use: cooling diuretics, expectorants, diaphoretics, nervines, astringents, laxatives, antispasmodics, alteratives, purgatives, febrifuges

INTERNAL DAMP
Cold Condition

Overall: Usually good spirits; pale; usually overweight or puffy and edemic; swollen appearance; less active, slow, lethargic; some energy but doesn't move much or easily; joyful to depressed; can feel stuck, sad, melancholic; immunity a little lowered; cold: chilled and heavy, slow, labored; possible aversion to coldness and dampness

Voice: can be mucusy but soft; less talkative

Mucus: copious; cloudy to clear or white; thick or runny; no odor

Digestion: lack of appetite and sensation of taste; poor digestion, gas, bloatedness, nausea; possible vomiting; discomfort, pressure

Chest and Abdomen: full, congested, distension, dull, watery; flacid and lax abdomen

Skin: pale, cold, puffy, edemic, moist

Arms and legs: feel heavy, hard to move; edema , swollen; possible numbness

Joints: heavy, stiff, sore, dull aches and pains

Head: feels heavy, dull, full; possible dull headache; sleeps well and a lot; face can be puffy

Lips: pale, moist; no thirst

Tongue: pale, swollen, flabby body; wet, thick white or runny coat

Breathing: labored, raspy, wet

Pulse: rapid and full; slippery

Urination: light to clear or cloudy; copious; no odor; night-time urination

Stool: watery; possible diarrhea that is clear and watery

Hands and feet: feel cold; poor circulation

Treatment Principle: clear Dampness and Cold

Herbal Energy to Use: warm, hot; drying

Herbal Properties to Use: warming diuretics, expectorants, diaphoretics, nervines, antispasmodics; carminatives, stimulants, laxatives, heat tonics

Herbal Properties, Constituents, Families and Formulas

Using herbs productively requires knowing their individual properties and knowing how to appropriately combine them into effective formulas. This may further be enhanced by an understanding of plant chemistry. When all of these are carefully matched with the symptoms of an illness, it is possible to heal it quickly and effectively and with less herbal treatment.

Herbal Properties

Herbs are usually referred to according to their properties. The property of an herb is its specific effect on one or more systems or general aspects of the body. For instance, herbs that clear mucus from the lungs are said to have an expectorant property, those that cause the urine to flow have a diuretic property and those that relax muscles have an antispasmodic property. Others, like ginseng, strengthen the energy of the entire body and so have a tonic property.

Since herbs have more than one effect on the body, they each have several properties. There are hundreds of terms to describe these properties, yet an understanding of the ones most frequently used is sufficient. These terms are defined as follows with Western and/or Chinese herb examples:

Alterative: improves or "alters" the condition of tissues, including enriching the blood flow to the tissues and purifying or detoxifying the blood; use for blood toxicity, infections, inflammations, arthritis, cancer and skin eruptions. Examples: *burdock root, dandelion, yellow dock, red clover, chapparal, oregon grape.*

Analgesic: relieves pain; use for any kind of pain, cramps, spasms and toothaches. Examples: *cloves, valerian, willow bark, yarrow root, mints.*

Anodyne: powerfully relieves pain. These can be very strong and addicting. Examples: *valerian, skunk cabbage, wild lettuce.*

Anthelmintic: kills intestinal worms. Examples: *garlic, prickly ash, black walnut, wormwood, fennel, fenugreek, bitter herbs in general.*

Antibiotic, antibacterial: stops the growth of and destroys germs, bacteria or amoebas (these often work by stimulating the body's own immune response); use for infections and inflammations. Examples: *chaparral, echinacea, garlic, goldenseal.*

Antidiarrhetic: alleviates diarrhea. Examples: *blackberry root, oak bark, witch hazel, mullein.*

Anti-inflammatory: clears inflammations and inflammatory conditions. Examples: *aloe vera, eyebright, marshmallow, slippery elm.*

Antiphlogistic: counteracts inflammation; use for infections and inflammation. Examples: *echinacea, goldenseal, garlic.*

Antipyretic: lowers or prevents fever; use for fevers, infections and inflammations. Examples: *boneset, chrysanthemum, yarrow, elder, catnip.*

Antirheumatic: alleviates rheumatic conditions; use for painful conditions of the joints and muscles with inflammation and stiffness. Examples: *motherwort, prickly ash, black cohosh, boneset.*

Antiseptic: kills or prevents the growth of bacteria and counters sepsis; use for wounds, cuts, sores, bites, stings and skin infections. Examples: *calendula, goldenseal, garlic oil.*

Antispasmodic: prevents or relaxes muscle spasms. Used internally or externally, some are usually included in most herbal formulas to relax the body, which allows for more rapid healing. Examples: *black cohosh, dong quai, lobelia, scullcap.*

Antitumor: prevents or helps alleviate tumors. Examples: *chaparral, red clover, astragalus, reishi, fu ling.*

Antitussive: helps stop coughs and coughing spasms. Examples: *coltsfoot, mullein, comfrey.*

Antiviral: prevents or helps eliminate viral conditions. Examples: *echinacea, garlic, St. John's wort.*

Aperient: mildly causes bowel movements; use for constipation and mildly sluggish bowels. Examples: *yellow dock, oregon grape, bitter herbs in general.*

Aromatic: has a sweet, spicy or fragrant aroma. Examples: *peppermint, fennel, cardamom, cloves, ginger, angelica.*

Astringent: dries up secretions and has a constricting or binding effect to the tissues which tones tissues and muscles; use for any undesired secretions, swollen tonsils and hemorrhoids. Examples: *bayberry bark, squaw vine, schisandra.*

Carminative: relieves gas and cramping in the bowels; use for stomach pains, gas, indigestion and lack of appetite. Examples: *cumin, fennel, ginger, peppermint.*

Cholagogue: stimulates the flow of bile; use for indigestion and constipation. Examples: *oregon grape root, yellow dock, gentian, dandelion root.*

Demulcent: soothes and moistens, usually with mucilage; use for kidney and urinary bladder irritations, mucus membranes and inflammations. Examples: *comfrey, licorice, marshmallow, slippery elm.*

Diaphoretic: induces sweating either by relaxing the pores or stimulating the blood circulation to the surface of the body; use for colds, flus and fevers. Drink the herb teas hot for this. Examples: *basil, chrysanthemum, ginger, lemon balm, peppermint.*

Digestant: helps the process of digestion; use for indigestion, feelings of stuck or congested food, overeating, gas and bloatedness. Examples: *hawthorn, pueraria, gentian, chamomile.*

Diuretic: causes and increases the flow of urine; use for water retention, obesity, lymphatic swellings, edema (tissue swelling), skin eruptions, kidney stones and bladder infections. Drink the herb teas cool for this. Examples: *parsley root, uva ursi, corn silk.*

Emetic: induces vomiting, usually when taken in larger quantities; use for food poisoning and stomach congestion. Examples: *lobelia, licorice, peppermint, mustard, Ipecac.*

Emmenagogue: promotes and sometimes regulates menstruation, usually causing it to come earlier, often with increased flow; use for any menstrual and related problems; normally not used when there is excessive bleeding. Examples: *angelica, black cohosh, dong quai, mugwort.*

Emollient: softens, soothes and protects the skin; use for dry and chapped skin, cuts and sores. Examples: *chickweed, comfrey, slippery elm.*

Expectorant: expels mucus from the lungs and throat; use for cough, lung congestion, asthma and bronchitis. Examples: *coltsfoot, elecampane, mullein.*

Febrifuge: reduces fevers; an antipyretic. Example: *honeysuckle, yarrow, boneset.*

Galactogogue: increases flow of mother's milk; use to improve nursing. Examples: *dandelion, fennel, milk thistle.*

Hemostatic: stops bleeding and hemorrhaging; use for bleeding from any body opening and for internal bleeding and hemorrhage. Examples: *bayberry, cayenne, tienchi ginseng, fresh shepherd's purse.*

Hepatic: cleanses and regulates liver function; use for liver congestion and toxicity, side and rib pain, bitter taste in the mouth, hepatitis, jaundice, enlargement of the liver, spasms and aches and pains that come and go. Examples: *barberry, dandelion root, oregon grape, gentian.*

Hypotensive: alleviates high blood pressure. Examples: *garlic, motherwort.*

Laxative: promotes bowel movements; use for constipation, irregularity and poor digestion. Examples: *cascara sagrada, dandelion root, psyllium seed.*

Lithotriptic: dissolves and eliminates urinary and gall bladder stones. Examples: *dandelion, parsley root, oregon grape root, turmeric.*

Nervine: calms, quiets, nourishes and strengthens the nervous system; use for nervousness, stress, restlessness, insomnia, crying and nervous tension. Examples: *lobelia, scullcap, valerian.*

Oxytocic: stimulates uterine contraction; use to assist and induce labor. Examples: *angelica, black cohosh, squaw vine.*

Parasiticide: destroys parasites and worms in the digestive tract or on the skin. Examples: *chaparral, garlic, rue.*

Parturient: helps prepare the uterus for childbirth during pregnancy. Examples: *raspberry, squawvine, black cohosh.*

Purgative: a strong laxative that causes increased intestinal peristalsis. Example: *rhubarb.*

Rejuvenative: renews the body and mind, increasing the quality of life and possibly counteracting the effects of aging; use for premature wrinkles and gray hair, loss of body strength and endurance, senility, general debility and dryness. Examples: *American ginseng, aloe vera, licorice, ho shou wu, reishi.*

Rubefacient: increases the flow of blood at the surface of the skin and produces redness where applied; use for inflammations, congestion in deeper areas, arthritis, rheumatism and sprains. Examples: *black pepper, cayenne, mustard.*

Sedative: strongly quiets the nervous system; use as you would nervines and antispasmodics. Examples: *scullcap, valerian, hops.*

Sialagogue: increases the flow of saliva. Example: *echinacea.*

Stimulant: stimulates blood circulation, breaks up obstructions, increases energy and warms the body; use for coldness, menstrual cramping, painful obstructions, colds, flus and lack of energy or vitality. Examples: *cayenne, black pepper, bayberry bark, cinnamon, ginger, prickly ash.*

Stomachic: promotes digestive ability; use for poor digestion, gas and lack of appetite: Examples: *codonopsis, elecampane, gentian.*

Tonic: strengthens and promotes the overall body processes or particular organs to function better; use to improve any organ or system function and to strengthen and build blood or energy. Examples:

bile tonics: *goldenseal, oregon grape root*
bitter tonics: *gentian, citrus peel*
blood tonics: *dong quai, lycii berries, rehmannia*
heart tonics: *hawthorn, motherwort*
energy tonics: *astragalus, ginseng, jujube dates, licorice*
immune tonics: *reishi, astragalus, schisandra*
liver tonics: *dandelion, fennel*
nerve tonics: *scullcap, valerian*
nutritive tonics: *comfrey, marshmallow, slippery elm*
sexual functions tonics: *dong quai, ginseng, licorice*
stomach tonics: *codonopsis, elecampane*
urinary tonics: *parsley, rehmannia*

Vermifuge: expels intestinal worms. Examples: *garlic, wormwood.*

Plant Chemistry

The active parts of a plant which have an effect on the body are called its active principles or chemical constituents. Learning about the functions of the various chemical constituents is very useful as it helps determine a plant's effects. However, it is not necessary information for using herbs, and when used out of context of the entire plant, can even be limiting and misleading.[1] The science and study of plant chemistry is called **Pharmacognosy.**

Plant chemistry covers all aspects of a plant's structure, growth, reproduction, active ingredients and nutrients. The primary compounds of a plant are the elements it needs to live on: its vitamins, minerals, sugars, starches and so forth. Yet, plants also produce secondary compounds in small quantities which have various biological effects. These are the active constituents of the plant that are studied for their therapeutic uses.

There are thousands of chemicals in plants. Here, we are only considering the main medicinal plant constituents. This is simply a brief reference list of a few of the more potent ones, and it is not intended to fully describe the details of plant constituents or plant chemistry. Consult the bibliography for further informational sources.

Acids: Weak acids are found in plants in many different forms. Acids cleanse and detoxify, astringe the tissues and stimulate pancreatic and bile secretions. Citric and tartaric acids, for example, are most concentrated in unripe fruit and have an antibacterial property. They stimulate the flow of saliva and are mildly laxative and diuretic. Citric acid provides Vitamin C to the body whereas oxalic acid, found in spinach, chard and sorrel, binds with calcium in the body and makes the calcium unavailable, ultimately causing kidney stones to form.

Salicylic acid, found in meadowsweet, willow bark, white poplar and wintergreen, has recognized analgesic effects and so has been synthesized into the drug, aspirin. Tannic acid is described under the category, Tannins. Acids are insoluble in vinegar. Examples: *red clover, yarrow, willow bark.*

Alkaloids: These organic substances contain carbon, hydrogen and especially nitrogen and, though very diverse, produce profound effects. They are found in some poisonous and hallucinogenic plants and include nicotine, caffeine, morphine, opium poppy and codeine. One alkaloid group, pyrrolizidine alkaloid, causes liver blockage in humans and cancer in mice. Usually this occurs when the plant is taken in very high doses over a long period of time, since this alkaloid is slowly accumulative in the body. However, many of the pyrrolizidine-containing plants have been used safely by traditional peoples around the world for thousands of years.[2]

Alkaloids act on particular organs, such as the liver, nerves, lungs and digestive system and especially influence the central nervous system. They usually have a bitter taste and are slightly alkaline. Some are anti-inflammatory and antibacterial. Plants normally contain several alkaloids in combination. Alkaloids are soluble in vinegar, have limited solubility in alcohol and are comparatively insoluble in water. Examples: *oregon grape root, goldenseal, barberry.*

Glycosides: This organic plant principle is a combination of a sugar with a non-sugar compound which makes them more water-soluble and transportable. They are found in many combinations and these are discussed separately. Glycosides are soluble in water and alcohol.

Cardiac glycosides: These have a marked effect on the heart and increase its efficiency by increasing the force and power of the heart beat without increasing the amount of oxygen needed by the heart muscle. Examples: *foxglove, lily of the valley.*

Anthraquinone glycosides: These irritate the large intestines and have a laxative effect. They should always be combined with a carminative like ginger or fennel to relieve the gripping pain they can cause. Examples: *rhubarb, senna, yellow dock, cascara.*

Flavones and Flavonoid glycosides: These are the compounds that most commonly cause yellow light to be reflected from plants. They have a wide range of activity and include antispasmodics, anti-inflammatories, antifungals, diuretics, heart and circulatory stimulants, antibacterials and antivirals. According to herbalist David Hoffman, the bioflavonoid Vitamin P is found with Vitamin C in plants and aids its absorption in the body. It also strengthens the capillary walls while reducing high blood pressure and aiding bruising and bleeding. Example: *hawthorn berries, raspberry, ginkgo.*

Phenols and Phenolic glycosides: Phenol is a basic building block of many plant constituents. Some have antiseptic, febrifuge, analgesic and anti-inflammatory activities; externally, antiseptic and rubefacient properties. Examples: *clove, thyme.*

Coumarins and their glycosides: These are best known for their aromatic components used in perfumery. Yet, they are also antibacterial and act as anti-blood clotting agents. Examples: *black haw, red clover, dong quai.*

Saponins: These are also glycosides which have an ability to dissolve in water and form a lather when shaken. Saponins have a structure similar to the human sex and stress hormones and so have been used in the synthesis of these types of drugs. Examples: *fenugreek, licorice, sarsaparilla, wild yam.*

Tannins: As the name suggests, these principles have been used to tan leather. In small amounts, tannins cause an astringent action, acting on protein to form protective skin on wounds and inflamed mucus membranes, promoting their rapid healing. They are used externally for minor burns, cuts, inflammations and infections, swellings, hemorrhoids and varicose ulcers. Internally they control diarrhea, peptic ulcers, colitis secretions and bleeding. Tannins are soluble in water, glycerine and alcohol. Examples: *oak bark, black haw, blackberry.*

Essential or Volatile Oils: These oils in various combinations provide the rich smells of plants. They are easily released from them, especially when the plant is crushed or exposed to the sun. Because they permeate and travel through the body quickly and easily, they have a wide range of use. They stimulate the production and activity of white blood cells, are antiseptic, carminative, antispasmodic, anti-fungal, analgesic, febrifuge, sedative, anti-inflammatory and/or rubefacient in action and stimulate sweating in colds, flus and fevers. They are also used in perfumes, aroma therapy and insect repellents. Most are soluble in alcohol and slightly soluble in water. Examples: *rosemary, thyme, mint.*

Bitter Principles: This is a group of chemicals that have a very strong bitter taste. They stimulate the secretion of all digestive juices and bile, thus activating digestion, bowel elimination and increasing appetite. Bitters, as some herbal combinations have traditionally been called, are often taken before a meal for just these reasons, although they are valuable after meals for indigestion. They are also antibiotic and antifungal in action. Bitter compounds are soluble in water and alcohol. Examples: *gentian, wormwood, goldenseal.*

Carbohydrates: These are found in the form of starches or sugars, giving basic nutrition and energy. They can also form mucilages, the slippery, stringy exudates from many plants. They serve as a soothing and healing gel on damaged mucus membrane linings in the lungs, digestive and urinary tracts, tissues and nerves. Examples: *marshmallow, comfrey, plantain, slippery elm.*

Alcohols: This vast class is often seen as constituents of volatile oils or in waxes which are found as the coating of leaves and other parts of plants.

Resins: This is a plant secretion or excretion that is usually transparent or translucent and yellowish to brown in color. They are soluble in alcohol, fixed oils and volatile oils and insoluble in water. Example: *myrrh.*

There are other plant components, such as vegetable oils, vitamins, trace elements, oleo-resins, gums, lipids, enzymes and other proteins, balsams and coloring matter. The myriad aspects that comprise a plant's chemistry truly give it a unique character which, when combined with the plant's energy, properties and special qualities, yield the unique healing ability of that plant.

Herbal Families

The study of plants is called **Botany** and the science of plant classification is termed **Taxonomy**. Herbs are arranged according to specific groupings for their identification. These are in order of the most general to the most specific (following the recent changes in classification): kingdom, division, class, subclass, order, family, genus, species and common name. The genus and species identify the specific plant. The family of an herb is also frequently referred to since it identifies specific commonalities it shares with other herbs contained in that family. An example classification is lemon balm:

Kingdom: Plantae (plant kingdom)
Division: Magnoliophyta (this is the angiosperms, including the flowering plants)
Class: Magnoliopsida (this is the dicots)
Subclass: Asteridae (gentian-aster subclass)
Order: Lamiales (mint order)
Family: Lamiacea (mint family)
Genus: Melissa
Species: officinalis
Common Name: lemon balm

These groupings are done according to their botanical classification, usually based upon the comparative study of the structure of their flowers, fruits and leaves. Other than identification, it is useful to know the family of a specific herb as this can give hints at what possible uses other herbs in that family might have.

For example, most herbs in the Rose Family Rosaceae, such as blackberry and agrimony, have an effect on the intestinal tract. On the other hand, Chinese ginseng and North American spikenard are both in the Araliaceae family, and both plants have saponins as major constituents. Thus, spikenard may have similar tonifying effects as ginseng does. Further exploration in these areas could be very valuable for learning the uses of less known herbs of North America.

On the following page is a list of the plant families listed in this book and their common names (this is not inclusive of all plant families). Recently, several family names have been changed. I have put these in parentheses next to the old family name. Both are used interchangeably, but because the old family names are the ones still commonly known, I have used them throughout the book.

Herbal Formulary

Herbs are often used individually and are very potent this way. Yet, when combined carefully with several other herbs, they can enhance each other's action and cover a broader range of application and effects. They also have less potential for causing side effects since the other herbs in the formula tend to balance and soften each other's effects.

Creating a formula this way is truly an art. There are no hard rules for formulating, which leaves room for creativity and individuality. There are some guidelines, however, which are valuable and will enhance the effectiveness of the herbs.

First, determine the effect you desire the formula to have, such as to clear mucus from the lungs, nose and sinuses from a cold, to aid digestion, or to strengthen a weak and lethargic system with low resistance. Each of these requires different herbs and a different herbal approach.

In the first condition, expectorants and diaphoretics are used; in the second, carminatives, cholagogues and a tonic that improves digestive ability are called for; in the third, energy and immune-enhancing tonics are specific. Therefore, the first step in creating a formula is deciding its major thrust and desired effects.

Once this is known, the energy of the condition needs to be determined. The chapter *The Energy of Illness* gives the necessary factors for figuring out if the illness is one from heat, from coldness, or a mixture of both. When the energy is determined, you can choose herbs with the specific properties indicated for that illness and with the appropriate cooling or warming energies.

For instance, if a person has a cold with thick yellow mucus congestion and a fever, then you want to clear mucus from the lungs and nose with cool expectorating and febrifuge herbs. If the person's indigestion is characterized by gas and bloating after eating with a feeling of food getting stuck or not moving well, then warming carminatives with a few cool cholagogue herbs are chosen. You may even want to add a warm digestive tonic. Lastly, if you desire to strengthen a weak system with low energy and immunity, then you want to combine warm energy tonics with warm immunity-enhancing herbs.

After this is determined, deciding which herbs to combine and their ratios and proportions is the next step. Standard guidelines exist for this and include combining herbs with main, supporting, assisting and conducting functions. Their ratios and proportions, or parts, are then decided by the function each herb has in the formula.

Main Herb: This category provides the major therapeutic effect desired and encompasses the bulk of the formula. Most of the herbs are included here, all of which have similar functions and treat the same area.

Assisting Herbs: A few herbs are added in smaller quantity to treat associated symptoms and bring out the effects of the main and supporting herbs.

Supporting Herbs: These herbs support the action of the main herbs and develop their functions. They are fewer in number than the main herbs and give subsidiary effects.

HERBAL FAMILIES

Family	Common Name	Example Herbs
Araliaceae	Ginseng Family	ginseng, tienchi, American ginseng
Berberidaceae	Barberry Family	barberry, oregon grape
Boraginaceae	Borage Family	borage, comfrey
Campanulaceae	Bellflower or Bluebell Family	codonopsis
Caprifoliaceae	Honeysuckle Family	black haw, honeysuckle
Caryophyllaceae	Pink Family	chickweed
Compositae (Asteraceae)	Sunflower Family	burdock, calendula, chamomile, coltsfoot, dandelion, echinacea, elecampane, mugwort, yarrow, atractylodes, chrysanthemum
Cruciferae (Brassicaceae)	Mustard Family	shepherd's purse
Cyperaceae	Sedge Family	cyperus
Dioscoreaceae	Wild Yam Family	Chinese wild yam
Ephedraceae	Ephedra Family	ephedra
Ericaceae	Wintergreen & Heath Family	uva ursi
Gentianaceae	Gentian Family	gentian
Ginkgoaceae	Ginkgo Family	ginkgo
Hypericaceae	St. John's wort Family	St. John's wort
Labitae (Laminaceae)	Mint Family	lemon balm, peppermint, motherwort, scullcap
Lauraceae	Laurel Family	cinnamon
Leguminosae (Fabaceae)	Pea Family	fenugreek, licorice, red clover, astragalus, pueraria
Liliaceae	Lily Family	aloe, garlic, sarsaparilla
Lobeliaceae (Campanulaceae)	Lobelia Family	lobelia
Malvaceae	Mallow Family	marshmallow
Myricaceae	Bayberry Family	bayberry
Piperaceae	Pepper Family	black pepper
Plantaginaceae	Plantain Family	plantain
Polygonaceae	Buckwheat & Dock Families	yellow dock, ho shou wu
Polyporaceae	Polypor Family	fu ling, reishi
Ranunculaceae	Buttercup Family	black cohosh, peony, goldenseal, aconite
Rhamnaceae	Buckthorn Family	cascara sagrada, zizyphus, jujube dates
Rosaceae	Rose Family	blackberry, wild cherry, raspberry, hawthorn
Rubiaceae	Madder Family	squawvine, gardenia
Rutaceae	Citrus Family	prickly ash, citrus
Schisandraceae	Schisandra Family	schisandra
Scrophulariaceae	Figwort Family	eyebright, mullein, rehmannia
Solanaceae	Nightshade or Potato Family	cayenne, lycii
Ulmaceae	Elm Family	slippery elm
Umbelliferae (Apiaceae)	Parsley or Carrot Family	angelica, fennel, parsley, bupleurum, dong quai
Urticaceae	Nettle Family	nettle
Valerianciae	Valerian Family	valerian
Vergenaceae	Verbena Family	chaste berry
Zingiberaceae	Ginger Family	cardamom, ginger, turmeric
Zygophyllaceae	Caltrop Family	chapparal

Conducting Herbs: These direct the power of the other herbs to the desired location in the body. They usually have descending, ascending, inward or outward actions. They also transport the entire herbal formula quickly so its actions aren't dissipated in the process of assimilation. Only one or two herbs in this category are included, usually in 1/4 part amounts.

A *part* for each of these herb functions is defined as the proportion for each herb to the entire formula in either weight or volume. Main herbs generally comprise one or more parts of the formula, assisting herbs include 1/2 to 1 part, supporting herbs usually make up 1/2 part and conducting herbs 1/4 part.

For instance, when adding up all the parts in this formula, there are 5-1/4 total parts. A main herb of one part, therefore, represents about 1/5 of the entire formula. An assisting or supporting herb is about 1/10 of the formula. Therefore, if you were to make up 5 total ounces of the formula, then 1 part is 1/5, or 1 ounce, and 1/2 part is 1/10, or 1/2 ounce (using proportions in weight).

As an example, let's look at a formula to clear thick yellow mucus from the lungs in a cold. There is also a lot of coughing, restlessness, a sore throat and slight fever. This cold is one of heat from the signs of thick yellow mucus, restlessness, sore throat and fever. The formula, therefore, is to clear the heated mucus, lower the fever, soothe the cough and throat and open the surface to let the cold out:

The main herbs, coltsfoot, mullein and comfrey, are all expectorants and astringents, well known for their usefulness in clearing heated mucus, alleviating cough and soothing inflamed conditions. Yarrow, as an assisting herb, is also astringent, but further opens the surface and causes a sweat through its diaphoretic action. In addition it has an anti-spasmodic effect which helps allay the cough. Honeysuckle is assisting because it also opens the surface and lowers fevers.

The supporting herbs, licorice and lobelia, aid expectoration of mucus, but have additional antispasmodic properties and soothe and heal inflammations. Licorice also adds a pleasant taste to the formula. Lastly, raw ginger is included as the conducting herb because it is stimulating and circulating and opens the surface to cause a sweat. The raw ginger has an upward energy and so moves the herbs to the upper part of the body and stimulates their activity. Because only 1/4 part is included, the warm energy will not aggravate the heat of the condition. Further, a little warm energy helps balance the predominantly cool formula.

In general, formulas for acute conditions contain fewer herbs, and most of them are main and supporting in function. This is so the formula quickly and strongly affects the acute ailment and is not diluted with other functions. The formula is generally taken frequently; for instance, 4 to 6 cups of tea per day.

Chronic conditions are better treated with a variety of herbs which support and complement one another. It is important in these cases to slowly and gradually affect changes in the body's condition because the energy is weak. As the chronic condition improves and the body gets stronger, it may eventually have the power to manifest the ailment as an acute disease. At this point the formula should be changed to target the acute condition. Formulas for chronic conditions are taken less frequently; for example, 2 to 3 cups of tea per day.

When choosing herbs, select those with an effect complementary to the formula. For instance, when a demulcent is needed in a diuretic formula, marshmallow is a good choice since it is also diuretic; yet in a tonic formula licorice is the preferred demulcent since it is a tonic itself and harmonizes the many herbs in that formula. Likewise, when choosing an

FORMULA TO CLEAR MUCUS

Herb	Function	Parts	Energy
coltsfoot	main herb	1 part	cool
mullein	main herb	1 part	cool
comfrey	main herb	1 part	cool
yarrow	assisting herb	1/2 part	neutral
honeysuckle	assisting herb	1/2 part	cool
licorice	supporting herb	1/2 part	neutral
lobelia	supporting herb	1/2 part	neutral
raw ginger	conducting herb	1/4 part	warm

antispasmodic, lobelia is used for acute ailments because of its strong direct action; valerian is better for treating superficial chronic ailments; whereas scullcap is best in treating deeper and more debilitating chronic ailments affecting the nerves.

Balancing herbs with each other to soften, enhance or counteract their actions is another art of creating formulas. If a formula needs to be strongly heating or cooling, do not dilute it with herbs of the opposite energy. It should predominantly contain either warming or cooling herbs. On the other hand, if a formula's heating or cooling energy is too strong for the patient or disease, it could possibly cause a reaction. In this case add small amounts of herbs with opposing energies and actions. For example, warming ginger or cinnamon may be added to a cold formula, or cooling and soothing marshmallow may be added to a hot formula.

Cold purgatives, such as rhubarb, can cause abdominal cramping and so need a small amount of a warming carminative, such as ginger or fennel, added to counterbalance possible griping. Carminatives further relax the stomach so the herbal properties are better assimilated.

A formula containing many bitter herbs is balanced by adding sweet herbs such as licorice, jujube dates and/or honey. These sweet herbs also protect the stomach from excess bitterness which can overly stimulate the secretion of hydrochloric acid and ultimately create chronic digestive weakness.

When using a majority of diuretic herbs, it is important to include some demulcents to soften the more irritating diuretics, such as uva ursi, and ease the process of releasing any possible kidney stones present. The same is true of a strongly spicy or laxative formula when demulcents may be added to buffer their irritating effects. Demulcent herbs also soften the internal tissues, thus making them more absorbent of the herbal properties. Marshmallow, slippery elm, comfrey and licorice are good choices.

Adding an antispasmodic herb to a formula is important to relieve any spasms or nervous tension associated with the ailment. This will further benefit the assimilation of the herbal formula. It also helps prevent a reaction to any strong effects of the formula; for instance, bitter herbs possibly causing stomach upset. Lobelia, valerian and scullcap are commonly used this way.

A well-balanced formula won't cause any side effects. Yet, some people can experience some gastrointestinal disturbance if they frequently take their herbs on an empty stomach. This occurs because the full dose of the herbs directly enters the stomach and intestines. Thus, if a reaction occurs, it can be prevented almost always by taking the herbs after a meal.

In general, herbs are more effective for treating certain conditions if taken at particular times. For intestine, bladder, liver, gall bladder and kidney conditions, take between meals or 1/2 hour before meals (take immediately before eating if you have a tendency to a gastrointestinal disturbance); for stomach, digestive problems, weight gain, stomach upset and related conditions, take with meals; and for lung, heart, sinus, head and related conditions, take 1/2 hour after meals.

While creating an herbal formula may seem complicated, it really can be rather simple and easy. Some formulas contain only three herbs. Others have just main herbs as their ingredients. The choice and what effect you want it to have are up to you. Be creative and have fun!

---

[1] When scientists began separating out one particular constituent and looked at it closely, they found out why plants had such strong effects on the body, and these effects corresponded to the way the whole plant was traditionally used. For instance, Digitoxin was created from a cardiac glycoside found in foxglove, an herb known to regulate the heart (though it is dangerous). Likewise, salicylic acid in meadowsweet was extracted to form aspirin, having the same analgesic effect as the herb. (Salicylic acid is also found in willow bark and poplar bark and buds.) Thus, active ingredients were extracted out separately, concentrated and given alone to treat specific conditions. Drugs, first created this way, were later synthetically produced in the laboratory, usually with a change of molecule to make the product stronger or "better."

Plants are a complex synergistic whole in which each of the chemical parts contribute to or buffer the other parts. In separating out one active part from the rest and concentrating it, this balance is lost, usually resulting in toxic side effects. Further, this perpetuates the symptomatic approach to treating illnesses rather than treating the person and his/her unique condition.

While seeking out the physical effects of a plant's constituents in the laboratory scientifically validates the traditional uses of plants and gives further understanding to them, it is not a holistic method for using herbs themselves. The map is not the territory; it is not the isolated components which are responsible for the healing action of a plant, but the whole plant itself.

[2] Comfrey is one of these pyrrolizidine alkaloid-containing plants and therefore has come under controversy. Because it has been used extensively for hundreds of centuries safely, it is hard to prove it has caused any problems. Michael Tierra's clinical observation has noted many individuals taking high doses of comfrey long-term without any ill effects. However, because the issue isn't clear, perhaps it is better to use comfrey and other pyrrolizidine-containing plants for short periods of time if taken internally and avoid giving them to children, pregnant or nursing women, those with liver disease or those with a differential diagnosis of a stagnant condition, since they are the most susceptible to problems from this alkaloid. Externally, comfrey can be used safely and without concern.

Knowing the Herbs

To begin knowing herbs, it is best to learn a few herbs very well. Because each herb has several uses, it can often cover a wide range of conditions and situations. With time you'll find favorites which work for you, and you'll use them over and over again. Start by learning the herbs' energies and tastes, then actions, properties and special uses. Experiment with them, then try several projects. Go out and identify, harvest or grow them. Observe their growth patterns throughout the seasons.

Each herb has a personality. It has a primary property or action, such as causing a sweat (diaphoretic). Then it has a secondary property, such as relaxing or calming (antispasmodic, calmative or sedative) or aiding digestion (carminative). Most herbs have several properties and all together they determine the unique personality of that herb.

For example, peppermint, pueraria and ginger are all diaphoretics. Yet, peppermint lowers fevers, pueraria relaxes the body and ginger aids digestion. If you are looking for herbs to alleviate a cold, first determine what energy the diaphoretic should be: cool, warm or neutral. Then decide what additional effects are needed. If there is a cold with a fever, choose a diaphoretic which lowers fevers; if there is tension, spasms or a tight neck and shoulders, choose one which is antispasmodic; or if the cold is accompanied by poor digestion, gas, bloatedness or stomachache, select one which is carminative. This is fine-tuning your herbal selection and leads to a deeper knowledge of each herb's personality and abilities. This differentiation is part of the art of herbalism.

The herbs included here are commonly used in Western and Chinese herbology. They represent a range of cool to warm energies and a variety of properties. Effective in treating several conditions, these herbs are basically mild and safe for general use. They are well known in Western usage and are easily obtained. In fact, many can probably be found along the roads or in vacant lots near your own home, if not in your own back yard.

Many of the herbs may seem to have broad indications for use. These are listed to reveal the many uses an herb can have. However, as stated in the chapter *The Energy of Illness*, this information needs to be modified according the person's constitution and circumstances. An herb that treats headaches, for instance, is not useful for every person's headache. Be sure to first identify the correct condition (type of headache), along with its energy, and then discriminate between the herbs to choose the appropriate ones. This comes more easily with experience.

The first section covers Western herbs, and the second covers several Chinese herbs valuable to know. A particular format is followed in describing each herb:

Name of herb: The herb's common name.

Latin name: Carolus Linnaeus in the 1700s first categorized herbs and used Latin names; if it says spp. it means any member of the species.

Family: A family is a group os plants that are related due to specific aspects they have in common—see the chapter *Herbal Properties, Constituents, Families and Formulas* for further information.

Part used: This covers what parts of the herbs are used, such as the whole herb, root, flowers, seeds or above-ground part. The root grows down into the ground; a rhizome grows horizontally under the ground; a root bark is the outer bark on the outside of the root; above-ground parts includes the entire herb growing above the ground—leaves, stems, seeds and flowers; the bark is the bark of a tree or shrub.

Energy and taste: The cooling, warming or neutral energy of the herb along with its sweet, sour, bitter, salty or pungent tastes is given. Refer to the chapter *The Energy of Herbs* for further information.

Active constituents: This outlines most of the active constituents in the herb. These are not meant to be all-inclusive or detailed, but to give a general idea. Refer to the chapter *Herbal Properties, Constituents, Families and Formulas* for descriptions of plant constituents and their effects.

Actions: This describes how the herb affects the body, including its action on specific organs as well as any general effects.

Properties: These are the ways in which the herb acts on the body, such as diaphoretic (causes sweating) or antispasmodic (stops spasms). A description of all the properties is included in the chapter *Herbal Properties, Constituents, Families and Formulas*.

Dose: The individual dosage for that herb is given in its most frequently used forms. Dosages for both acute and chronic states are given when appropriate, as are the best times and ways for the herb to be taken. Refer to the chapter on *Herbal Preparations* for definitions and instructions on the various ways to make and take herbs.

In general, herbs to treat the lower part of the body, such as the bladder, kidneys, intestines, genital area, lower body conditions and sometimes the liver and gall bladder are taken between and up to 1/2 hour before meals. Herbs to treat the middle of the body, stomach, spleen, liver, gallbladder and digestive disorders are taken with meals. Herbs to treat the upper part of the body, heart, lungs and upper body ailments are taken 1/2 to several hours after eating. When a diaphoretic or tonic effect is desired, take the herbal tea warm. When a diuretic effect is wanted, take it cool.

Dosages are calculated for a person weighing about 150 pounds. However, even if weighing this, each body responds differently to herbs; and therefore, a particular dosage given may be either too high or too low for your own needs and reactions. Start with the dosage given and then increase or decrease according to how your body responds.

For children, there is a convenient rule of thumb for figuring herb dosages from ages birth to 12. Calculate according to the child's body weight as compared to the adult dosage, as follows:

$$\frac{\text{Child's weight in pounds}}{150 \text{ pounds}} = \text{the fraction of the adult dose to use}$$

For example, if a child weighs 50 pounds:
$$\frac{50}{150} = .33 = 1/3 \text{ of the adult dose is used for this child}$$

A good way to give herbs to young children is to put the herbal tea into a dropper bottle, then give several dropperfuls throughout the day. Not only is this convenient, but it is a fun way for children to take herbs. They also take herbal pills easily, especially if licorice or slippery elm is added for taste.

The general doses follow: teas—1 ounce herb per pint water, 2-3 cups/day; capsules—2 "00" capsules 3 times/day; tincture—10-30 drops 3 times/day. The grams given for formulas vary per herb and are individually indicated where appropriate. For those who are sensitive to herbs, start with the lower dosage and increase or decrease as appropriate.

Precautions: These are the conditions in which you should not take the herb, along with possible warnings or side effects.

Other: Any other important or interesting details about the herb are included here.

The section includes the detailed information of the herb's common use along with some ancient or exotic uses, including those by Western, Chinese and Ayurvedic (East Indian) medicines, where appropriate. Any precautions for its uses are outlined. This information is gleaned from the author's and other herbalists' experiences and training along with the common uses herbal literature describes. Refer to the Bibliography for herbal book references.

Various ways the herb is applied are also given, all of which are described in the chapters on *Herbal Preparations*, *Home Remedies* or *Home Therapies*. Be sure to look up the applications in one of these chapters as more information on them is given there. For example, if you read that a ginger fomentation is good for sore joints, then see the chapter on *Herbal Preparations* to learn how to prepare and apply fomentations.

Indications: This summarizes the most common ailments for which the herb is used. It is not exhaustive by any means, but a quick reference and guideline.

Projects: The most common methods of application for the herb are outlined, all of which are described in the chapters on *Herbal Preparations*, *Home Remedies* and *Home Therapies*. I highly recommend that several of these projects be done, as personal experimentation and application is one of the best ways to learn about herbs.

WESTERN HERBS

Aloe

Aloe barbadensis, A. vera; Liliaceae

Part used: gel; powder of the leaf

Energy and taste: cold; bitter

Actions: clears heat; liver, heart, spleen, large intestine, female reproductive

Active constituents: barbaloin, isobarbaloin, amorphous aloin, aloiemodin, polysaccharides, anthraquinone glycosides, glycoproteins, sterols, saponins, organic acids and resin

Properties: purgative, cholagogue, emmenagogue, anti-inflammatory, alterative, bitter tonic, vulnerary, demulcent, emollient, rejuvenative

Dose: gel—2 tsp mixed in apple juice or water 3 times/day; 1/2-1 tsp of powdered root in capsules or steeped in a cup of boiling water (be warned—it has a nauseating taste!)—2 "00" caps 3 times/day

Precautions: powder and large doses of gel: pregnancy and during menstruation; hemorrhoids, uterine or rectal bleeding

Aloe gel is best known for its use in healing burns, skin rashes and itch, injuries, sores, insect bites and stings, poison oak and ivy, acne, herpes and wounds. I have several times seen it successfully stop the pain of burns and promote their quick healing without blisters or scars forming.

Aloe plants are easily obtained and grow well in the home. They are good to keep on hand as a first aid remedy for burns and irritations. To use, break off the green leaf and cut off any yellow sap under it. Slice the leaf open and apply the gel found inside liberally over the hurt area. Alternatively, the bottled gel may be used this way.

In Ayurvedic medicine aloe gel is one of the most important tonics for the female reproductive system, the liver and for cooling excess fire in the body. It imparts a youthful energy, rejuvenates the uterus, benefits premenstrual syndrome and prevents wrinkles from forming. It is rich in vital enzymes and is pleasant tasting. Ayurveda says that women undergoing menopause, who have had hysterectomies, and age 40 or over should take aloe daily. For this tonic effect take 2 tsp in water with a pinch of turmeric two or three times a day.

The powder of aloe is a very strong purgative, more so than rhubarb, and so is not used frequently. In large doses aloe stimulates strong blood circulation and so should be avoided in pregnancy. Since it is a very cold herb, it should be used sparingly by those with coldness or indigestion with gas and bloatedness.

Indications: gel: burns, inflammatory skin problems, PMS and gynecological conditions; powder: constipation

Projects: capsules, gel water, poultice, wash, first aid, pills, wine

WESTERN HERBS

American Ginseng

Panax Quinquefolium; Araliaceae
Chinese: *xi yang shen; say yang sum*

Part used: root
Energy and taste: cool; sweet, slightly bitter
Active constituents: triterpenic saponosides (known as ginsenosides), traces of essential oils, traces of germanium (which may be partially responsible for its remarkable action)
Actions: lung, stomach, spleen, kidney
Properties: tonic, demulcent, rejuvenative
Dose: 3-9 gm in decoction
Precautions: avoid when there is poor digestion with watery diarrhea

American ginseng is used widely by the Chinese as a tonic for the substance and fluids of the body. It moistens and lubricates while clearing deficient heat such as chronic, unabating fevers, irritability, thirst, night sweats, dryness and coughing up of blood, all with weakness, deficiency and debility. As such, it is valuable for AIDS.

Indications: fevers, thirst, night sweats, coughing up blood (all with weakness and deficiency), AIDS
Projects: tea, soup, wine, congee

Angelica

Angelica archangelica; Umbelliferae

Part used: root
Energy and taste: warm; spicy, bitter
Actions: removes stagnation; lungs, stomach, intestines, circulation
Active constituents: volatile oil, coumarins, acids, resins, starches, flavonoids and sterols
Properties: carminative, stimulant, emmenagogue, diaphoretic, expectorant
Dose: infuse 1 ounce bruised root/1 pint boiled water, drink 1 cup 3 times/day; 2 "00" capsules 3 times/day; tincture, 10-30 drops 3 times/day; 3-9 gm in formula
Precautions: pregnancy, diabetes, bleeding

Angelica stimulates blood circulation and warms the body. Daily doses can help those with coldness stay warm in winter. Because it induces sweating, it is useful for treating colds, flu, pleurisy and all lung diseases. Being a strong emmenagogue, it also promotes menstruation and helps menstrual disorders occurring from coldness. In fact, it is similar to dong quai (*Angelica sinensis*) in moving the blood and promoting menstruation, but doesn't have its blood building properties.

Angelica aids indigestion due to coldness, relieves spasms of the stomach and intestines, helps stomach ulcers and anorexia and dispels gas. It is said that its regular use creates a distaste for alcohol. Because it can increase sugar in the blood, diabetics should avoid using this herb.

Externally angelica may be applied as an oil, poultice or liniment to treat rheumatism, arthritis and skin disorders. The root oil prevents bacterial and fungal growth. Frequently used as a flavoring and bitter digestive, angelica oil is used in various liqueurs such as Benedictine and Chartreuse, the leaves as a garnish or in salads and the stems in candies.

Indications: colds, flus, pleurisy and other lung diseases, menstrual disorders from coldness, indigestion, spasms, ulcers and gas from coldness, arthritis, rheumatism
Projects: tea, oil, poultice, liniment, tincture, capsule, cider, sweating

Barberry

Berberis vulgaris; Berberidaceae

Part used: root
Energy and taste: cold; bitter
Actions: liver, gallbladder, stomach, colon
Active constituents: berberine and other alkaloids, chelidonic acid, resin, tannin, wax

WESTERN HERBS

Properties: alterative, hepatic, laxative, anti-inflammatory, bitter tonic

Other: Many species of this plant are found throughout the world, such as the Pacific Northwest varieties called Oregon Grape (*Berberis aquifolium* and *Mahonia repens*)

Dose: decoct 1 ounce/pint water, drink 3 cups/day; 2 "00" caps, 3 times/day; tincture, 10-30 drops, 3 times/day; 3-9 gm in formula

Precautions: pregnancy

Barberry is one of the mildest and best liver tonics known. It cleanses and regulates the liver's function and so is especially useful for jaundice, hepatitis and enlargement of the liver and spleen. Its detoxifying action helps heal acne, boils, conjunctivitis and fevers. Because it clears excess as well as deficient heat, it is milder and safer to use than other herbs in this category, such as golden seal or gentian.

As a bitter tonic barberry stimulates digestion, acts as a mild laxative, and clears the heat and toxins in arthritis and rheumatism. It is also useful for amoebic and bacillary chronic dysentery and diarrhea. Because it stimulates the uterus, it should be avoided in pregnancy.

Ayurveda combines barberry with turmeric to reduce fat, and with twice the amount of turmeric, for diabetes. This combination also regulates liver energy similar to bupleurum in Chinese medicine.

Indications: hepatitis, jaundice, enlargement of liver and spleen, acne, boils, chronic diarrhea and dysentery (amoebic, bacillary), fever, conjunctivitis, arthritis

Projects: tea, eye wash, capsule, bitters

Bayberry

Myrica cerifera; Myricaceae

Part used: bark of the root
Energy and taste: warm; spicy, astringent

Actions: spleen, lungs, liver, circulation

Active constituents: triterpenes, flavonoids, tannins, phenols, resins and gums

Properties: stimulant, astringent, expectorant, diaphoretic

Dose: decoct 1 ounce/pint water, drink 1/2 cup 2-3 times/day; powder—1 tsp per cup boiling water, or 2 "00" capsules 3 times/day

Precautions: in large doses it is emetic

Bayberry is a powerful stimulant. It raises vitality and resistance to disease, especially in the initial stages. It clears mucus, dispels colds, flus and coughs, cleanses the lymphatics and, in general, eliminates cold mucus conditions in the body. For any of these situations, take in a capsule or as a tea, gargle for sore throats, smoke to clear the lungs and snuff to clear the sinuses.

The astringency of bayberry stops persistent diarrhea, bowel inflammation, excessive menstrual bleeding, uterine prolapse and uterine and vaginal discharges. Its stimulant action warms and circulates energy and blood. Thus, it promotes the healing and toning of tissue after checking the undesired discharge.

Externally, the powdered bark may be made into a paste, poultice or wash to help old wounds, ulcers and sores that do not heal. It makes an excellent toothpowder, astringing and cleansing receding and bleeding gums. For this it combines well with powders of cinnamon, myrrh, echinacea and salt. A fomentation made from the tea can be applied nightly to relieve, cure and prevent varicose veins. In the past wax from the berries was used for making candles.

Indications: colds, flus, sore throat, sinus and lung congestion, diarrhea, excessive menstrual bleeding, uterine prolapse, vaginal discharge, sores, ulcers

Projects: tea, powder, capsule, paste, fomentation, toothpowder, gargle, poultice, wash, smoked, bolus, sweating, pill, cider

WESTERN HERBS

Blackberry

Rubus villosus; Rosaceae

Part used: leaves, root bark, fruit
Energy and taste: neutral; leaves, root bark: bitter, astringent; fruit: sweet, sour
Active constituents: leaves, root bark: both are high in tannins; fruit: isocitric and malic acids, sugars, pectin, momoglycoside of cyanidin and Vitamins A and C
Actions: leaves, root bark: stomach, intestines; fruit: liver, kidney
Properties: leaves, root bark: astringent, hemostatic; fruit: blood and nutritive tonic, refrigerant
Dose: leaves—infuse 1 ounce/pint water; root bark—decoct 1 ounce/pint water; both—drink 3 cups/day or use 3-9 gm in formula; fruit—9-15 gm

Blackberry root bark is perhaps one of the best remedies for diarrhea and dysentery, even in infants. For this, simmer 1 tbsp with 1 tsp cinnamon powder in 1 cup milk for 5 minutes on low heat or take powdered in capsule form. The leaves also work for this but are less astringent and so better for milder cases. They are better as a uterine tonic and, along with the root, help inhibit excessive menstrual bleeding.

The berries and juice build blood, aid anemia, cool the blood and regulate menses. In excess, however, they cause loose stools, which is interesting since the leaves and root firm loose stools. The Chinese use blackberries to strengthen vitality and virility, promote fertility and hair growth, improve the complexion and cure fevers and colds.

Indications: diarrhea, dysentery, excessive menstrual bleeding, building blood
Projects: tea, capsule, food, bolus, sun tea, juice

Black Cohosh

Cimicifuga racemosa; Ranunculaceae

Part used: root
Energy and taste: cool; sweet, spicy, slightly bitter

Active constituents: various glycosides such as actaeine, cimicifugin, bitter principles, racemosin, estrogenic substances, triterpene glycosides, isoferulic acid, tannin
Actions: liver, spleen, stomach, large intestine
Properties: antispasmodic, expectorant, emmenagogue, diaphoretic, alterative, parturient
Dose: decoct 1 ounce root/pint water, take 3 cups/day; 2 "00" caps 3 times/day; tincture, 10-60 drops, 3 times/day; 3-9 gm in formula
Precaution: too large a dose will cause nausea, dizziness and dimness of vision; avoid in first and second trimester of pregnancy

Western herbalism primarily uses black cohosh as an antispasmodic useful for nervous conditions, hysteria, neuralgia, cramps and pains. It treats delayed and painful menses and, combined with lung and cough herbs, it eases whooping cough, asthma and bronchitis. Black cohosh facilitates childbirth, especially when combined with raspberry and squaw vine and taken daily for the last two weeks of pregnancy. Native American women also used it to relieve pains associated with childbirth and menses. It is used in Europe for rheumatism, arthritis and feelings of heaviness in the limbs.

Chinese herbalism uses *Cimicifuga foetida* as a cooling diaphoretic for colds, flus, fever, headache and sore throat and to bring out skin rashes such as measles. It also raises the energy of the body and so lifts up a prolapsed stomach, intestines, bladder or uterus.

Indications: nervous conditions, cramps, delayed and painful menses, childbirth, measles, prolapsed organs, rheumatism, arthritis
Projects: tea, tincture, capsule

Black Haw

Viburnum prunifolium; Caprifoliaceae

Part used: dried bark of root or stem
Energy and taste: cool; bitter

WESTERN HERBS

Active constituents: coumarins including scopoletin, viburnin, salicin, volatile oil, acids, and tannin
Actions: liver
Properties: antispasmodic, analgesic, uterine tonic, sedative, nervine
Dose: infuse 1 ounce/pint water, drink 3 cups/day; 3-9 gm in formula
Precaution: avoid if blood doesn't clot easily

Black haw is a useful antispasmodic and analgesic for treating all nervous conditions, including convulsions, hysteria and spasms. It is reliable for dysmenorrhea, PMS, irregular menstruation, menstrual cramps, spasms and all painful conditions. It helps to control morning sickness and can change the mental attitude of an expectant mother from depression to cheerfulness.

Being a uterine tonic, it is indicated in habitual miscarriage any time during pregnancy, although for it to be effective it should be taken several weeks before the miscarriage usually occurs. It is used after childbirth to check pain and bleeding. Cramp bark (*Viburnum opulis*) can be used as a substitute for black haw but is stronger in action.

Indications: nervous conditions, convulsions, hysteria, spasms, cramps, pains, menstrual difficulties, PMS, threatened miscarriage, postpartum pain and bleeding
Projects: tea, capsule, tincture, pill

Black Pepper

Piper nigrum; Piperaceae

Part used: fruit
Energy and taste: hot; spicy
Active constituents: essential oil that contains phellandrene, two acrid resins, hot tasting amides, 5-9% peperine, peperidine and aromatic acids
Actions: kidneys, spleen, stomach
Properties: stimulant, expectorant, carminative
Dose: 1/4 to 1/2 tsp powder as needed; 2-5 gm infused in formula; as a seasoning with food

Precautions: inflammatory conditions of the digestive organs, excessive heat in the body; prolonged daily use of black pepper can cause the tendons to contract, thus injuring flexibility

While predominantly used as a spice, black pepper is an important metabolic stimulant and expectorant. It is one of the best herb foods for weak digestion, gas, stagnant food in the stomach, bloatedness and mucus in the colon. It also dries cold mucus in the lungs, throat and sinuses, clearing out colds, coughs and other mucus conditions. It counteracts cold damp symptoms, dries up secretions and gives warmth to the body. It is a good antidote to cold and raw foods.

One of the best ways of taking black pepper is in its traditional Ayurvedic combination ground together with pippli long pepper and ginger root and mixed with a little honey to form a paste. This paste is taken in quarter to full teaspoon doses with a little hot water three times a day. If the pippli long pepper cannot be located (try Indian food stores), use anise seed instead. At the first signs of a cold or mucus congestion, I give this paste with great results.

Indications: weak digestion, gas, bloatedness, colds, cough, mucus from coldness, sinus congestion
Projects: spice, paste, capsule, powder, chai

Borage

Borago officinalis; Boraginaceae

Part used: leaves
Energy and taste: cool; bitter, sweet
Active constituents: mucilage, tannin, traces of essential oil, pyrrolizidine alkaloids in small amounts
Actions: lungs, heart
Properties: refrigerant, diaphoretic, febrifuge, aperient, galactagogue, diuretic, demulcent, emollient
Dose: infuse 1 ounce/pint water, drink 3 cups/day; 3-9 gm in formula

As borage is very cooling, it is valuable for lowering high fevers and clearing excess heat. It also decongests the lungs and so is beneficial for chronic mucus, bronchitis and pneumonia. The mucilage content increases the production of mothers milk. Because borage is a restorative agent for the adrenal cortex, it helps heal the adrenal glands after medical treatment with cortisone and other steroids and regenerates the adrenals when under stress.

Externally, borage is used as a soothing and anti-inflammatory poultice, tincture, salve or liniment on inflammatory swellings, rheumatism and all irritations of the skin and mucous membranes. Traditionally it has been used as a galactagogue, but because of its pyrrolizidine alkaloid, it is best avoided by pregnant women, nursing mothers and children. The beautiful star-shaped blue flowers can be eaten and are a delightful garnish in salads. Traditionally, the leaves have also been eaten.

Indications: fever, pneumonia, bronchitis, skin and mucous membrane inflammations, stress

Projects: tea, tincture, poultice, liniment, salve, salad, sun tea

Burdock

Arctium lappa; Compositae

Parts used: root and seeds

Energy and taste: cool; bitter, slightly sweet

Active constituents: up to 50% inulin; a bitter glycoside—arctiin, 2 ligans, volatile oil, tannin, resin, mucilage, sugar, acids, iron, calcium, Vitamin C

Actions: clears heat, detoxifies blood; kidneys, spleen, stomach, liver, skin; general effects on the whole body

Properties: alterative, diuretic, diaphoretic, nutritive

Dose: decoct 1 ounce/per 1 pint water; drink 3 cups/day; 3-10 gm in formula

A good blood and lymphatic cleanser, burdock root is an excellent remedy for all skin diseases. It clears rashes, boils, eczema, styes, carbuncles and canker sores. For skin diseases it may be combined for further effectiveness with yellow dock and sarsa-

parilla. Because burdock provides an abundance of iron, it strengthens as well as cleanses the blood.

Burdock also detoxifies the liver, clearing heat, anger, irritability and restlessness. This has beneficial effects on arthritis, rheumatism, gout, infections and inflammations. It further has a diuretic action on the kidneys which helps clear the blood of harmful acids and aids low back pain, fluid retention and sciatica. Lastly, it causes sweating and lowers fevers—uses to which the Chinese put it. Burdock seeds are very effective in healing skin disorders, such as psoriasis and alopecia. For this it is used as a wash, tincture or oil.

The raw root may be used as a food. The Japanese first thinly slice and soak it for 15 minutes in vinegar water and then boil it in salt water. This is a cleansing and strengthening food for the body and, eaten in this way in the morning, has helped lessen sweet cravings in some instances. It is a good food to incorporate into our diets as the bitter taste aids digestion and is so rarely included in meals. The roots may be roasted and added to roasted dandelion for a coffee substitute beverage. The Chinese eat the leaves as a potherb.

Indications: all skin diseases, fever, stye, boils, rash, canker sore, arthritis, rheumatism, toxicity of blood, kidney inflammation

Projects: tea, oil, tincture, poultice, wash, capsule

Calendula

Calendula officinalis; Compositae

Parts used: flowers

Energy and taste: neutral; spicy, bitter

Active constituents: essential oil containing carotenoids, saponin, resin and bitter principle

Actions: removes blood stagnation, aids blood and skin; liver, heart, lungs

Properties: vulnerary, astringent, diaphoretic, antispasmodic, stimulant

Dose: infuse 1 ounce herb/pint water; acute—drink 1 cup tea every hour until symptoms lessen, then drink 1 cup 2-4 times/day until problem is gone; other—

WESTERN HERBS

drink 3 cups/day; tincture, 10-30 drops; 3-6 gm in formula

Other: often known as marigold instead of calendula

Calendula is an ancient herb, having been used since the 12th century in Europe and even earlier in Egypt, where it originated. It is often used as a dye; in fact, cheese was originally dyed yellow by its flower. Many varieties of calendula exist, and one of them is the common marigold, by which name it is often known. The larger flowers are more medicinal and make beautiful garden plants.

The volatile oils of calendula stimulate blood circulation and cause sweating, thus aiding fevers to break and skin eruptions to come out faster. For this reason it is specific for measles, rashes and related eruptive diseases. When my son had the chicken pox, I had to apply calendula tincture (oil would work as well or even a wash from the tea) only once to each pox for the itching and eruption to stop. Within the day he was feeling much better and the chicken pox rapidly cleared up.

Calendula is actually specific for any skin problems, and I have seen it useful for fungus. Many mothers find it wonderful for diaper rash. It promotes the rapid healing of wounds and aids persistent ulcers, burns, bruises, injuries, varicose veins and bleeding, including bleeding hemorrhoids. In all these cases it is applied as a salve, oil or poultice.

Like mullein, calendula flowers can be made into an oil and used for earaches and other infections; as a natural antiseptic it prevents the growth of harmful bacteria. It is a good first aid remedy since it can be easily found and has so many uses.

Calendula flowers are also specific for any blood stagnation problems, such as bruises, sprains and wounds and their associated pain. Again, it can be applied externally to the wound itself or taken internally as a tea. Calendula tea stimulates the blood circulation, cleanses the blood, eases cramps and regulates the menses. It also helps stomach disorders and gastric and duodenal ulcers. Cooled calendula tea can be used as an eye wash for sore, red and irritated eyes.

Indications: cuts, sores, wounds, burns, fevers, earaches, irritated eyes, burns, fevers, cramps, bruises, measles, chicken pox and other eruptive skin diseases, bleeding wounds or hemorrhoids

Projects: oil, tincture, poultice, salve, tea, dye, foot bath, wash, first aid, fomentation, potpourri, sweating, sun tea

Cardamom

Elettaria cardamomum; Zingiberaceae

Part used: seed

Energy and taste: warm; spicy

Active constituents: essential oil including D-borneol, bornylacetate, d-camphor, nerolidol, linalool

Actions: spleen, stomach, lungs, kidney

Properties: stomachic, carminative, expectorant, tonic

Dose: 1/4 to 1 tsp powder as needed; 3-6 gm steeped in formula

Cardamom is a delicious spice that aids digestion and eliminates gas, bloatedness, diarrhea, colic, nervous digestive upset, belching, vomiting, acid regurgitation, abdominal distention, stagnant food in the stomach and headaches due to indigestion. It also counteracts mucus congestion in the lungs and sinuses, helping colds, cough, bronchitis, asthma, and hoarse voice. When added to milk or fruit it neutralizes the mucus-forming properties. For a lung tonic recipe, core a hard winter pear, stuff it with honey and 1/2 to 1 teaspoon cardamom powder and bake.

Indications: indigestion, gas, bloatedness, diarrhea, colic, belching, vomiting, colds, cough, bronchitis, asthma

Projects: paste, spice, powder, chai, tea

WESTERN HERBS

Cascara Sagrada

Cascara sagrada; Rhamnus purshiana; Rhamnaceae

Part used: bark of tree, dried and aged at least a year

Energy and taste: cold; bitter

Active constituents: anthraquinone and emodin glycosides, aloins, bitter principle

Actions: spleen, stomach, liver, gallbladder, large intestines

Properties: laxative, bitter tonic, nervine, emetic

Dose: infuse 1-2 tsp in cup of boiling water for 10 minutes, taken at bedtime; tincture, 20-40 drops 3 times/day, or 1/2-3/4 teaspoon for faster action; 3-9 gm in formula

Other: also known as California buckthorn; called the sacred bark

The cold bitter properties of cascara stimulate secretions of the entire digestive system, including the liver, gallbladder, stomach and pancreas. Such secretions cause a laxative action and aid digestion. Thus cascara is good for chronic constipation, colitis, hemorrhoids due to poor bowel function, liver congestion, cirrhosis, jaundice, indigestion and poor appetite. It tones the entire intestinal tract.

Cascara is mild and so suitable for delicate and elderly people and constipation during pregnancy. It can be used safely on a daily basis without becoming habit-forming. It is usually taken in capsule or tincture form since it is too bitter for most people to drink as a tea. For those with sensitive bowels, it should be combined with a little ginger, anise or fennel seed to prevent griping or cramping. Only the dried bark which is 1 year or older should be used. The fresh is too irritating.

Indications: constipation, indigestion, poor appetite, sluggish bowels, hemorrhoids, colitis, liver congestion, jaundice, cirrhosis

Projects: tea, tincture, capsule

Cayenne

Capsicum anuum; Solanaceae

Parts used: the ripe fruit (peppers)

Energy and taste: hot; spicy

Active constituents: a pungent phenol compound (capsaicin), a red carotenoid pigment (capsanthin), several vitamins including Vitamins A and C

Actions: stops bleeding, activates blood; kidneys, lungs, spleen, stomach, heart

Properties: stimulant, astringent, carminative, hemostatic, antispasmodic

Dose: two "00" capsules 2-3 times/day; 1/4-1 tsp/cup warm water, 2-3 times/day

Precaution: avoid if there's a tendency toward nosebleeds or if there is nervousness, a flushed face, AIDS or other wasting disease, or if there is any dryness or internal inflammation; use carefully as it is very spicy; large doses cause vomiting

Since cayenne is so hot, the idea that it is harmless is sometimes hard to believe, yet it is not irritating when uncooked. Its hot stimulating properties make it perfect for breaking up congestion in the body, clearing mucus, moving the blood, helping to eliminate headaches, cramping and diarrhea and dispelling internal and external cold and cold dampnesss. It will also give more energy and stimulate vitality.

Cayenne is considered a superior crisis herb, useful as a first aid remedy for most conditions. At the first sign of colds, flus, indigestion, bleeding or that "low" feeling, it is a perfect remedy to take and will ward off diseases due to cold and damp. It is useful for pains of the stomach, bowels and cramps. For any type of external bleeding, sprinkling cayenne powder on the wound will stop it without burning the skin or causing pain. It will further stop hemorrhaging internally and externally in acute conditions because it

WESTERN HERBS

normalizes circulation. For the same reason, it is well suited for those who have either high or low blood pressure.

Cayenne is a terrific stimulant for the heart, circulation and preventing heart attacks and strokes. It can be taken as a daily tonic for the heart and blood. It will also increase body vitality and arrest depression. The Chinese use it for rheumatism. Cayenne helps digestion, stimulates the appetite and dispels gas. If used carefully, starting with small doses and gradually increasing tolerance, it can heal stomach ulcers.

Like ginger in Chinese medicine, cayenne is often added to Western formulas as a stimulant to carry the herbs quickly and effectively throughout the body to their specified locations, making the other herbs more potent. Cayenne, however, opens the pores and causes a sweat. It ultimately eliminates body heat. Dried ginger, on the other hand, heats the inside of the body without the loss of body heat.

Therefore, those who tend to feel colder should use smaller amounts of cayenne. Those who tend to feel very warm should use cayenne sparingly and with care internally as it could aggravate an already internal hot condition. In general, cayenne may be taken in larger doses for a beneficial short-term effect in acute conditions, but in small doses for a long-term tonic.

Cayenne may be taken as a powder diluted in water which gives fairly immediate results. It is quite hot and spicy to taste, however, and takes getting used to. Begin with a small amount and slowly work up to more. At first one may feel nauseous, but the feeling will soon pass and a wonderful sense of well being follows. It may alternatively be taken in capsule form.

Externally, cayenne tincture or oil rubbed on toothaches, cramps, sprains, muscle pain and stiffness, swellings and sore joints will heal and stop pain. For arthritis, it is very beneficial when applied to the painful areas, then wrapped in flannel cloth and kept in place throughout the night. Cayenne powder may be used as a gargle in laryngitis and sore throat, and, in very small amounts (a pinch) diluted in water, as an eye wash to improve circulation and vision.

Indications: heart tonic, poor circulation, colds, flu, indigestion, loss of appetite, joint aches and pains, lowered vitality and energy, diarrhea, cramps, toothaches, swellings, headaches, depression, bleeding, sprains, arthritis

Projects: powder, capsule, tea, tincture, oil, liniment, first aid, gargle, eye wash, spice

Chamomile

Anthemis floes; A. nobiles; Matricaria chamomilla; Compositae

Parts used: flowers

Energy and taste: neutral; bitter, spicy

Active constituents: volatile oil, bitter principle (anthemic acid), coumarins, flavonoids, phenolic acids, tannin, resin

Actions: nerves, stomach, liver, lungs

Properties: nervine, carminative, tonic, diaphoretic, sedative, antispasmodic, vulnerary, antiseptic, emmenagogue

Dose: infuse 1 ounce/pint water; drink 4 cups tea/day or more as needed; 10-30 drops tincture

Precaution: some say that large doses are emetic

Chamomile has a high concentration of easily assimilable calcium which makes it particularly useful for soothing the nerves in nervous conditions such as nervousness, irritability, restlessness, hypertension, insomnia, cramps and spasms. It is also calming to the gastric system, soothing nervous stomachs and aiding indigestion, gas, pain and other stomach disorders.

Chamomile is a common European beverage used to promote digestion. The tea also benefits fevers, colds, flu and headaches, especially those due to indigestion. Further, it is a gentle laxative, brings on the menses and eases menstrual cramps, especially when combined with ginger. With scullcap it is a good safe daily nervine. Externally, a poultice, bath or herbal wash helps heal burns, cuts, sore muscles, painful joints, ulcers and rashes.

WESTERN HERBS

Chamomile has many uses for children. Because it is so calming, it is one of the best herbs to use for crying, whining and restlessness. It is also invaluable in teething, both for aiding the teeth to come in as well as for calming the irritation and restlessness this causes. Used in baby's bath water or as a wash, it will help diaper rash or burns, cuts and abrasions. The tea helps children's colic, gas and constipation and the oil can be combined with mullein or calendula for earaches.

Indications: nervousness, hypertension, restlessness, insomnia, nervous stomach, indigestion, gastric ulcers, gas, colic, stomachache, teething and related problems such as earache, neuralgic pain, stomach upset, stomach disorders, infantile convulsions, menstrual cramps and to bring on menses

Projects: tea, bath, wash, salve, oil, tincture, sun tea, potpourri

Chaparral

Larrea divaricata; Zygophyllaceae

Parts used: leaves

Energy and taste: cold; bitter, spicy, slightly salty

Active constituents: NDGA (nordihydroquaiaretic acid) which is vasodepressant and increases ascorbic acid levels in the adrenals, flavonoids, acids, free steroidal compounds, volatile oils, resin

Actions: clears heat; general effects on whole body, stomach, intestines, lungs, liver, kidneys

Properties: antiseptic, antibiotic, parasiticide; alterative, expectorant, diuretic, antitumor, laxative

Dose: infuse 1 tsp to 1 tbsp/cup water, drink 1/2 to 1 cup tea 2-3 times/day; 2 "00" capsules 2-4 times/day; 10-30 drops tincture; 3-6 gm in formula

Often known by the name greasewood, chaparral grows bountifully as a tall yellow flowering bush in a ring formation in desert areas. It is the oldest living thing on earth; some rings having been found to be 7500 years old! The small, sticky hard leaves are strongly bitter, and it is partly this taste which makes it a valuable antibiotic, laxative, liver tonic and heat-clearing herb.

Chaparral contains NDGA (nordihydroquaiaretic acid) as its primary constituent. This acid has a pronounced antioxidant effect, making it valuable for cancer, tumors, bacteria, viruses and parasites. It also has an anti-inflammatory or heat-clearing effect on the respiratory, intestinal and urinary tracts. Externally it is applied to heal wounds, itching eczema, scabies and dandruff, and a concentrated extract can be applied to reduce warts. A mouthwash used on a daily basis will prevent dental caries.

Eating the leaf straight off the bush is a great way to acclimate oneself to the desert. It will also keep the body cooler there and clean out toxins. Usually it is taken in capsule or tincture form, however. Chaparral is often combined with goldenseal and echinacea for an antibiotic effect in infections, inflammations, tumors and cancer.

Indications: cancer, tumors, parasites, constipation, diarrhea, skin diseases, scabies, dandruff, itching, eczema, warts, bacterial and viral infections

Projects: tea, capsule, tincture, liniment, bath, mouthwash

Chaste Berry

Vitex agnus-castus; Verbenaceae

Parts used: berry

Energy and taste: neutral; sweet, bitter

Active constituents: essential oil, fatty oil, the flavone casticin, iridoid glycosides

Actions: liver, spleen

Properties: emmenagogue, vulnerary, galactagogue

Dose: infuse 1 ounce/pint water; drink 3 cups/day; 3-4 capsules once/day in the morning on an empty stomach; 25-40 drops tincture, same way as capsules; 3-6 gm in formula; this herb should be taken long-term, 6 months or longer, for optimum effects, although benefits may be felt after 10 days

Precaution: pregnancy after the third month as it could bring on the flow of milk too soon

WESTERN HERBS

Chaste berry, also referred to as vitex, is a supreme female herb. It stimulates the pituitary gland and the secretion of luteotropic hormone which increases the output of progesterone. Thus, it regulates hormonal balance and the menstrual cycle, including normalizing estrogen. It treats PMS and its associated symptoms of migraines, depression, cramps, edema in legs, sensitive breasts and allergies. It also aids problems associated with menopause such as dry vagina, hot flashes, dizziness and depression.

Vitex treats amenorrhea, irregular menstruation, heavy bleeding or too short a menstrual cycle, withdrawal after the pill and fibroid cysts. It also treats acne in male and female teenagers. It is gentle with no side effects. Vitex increases mother's milk.

Indications: PMS, menopause, depression, irregular menstruation, amenorrhea, acne, promoting mother's milk

Projects: tea, tincture

Chickweed

Stellaria media; Caryophyllaceae

Part used: above-ground portion

Energy and taste: cool; bitter, sweet

Active constituents: saponins, coumarins and hydroxycoumarins, flavonoids, carboxylic acids, triterpenoids, Vitamins A and C and most of the B-complex, and lots of calcium and iron

Actions: lungs, stomach

Properties: expectorant, demulcent, emollient, antitussive, antipyretic, alterative, vulnerary

Dose: infuse 1 ounce/pint water; drink 3 cups or more as needed per day; 6-15 gm in formula; this herb is often eaten abundantly as a food for its therapeutic effects

This very commonly found "weed" is one of the best herbs to stop itching. It is wonderful for alleviating mosquito bites, eczema, scaly scalp, dandruff, hives, seboreia, hemorrhoids and other itchy skin conditions. Further, it can be used as a drawing poultice for boils, ulcers and abscesses. For these it is applied externally as an oil or salve (especially with olive oil), juice, ointment or poultice. The juice directly expressed from the leaves is especially effective for healing scalp problems.

Chickweed's moistening action relieves sore throats and soothes stomach and duodenal ulcers. It will further aid mucus expectoration from the lungs and lower fevers. It treats blood toxicity, inflammation and other "hot" diseases. Chickweed may also be used to reduce excess fat, being both mildly diuretic and laxative.

Indications: any itching conditions, rheumatism, boils, ulcers, abscesses, sore throat, fevers, excess fat

Projects: tea, bath, poultice, oil, juice, salve, ointment

Cinnamon

Cinnamomum verum; Lauraceae

Part used: dried inner bark of the shoots of the cinnamon tree

Energy and taste: hot; sweet, spicy

Active constituents: essential oil, mucilage, tannin, sucrose, resin, gum

Actions: spleen, kidney, liver, urinary bladder

Properties: stimulant, astringent, diaphoretic, demulcent, carminative, antiseptic, expectorant, hemostatic

Dose: infuse 1 tsp bark/cup water; drink 1 cup tea 3 times/day; 2 "00" caps 3 times/day; 10-30 drops tincture 3 times/day; 3-9 gm in formula

Precautions: pregnancy; individuals with wasting and dryness; signs of heat and fire; many children can only tolerate it in small infrequent doses

A deep acting stimulant, cinnamon warms the internal body, raises vitality, stimulates circulation and clears congestion. It aids many problems which are due to coldness, such as cold hands and feet, feelings of coldness, chronic diarrhea, cramps, spasms,

WESTERN HERBS

indigestion, nausea, vomiting, gas, coughs, mucus, abdominal pains and heart and lower back pain. It also warms the kidneys and strengthens the adrenals, which helps enhance the immune functions and the body's ability to handle stress.

In the form of cinnamon milk, it is especially good for diarrhea in elderly people. This delicious drink is actually a good way to drink milk in general as the cinnamon warms up the milk's cool energy and the little honey added helps stop mucus from forming. Cinnamon can also be made into a paste by mixing the powder with honey. This is good to eat in winter to keep one warm and at other times to improve digestion, eliminate gas and clear up mucus in the chest. Cinnamon powder may be effectively added to fruits, milk and desserts to balance their cooling energy.

Chinese cinnamon, *C. cassia*, can often be found in many herbal stores. It is a stronger variety of cinnamon and is commonly used for impotence, spermatorrhea, cold and weak legs, backache, diarrhea, nausea and vomiting. It is also commonly used to promote menses and alleviate menstrual pain from coldness and in cases when the upper part of the body is hot (dry mouth, sore throat, toothache) and the lower part is cold (lower back pain, diarrhea, cold lower extremities).

The twigs of cinnamon are also used by the Chinese and are most specific for causing sweating to eliminate chills, fever, colds, flus and other respiratory conditions in those who have coldness. Traditionally, a small bowl of rice is eaten after sweating therapy with cinnamon tea to replenish the strength.

Indications: indigestion, gas, vomiting, circulation, arthritis, rheumatism, colds, flus, coughs, mucus, diarrhea, cramps, spasms, pain, warming the internal organs and hands and feet, impotence, spermatorrhea
Projects: tea, tincture, paste, milk, pills, spice, powder, capsule, tooth powder, first aid

Coltsfoot

Tussilago farfara; Compositae

Parts used: leaves, flowers
Energy and taste: neutral; bitter, sweet
Active constituents: leaves—mucilage, tannin, flavonoids, inulin, a glycosidal bitter principle, pyrrolizidine alkaloids in very small amounts; flowers—flavonoids, triterpenoid saponins, tannin, essential oil
Actions: lungs
Properties: antitussive, expectorant, demulcent, antiinflammatory, astringent
Dose: infuse 1 ounce/pint water, drink 3 cups/day; 2 "00" caps 3 times/day; 10-20 drops tincture; 3-9 gm in formula
Precautions: since it contains pyrrolizidine alkaloids, it should be avoided in pregnancy, nursing, liver disease and for prolonged use in very young children

The Latin name of coltsfoot, *Tussilago*, means cough dispeller, and coltsfoot is one of the best cough remedies available. It aids the relief of dry, irritating or persistent cough, wheezing, asthma, bronchitis, emphysema, whooping cough and difficulty of breathing. It is especially useful in chronic conditions and for persistent or acute episodes of spasmodic cough.

Additionally, coltsfoot has a demulcent and antiinflammatory action and so may be used effectively to soothe sore throats, laryngitis, hoarseness, flus and colds. For these it may be taken as a tea, smoked or in cough syrup. A cup of hot coltsfoot tea first thing in the morning is especially valuable for clearing the air passages in chronic cases. Chinese medicine also uses it for cough and lung disorders.

Indications: cough, asthma, bronchitis, whooping cough, emphysema, laryngitis, hoarseness, flu, cold, sore throat, difficulty in breathing
Projects: tea, syrup, smoked, tincture

WESTERN HERBS

Comfrey

Symphytum officinale; Boraginaceae

Parts used: leaves and root
Energy and taste: cool; bitter, sweet
Active constituents: allantoin, pyrrolizidine alkaloids, tannins, mucilage, starch, phenolic acids
Actions: general effects on the whole body, clears heat; lungs, stomach, bones, muscles
Properties: demulcent, vulnerary, expectorant, nutritive tonic, alterative, astringent, antitussive
Dose: infuse leaves, decoct root 1 ounce/pint water; acute—drink 1/2 to 1 cup tea/hour until condition lessens, then drink 2 cups/day until problem is gone; other—3 cups 3 times/day; 2 "00" caps 3 times/day; 10-30 drops tincture; leaves 3-9 gm, root 6-15 gm in formula
Precautions: Because of its pyrrolizidine alkaloids, it should be avoided in pregnancy, nursing, for prolonged use in children and liver disease (see endnote 2 in *Herbal Properties, Constituents, Families and Formulas*).

Comfrey's nickname, knitbone, is highly appropriate since one of its constituents actually causes cells to proliferate. Due to this, it helps heal broken bones, fractures and broken skin (try it on torn perineums after childbirth, using the fresh herb poultice daily), and it strengthens tendons. It is both taken internally and applied externally for these conditions.

Because comfrey has the highest mucilage content of any herb, it is very moistening and lubricating. It soothes burns, inflammations and other skin irritations, psoriasis, eczema, ulcers, healing wounds and varicose veins and draws out poisons from boils and insect bites or stings. I have found comfrey, along with perhaps plantain and echinacea root powder, to be incomparable in drawing out the poison from spider bites, healing them quickly and painlessly. Comfrey can be applied as a poultice or salve for these.

A wonderful herb for the lungs, comfrey's cooling moistening effects heal bronchitis, tonsillitis, pharyngitis, pleurisy, pneumonia and consumption and coughs, including whooping cough; they also expel phlegm, soothe the throat, lower fever and, overall, rejuvenate the lungs and mucous membranes. They help the pancreas regulate blood sugar levels and promote the secretion of pepsin, thus aiding digestion.

Comfrey also stops bleeding from the stomach, lungs, bowels, kidneys, ulcers and piles. For this take a strong decoction of the root, using 1/2 to 1 ounce of root every 2 hours until the bleeding has stopped, or boil 2 tsp powder in 1 cup milk. Comfrey can also be eaten directly in salads, steamed, or blended into fruit or vegetable drinks for added nutrition and chlorophyll.

The root can be used as well as the leaf and is stronger in tonic properties for healing the lungs and mucous membranes, especially in cases of dryness, heat and inflammation. The leaves are more astringent and anti-inflammatory. Comfrey is a powerful and true tonic for nourishing and promoting tissue growth in the body.

Indications: skin wounds and tears, bites, stings, boils, inflammatory lung conditions, coughs, fevers, bleeding, fractures, broken bones
Projects: salve, poultice, tea, syrup, potherb, capsule, milk, fomentation

Dandelion

Taraxacum officinale; Compositae

Parts used: leaves and root
Energy and taste: cold; bitter, sweet
Active constituents: an acrid bitter resin (taraxacerin), inulin (25%), phytosterols, saponins, glutin, gum potash, Vitamins A and C (the Vitamin A content is higher than in carrots)
Actions: clears excessive heat, detoxifies liver, kidney, gallbladder, bladder, spleen, stomach, pancreas
Properties: bitter tonic, diuretic, lithotriptic, astringent, cholagogue, galactogogue, laxative, alterative
Dose: decoct 1 ounce cut root/pint water; drink 1 cup tea 3 times/day; 2 "00" caps 3 times/day; 10-30 drops tincture; 3-9 gm in formula

WESTERN HERBS

This notable "weed" is often needed most by those who love to pull it—excitable, fiery and angry people—because it clears the heat and congestion from the liver which usually causes this. It is one of the best herbs for the liver, cleansing the blood and strengthening this organ, even curing hepatitis, jaundice and cirrhosis. I have seen dandelion effectively heal hepatitis when 6 cups of tea from the raw root are taken each day for a week or two. It stimulates the secretion of bile, thus aiding digestion, acting as a laxative and breaking up gall and kidney stones.

Its blood cleansing properties treats skin rashes, measles, chicken pox, eczema, poison oak and ivy and other skin eruptions. The Chinese use it for infections, inflammations, boils, abscesses, swellings, carious teeth, red, swollen and painful eyes, fever and other heat-related conditions. Externally, it's juice is applied to snake bites.

Dandelion's action on the digestive system is also notable. It stimulates and strengthens the digestive process and is valuable for diabetics and hypoglycemics. It is useful for detoxification from over-eating meat and fatty and fried foods. Its diuretic effect cleanses the kidneys and lowers blood pressure. For the breasts, dandelion's effects reduce sores, tumors, swollen lymph and cysts and are possibly preventative of breast cancer. It also stimulates the production of mother's milk. Dandelion leaf tea, taken cool, is one of the most effective diuretics.

The leaves are very high in iron, vitamins and minerals, especially Vitamin A and potassium, and are useful for treating anemia. Eaten when young in the spring, they help clear out any excesses from winter, aiding in the prevention of spring colds. The root can be roasted and made into a strong tea which Europeans call Dandelion Coffee. It actually is an excellent coffee substitute, since its full-bodied bitter flavor is satisfying and counteracts the effects of previous caffeine by cleansing the injured liver. It combines well with chicory and burdock roots for a closer coffee flavor. In general, the roasted roots can be used by those with coldness and the raw roots by those with heat.

Indications: indigestion, liver congestion, hepatitis, jaundice, cirrhosis, constipation, skin eruptions, breast sores, tumors, cysts, promotion of lactation, urinary bladder and kidney infections, kidney and gallstones, diabetes, hypoglycemia

Projects: tea, potherb, tincture, salve, "coffee"

Echinacea

Echinacea spp.; Compositae

Parts used: root

Energy and taste: cool, spicy, bitter

Active constituents: echinacoside, unsaturated isobutyl amides, polysaccharides, polyacetylenes, essential oil, fatty acids

Actions: clears heat; blood, lymph, lungs, stomach, liver

Properties: alterative, antibiotic, vulnerary, stimulant, antiseptic, antibacterial, antiviral

Dose: acute conditions—take 1 dropperful of tincture or 2 "00" capsules every 1/2 hour; as symptoms lessen, take same dosage every two hours and taper off until problem is gone; other—decoct 1 ounce/pint water; 2 "00" caps 3 times/day; 10-30 drops tincture; 3-9 gm in formula

Echinacea is Nature's natural antibiotic and works by activating leukocytes (white blood cells which fight infections) and (according to Tierra in *Planetary Herbology*) T-cell formation that assist the healing process, raise the body's immune level and encourage wounds to heal. It also inhibits the hyalurinodase enzyme which causes the spread of bacteria. Thus, it is one of the most powerful and effective remedies against all kinds of bacterial and viral infections and inflammations. Large doses can be taken because it is not toxic, although it has been found that after taking echinacea continuously for about 10 days its effectiveness lessens. (It is often wise to take herbs only as they are needed and then "rest" from them for several days before taking more.)

WESTERN HERBS

Echinacea is a wonderful blood cleanser, effective for blood poisoning and toxicity, cancer and other poisonous conditions. It further helps alleviate the effects of vaccination, lowers fevers, including typhoid fever, and is useful in helping prevent and cure colds, flus and sore throats. For those with internal heat, echinacea is fine alone, but for those with coldness or any deficiencies, it works better when combined with panax or Siberian ginseng or astragalus.

Externally, echinacea is excellent for all venomous bites (such as snake, insect and spider), poison oak and ivy, boils, cuts, wounds and other skin infections and for teething. It is even more effective when taken both externally and internally, the more frequently the better, or when combined with other remedies, such as salves, washes, baths and poultices. It is such a valuable herb, in fact, I always carry echinacea tincture in my purse for first aid and emergencies.

Indications: all infections and inflammations, bites, wounds, immune enhancing, colds, blood poisoning, fevers, poison oak and ivy, boils and other skin infections, cancer

Projects: tincture, salve, wash, capsule, first aid, tea, powder, poultice, bath

One of the best rejuvenative tonics for the lungs, elecampane tones and strengthens the digestive and respiratory organs and the nutritive functions of the body. It gives the lungs and spleen/stomach more energy and digestive ability. It also clears and inhibits the formation of mucus due to poor digestion and assimilation and clears mucus created by coldness from the lungs, aiding bronchitis and asthma. It remedies chronic coughs where the general condition and appetite are reduced. It is especially indicated in general debility from prolonged disease, overwork or old age.

For chronic lung ailments combine with wild cherry bark, comfrey root and licorice or extract 1 ounce of the bruised root in a pint of red wine and take 1 tbsp every several hours. To increase its tonic properties, roast the roots in a dry pan with honey. The root contains a starch-type carbohydrate, called inulin, which has a sweetish taste and is used as a sugar substitute for diabetics. This is **NOT** insulin, however.

Chinese medicine uses the root as an expectorant and stomachic and the flowers to bring down the energy of the lungs, thus stopping coughs, wheezing, hiccoughs, nausea and vomiting.

Indications: colds, cough, asthma, bronchitis, poor or weak digestion, nervous debility

Projects: tea, syrup, wine, pills, capsule

Elecampane

Inula helinium; Compositae

Part used: root, flower

Energy and taste: warm; spicy, bitter

Active constituents: essential oil, bitter principles, resin, inulin (up to 44%)

Actions: removes excess dampness; lung, spleen

Properties: energy tonic, expectorant, carminative, stimulant, diuretic, cholagogue, astringent, antiseptic, diaphoretic, rejuvenative

Dose: decoct root and infuse flowers 1 ounce/pint water, drink 3 cups/day; 1 "00" cap 3 times/day; 10-30 drops tincture 3 times/day; 3-9 gm in formula

Eyebright

Euphrasia officinalis; Scrophulariaceae

Part used: above-ground portion

Energy and taste: cool; spicy, bitter

Active constituents: glycosides, tannins, substances similar to aucubine, phenolic acids and volatile oil

Actions: clears heat; eyes, liver, lung, blood

Properties: astringent, anti-inflammatory, expectorant, alterative

Dose: infuse 1 ounce/pint water, drink 3 cups/day; 2 "00" caps 3 times/day; 10-30 drops tincture 3 times/day; 2-5 gm in formula

WESTERN HERBS

Eyebright is well known for treating eye problems, including conjunctivitis, blepharitis, scrofulous eye conditions in children, other eye infections, superficial eye problems, eye weakness and *ophthalmia*. It aids the liver to clear heat and toxins from the blood, which then affects clarity of vision. It is also useful for inflammations of the nose, throat and bronchials, especially if the discharge is thin and watery. It decongests the upper sinuses. A specific for "snuffles," even in infants, place 5-10 drops tincture in 1/2 glass water and administer 1 tsp every 15-30 minutes for this.

Externally, the tea is used as an eyewash for eye problems when it is frequently combined with goldenseal or fennel. It may also be used as a compress to give rapid relief of redness, swelling and visual disturbances in acute inflammations and eye injuries.

Indications: conjunctivitis, eye infections, eye weakness, ophthalmia, inflammations of nose, throat and lungs

Projects: tea, eye wash, tincture, capsule

Fennel

Foeniculum vulgare; Umbelliferae

Parts used: seed

Energy and taste: warm; spicy, sweet

Active constituents: volatile oil (up to 8%) consisting mainly of anethole, flavonoids, coumarins, fixed oils, sugars

Actions: regulates energy; spleen, stomach, liver, kidney

Properties: stimulant, carminative, antispasmodic, diuretic, expectorant, galactagogue

Dose: Infuse 1 tsp/cup water, drink 3-4 cups/day; 2 "00" caps 3 times/day; 10-30 drops tincture 3 times/day; 3-9 gm in formula

In medieval times, the fennel plant, along with St. John's wort and rosemary, were hung over the door on Midsummer's Eve to ward off evil spirits. Today the delicious taste of fennel makes it a wonderful after-meal tea as it eases gas, indigestion, abdominal pain and spasms of the gastrointestinal tract. In India the roasted seeds are eaten after meals as a sweet digestive aid. Fennel is also excellent for digestive weakness or colic in children or in the elderly as its warm energy will not over-stimulate.

Fennel regulates liver energy, smoothing the flow of energy, calming the nerves, easing cramps and spasms and aiding bowel movements. It is often combined with purgatives to prevent any attendant griping. It helps clear mucus from the lungs and promotes the production of mother's milk. It is used in Chinese medicine for lower abdominal pain, indigestion, decreased appetite, vomiting, gas and intestinal spasms due to coldness. Fennel stalks may be eaten raw like celery and are a delicious and beneficial addition to any meal.

Indications: indigestion, abdominal pain, gas, cramps and spasms, colic, promotes lactation

Projects: tea, roasted seeds, syrup, compress, tincture, sun tea, food

Fenugreek

Trigonella foenum-graecum; Leguminosae

Part used: seeds

Energy and taste: warm; bitter

Active constituents: volatile and fixed oils, alkaloids, saponins, flavonoids, mucilage, Vitamins A, B1 and C and minerals (including calcium and iron)

Actions: liver, kidney

Properties: heat and energy tonic, nutritive, carminative, stimulant, demulcent, alterative, expectorant, antipyretic, rejuvenative

Dose: decoct 1 ounce/pint water, drink 3 cups/day; tonic—1 tsp powder/cup heated milk, take once/day; 3-9 gm in formula

Precautions: pregnancy (can stimulate contractions due to its oxytocic activity), conditions of heat or infections

WESTERN HERBS

One of the oldest known medicinal herbs, fenugreek seeds were used by the ancient Egyptians, Romans and Greeks for medicinal and culinary purposes. The seeds greatly benefit the nervous, digestive and respiratory systems, clearing mucus, preventing fever and treating stomach and digestive disorders. They restore the blood sugar balance, regulate insulin in diabetes and reduce cholesterol. They are also very nourishing for wasting diseases, such as tuberculosis, anemia, debility, neurasthenia and convalescence as they heal and strengthen. Made into a gruel the seeds stimulate mother's milk and promote hair growth.

In Chinese medicine fenugreek is used as a tonic to heal kidney disease where there is a sense of cold and pain in the lower back, abdomen and/or extremities and for hernia, gastric problems and morning sickness. The seeds may be sprouted and eaten to aid digestion and seminal debility. A poultice treats sores, ulcers and boils. They are included in curry powders and used as a flavoring.

Indications: indigestion, mucus, tuberculosis, anemia, convalescence, promotes lactation and hair growth, regulates blood sugar balance, low back pain

Projects: tea, poultice, sprouts, paste, gruel, milk

Feverfew

Chyrsanthemum parthenium; Compositae

Part used: leaves, flowers
Energy and taste: cool; bitter
Active constituents: volatile oils (camphor, terpene, borneol), various esters, bitter principle
Actions: stomach, liver
Properties: antipyretic, carminative, purgative, bitter tonic
Dose: infuse 1 ounce/pint water, drink 2-3 cups/day; 3-9 gm in formula
Precautions: do not use for migraines resulting from a weak or deficiency condition

Feverfew is specific for headaches, especially migraines, usually caused from excess heat in the liver. It also treats colds, flu, fevers and digestive problems.

Indications: headaches, migraines, colds, flu, fever, digestive problems
Projects: tea

Garlic

Allium sativum; Liliaceae

Part used: bulb
Energy and taste: hot; spicy
Active constituents: volatile oil (about 0.2%) including aliin (which breaks down to allicin), B Vitamins, minerals
Actions: lungs, kidney, spleen, stomach, large intestines
Properties: increases internal heat; stimulant, diuretic, diaphoretic, hypotensive, alterative, digestant, carminative, expectorant, antiseptic, antispasmodic, parasiticide, antibiotic
Dose: acute conditions—1 tsp/hour syrup, oil or juice; 3-5 cloves in decoction, raw, toasted or as paste/day; 3-6 gm in formula
Precautions: pregnancy—garlic is a mild emmenagogue, so use in very small amounts; yogis use it as medicine, but not as a food or spice because it can be too stimulating for some; prolonged direct contact to the skin of fresh garlic can cause irritation

Garlic is said to be a cure for every ailment but the one it causes: bad breath. It is a powerful rejuvenative herb, strengthening along with detoxifying. It is absorbed by the body so quickly that I and others have noticed that if we rub our feet with a clove we can taste or smell it on the skin within seconds. Its history is quite fascinating. It was invoked as a deity by ancient Egyptians at the taking of oaths, left as a supper at crossroads for Hecate in

WESTERN HERBS

Greece and more recently, used externally as a diluted juice in World War I to control suppuration in wounds, saving the lives of thousands of men.

Garlic is used in the treatment of all lung ailments, and I have seen the juice quickly heal lung debilitation and walking pneumonia. It treats colds, flus, fevers, infections, earaches and sore throats. It regulates blood pressure and so is beneficial for both high and low blood pressure. Take 1 clove each morning for this. Because it stimulates metabolism, it is used both for chronic and acute diseases. It treats weak digestion, improves circulation, arthritis, rheumatism, lower back and joint pains, genito-urinary diseases, nervous disorders, cramps and spasms and heart weakness and reduces cholesterol. Take the syrup in tablespoon doses 3 times a day before meals for any of these.

It is a preventative and treatment for all intestinal worms. For this one can insert an oiled garlic clove in the rectum, use garlic enemas, eat 3-5 raw cloves of garlic 3-6 times daily and in general, heavily dose oneself with it! Chinese medicine also uses it for this and ringworm, in which the paste is applied topically. It is also good for amoebic dysentery and is an effective antibiotic for staphylococcus, streptococcus and bacteria resistant to standard antibiotic drugs. It is an antifungal for the treatment of candida albicans yeast infections.

Many preparations of garlic are useful. It may be juiced and taken directly, or minced and combined with a little sesame or olive oil or honey and taken in teaspoon doses every 2 hours for respiratory conditions. The cloves may be coated in oil and wrapped in muslin for direct insertion into the vagina for vaginitis and leucorrhea, or the anus for pinworms. Enemas are made of garlic tea, and, of course, eating the cloves directly or cooked in food is also effective. Which form is chosen depends on the ailment being treated and the preferred form for ingestion. To preserve the beneficial effect of garlic, it should not be boiled.

Indications: colds, flu, coughs, bronchitis, pneumonia, lung ailments, infections, fevers, sore throats, ear aches, high or low blood pressure, indigestion, circulation, arthritis, rheumatism, pains, cholesterol, worms, dysentery, fungus, candida, vaginal infections, leukorrhea

Projects: juice, oil, bolus, douche, paste, enema, tincture, syrup, salve, cider, food, first aid, plaster

Gentian

Gentian spp.; Gentianaceae

Part used: root

Energy and taste: cold; bitter

Active constituents: the glycoside gentiopicrin, iridoids, alkaloids, phenolic acids

Actions: liver, urinary and gallbladder

Properties: alterative, antipyretic, bitter tonic, antibacterial, laxative

Dose: before meals, decoct 1 ounce/pint water, drink 1/2 cup 3 times/day; 2 "00" caps 3 times/day; 10-30 drops tincture/4 ounces water 20 minutes before meals as a bitter tonic; 3-9 gm in formula; 1 tsp bitters or brandy

Precaution: hyperacidity; irritable, sensitive stomach; indigestion with diarrhea

Gentian makes a wonderful digestive bitter tincture, taken in small doses before meals (although it may be tastier if combined with orange peel or cardamom seeds). The gastric juices increase as soon as the plant acts on the mucous membrane lining the mouth. Thus, it improves digestion, appetite, gastritis, heartburn, nausea, gas, diarrhea, constipation and gastric tone so that heavy food is more easily digested.

Gentian clears heat from the middle and lower parts of the body. This is useful in treating hepatitis, jaundice and most liver disorders and helps clear discharges, anal itch, herpes, rash, vaginal discharge and itch and urinary tract infections. For those with coldness or weakness, it is better used in combination with warming herbs. Chinese medicine also gives it for general debility and to strengthen the liver and memory.

Indications: indigestion, poor appetite, gas, nausea, heartburn, gastritis, diarrhea, constipation, hepatitis,

jaundice, anal itch, herpes, rash, vaginal discharge and itch, urinary tract infections
Projects: tea, tincture, herbal brandy, capsule, douche, powder, bitters

Ginger

Zingiber officinale; Zingiberzceae

Parts used: the rhizomes after a year's growth
Energy and taste: warm; spicy
Active constituents: volatile oil (1-2%) pungent principles (gingerol and shogaols)
Actions: stimulates circulation, warms the inside of the body; lungs, stomach, spleen, heart, kidney
Properties: stimulant, diaphoretic, carminative, emmenagogue, expectorant, antiemetic, analgesic, antispasmodic
Dose: fresh—steep 2-6 thin slices or 1" root grated/cup, drink 2-4 cups tea/day; acute—drink 1/2 cup every 2-3 hours until symptoms lessen, then decrease frequency until the problem is gone; dried—10-30 drops tincture; 3-9 gm in formula
Precautions: high fever, bleeding, ulcers, inflammatory skin diseases; use minimally during pregnancy

Most people associate ginger root as an herb-food used as a spice in cooking, such as gingerbread or pumpkin pie, or in the form of candied ginger, which the Chinese especially like. In addition, some know that when ginger is cooked with meat it helps the body to digest and assimilate the meat better, thus detoxifying it. However, ginger has tremendous multi-healing applications beyond its use as a spice. In fact, in Oriental medicine ginger is so highly regarded that it is included in about half of all multi-herb formulas.

Internally, ginger's warming and stimulating energy aids stomach upset, nausea, motion sickness, poor digestion, gas and excessive mucus accumulation, and it picks up the energy. It also alleviates colds, flus, lung complaints, cramps, pains, spasms, sore throat, diarrhea and general coldness. It combines well with chamomile for menstrual cramps. Because it is very warming, ginger powder will bring on and regulate menses suppressed by coldness. It will further help to warm those who generally eat more cooling foods, thus aiding their digestion.

External applications of ginger are a most valuable household remedy. Ginger juice rubbed into the skin relieves muscle pain. Ginger oil applied to the scalp eases dandruff and placed into the ear treats earaches. A hot foot or body bath can stop the onset of a cold, warm up cold feet and stop body pains. Ginger tea or tincture can be made into a gargle for sore throats.

A ginger fomentation placed on sore joints or muscles can ease pain, arthritis and rheumatism; and when put on a sore throat, it can relieve pain rapidly. Over the lungs it breaks up congestion and expels mucus. Over the lower abdomen and perineum during childbirth it speeds delivery and eases tearing. Chinese medicine recommends the fomentation be put over the kidneys (located on either side of the spine at waist level of the back) to help keep the body warm and activate the immune system. Often both internal and external methods are used together. For instance, a person with a cold, flu or sore throat might first drink a cup of ginger tea, then either place a ginger fomentation over the throat or lungs, take a bath in hot ginger water, and/or soak the feet in ginger tea.

One of ginger's special properties is its carrier function. Because of its stimulating action, ginger helps move other herbs through the blood, increasing their effectiveness and absorption rate. For this reason, ginger is frequently combined with most formulas, though in small amounts (1/4 part).

Both the fresh and dried roots can be used, and they have slightly different purposes. The fresh root is dispersing and diaphoretic. The dried root is hotter and drying and is used to warm and stimulate.

Fresh ginger is used for the following: colds, flus, coughs, sore throats, nausea, cramps, vomiting, colic, gas, indigestion, abdominal ache and fevers from coldness. Dried ginger is used to dissolve phlegm and disperse coldness as well as for cold extremities, diarrhea, coughs from coldness, rheumatism/arthritis and warming the stomach.

WESTERN HERBS

Ginger tea is usually made with fresh ginger root. Begin by bringing a pint of water to a boil. Cut off a one-inch section of fresh ginger root and grate finely. When the water boils, turn off the heat and put in the grated ginger root. Let steep for 15-20 minutes. Strain, cool and drink.

Indications: colds, flus, lung complaints, sore throat, diarrhea, pains, cramps, spasms, indigestion, nausea, gas, mucus conditions, poor circulation, earache, dandruff, diarrhea, menstrual difficulties due to cold

Projects: oil, fomentation, foot or body bath, tea, gargle, liniment, tincture, paste, soup, composition powder, cider, milk, powder, capsules, tincture, pill, spice, juice, first aid, sweating therapy, chai

Ginkgo

Ginkgo biloba; Ginkgoaceae

Part used: nut and leaf

Energy and taste: neutral; bitter, astingent; nuts are mildly toxic

Active constituents: nut—volatile oil, tannin, resin; leaf—lignans, glavonoids, mainly flavone glycosides, traces of essential oil and tannins

Actions: nut—lung, kidney; leaves—brain

Properties: nut—expectorant, antitussive, antiasthmatic, sedative, mildly astringent; leaves—improves circulation to the brain

Dose: nut—3-9 gm in formula, less if fresh; leaf—1 ounce herb/pint water in a 5 min. decoction; 40 drops tincture 1-3 times/day; 40 mg of the 24% standardized extract 3 times/day for a minimum of 3 months

Precaution: nut—since it is slightly toxic, it should not be taken in large doses over a long period of time; toxic symptoms include headache, fever, tremors, irritability and dyspnea. Licorice may be used antidotally with this herb.

The ginkgo nut expels mucus from the lungs, stops wheezing and cough, regulates urination, aids allergies and asthma and stops leucorrhea and spermatorrhea. It is used in Chinese medicine to add heat to the body, increase sexual energy and stop bedwetting and nocturnal emission.

The ginkgo leaf is effective for peripheral blood circulation, especially that to the brain. It improves memory, mental efficiency, concentration, mental confusion and senility. It also decreases anxiety tension, headaches, vertigo, visual problems, ringing in the ears, coldness, arthritis, rheumatism and hearing loss. It is especially good for the elderly. It is a powerful anti-oxidant and prevents damage caused by free-radicals. Because it does not affect the sugar metabolism of the body, it is safe for diabetics who often suffer from poor circulation.

Gingko leaf is commonly found in standardized extract form (the 24% concentration of the glycosides is the strongest). It can be taken in tincture and tea form also. Whatever form is used, it needs to be taken for a minimum of 3 months to realize its benefits.

Indications: nut—cough, allergies, asthma, leucorrhea, spermatorrhea, bed-wetting, nocturnal emission; leaf—poor memory and concentration, senility, headache, vertigo, tinnitus, coldness, arthritis, rheumatism, hearing loss, poor circulation

Projects: tea, tincture, standardized extract

Goldenseal

Hydrastis canadensis; Ranunculaceae

Part used: root

Energy and taste: cold; bitter

Active constituents: isoquinoline alkaloids (including hydrastine and berberine), resin, traces of essential oil, chologenic acid, fatty acids, sugar, starch

Actions: clears heat; mucous membranes, stomach, intestines, heart, liver, eyes

Properties: bitter tonic, alterative, anti-inflammatory, astringent, diuretic, laxative, antibiotic, antibacterial, antiseptic

Dose: infuse 1 tsp/cup boiling water; 10-30 drop tincture; 3-6 gm in formula; 2 "00" capsules 1-3 times/day or more for short-term use in acute conditions

WESTERN HERBS

Precautions: pregnancy; emaciation, neurasthenia, chronic debilitation, dizziness; long-term use can weaken the flora of the colon and diminish Vitamin B absorption

A wonderful cooling anti-inflammatory herb with antibiotic and antiseptic properties, goldenseal is good for infections and inflammations caused by heated conditions. It cleanses the mucous membranes and lymph glands throughout the body and dries yellow discharges in heated leukorrhea and vaginal yeast and bladder infections. It kills yeast and bacteria in the gastrointestinal tract and clears the flora when used moderately. If taken in excess, however, such as 1-2 gm a day for several weeks or months, it can destroy the beneficial bacteria and flora altogether.

Goldenseal detoxifies the liver and blood, stimulates bile, treats liver disease, tumors, cancer, indigestion, gas, hemorrhoids, heartburn, colitis, constipation and ulcers. It has a laxative action, stimulates the uterine muscles, contracts the blood vessels and inhibits excessive bleeding. It is effective against flu, fevers and infections of all kinds and treats amoebic dysentery (giardia) when used continuously for 10 days.

Taken with any herb, goldenseal increases the tonic properties for the specific organs being treated. Externally, it may be used in eyewashes for inflamed eyes or in salves, powders and tinctures for eczema, inflammation of the ear and other infections. I successfully used the powder on my baby's umbilicus after birth to prevent infection until the cord fell off.

For people who have coldness, goldenseal should be combined with warming herbs because of its cold, bitter properties, or used only short-term during acute heated conditions. Nourishing therapy should be given afterwards, such as rice cooked with tonic herbs.

Indications: infections, inflammations, ulcers, flus, fevers, hemorrhoids, leucorrhea, bladder infections, dysentery, constipation, colitis, heartburn, indigestion, liver congestion, cancer

Projects: tea, capsule, salve, douche, bolus, wash, tincture, poultice, liniment, powder, gargle

Hawthorn

Crataegus oxyacantha; Rosaceae

Part used: berries, flowers and leaves
Energy and taste: slightly warm; sour, sweet
Active constituents: amygdalin, crategolic acid, citric acid, tartaric acid, saponins, sugars, flavonoid glycosides, Vitamin C
Actions: heart, spleen, stomach, liver, circulation
Properties: cardiac tonic, digestant, antispasmodic, antidiarrhetic, astringent, sedative
Dose: infuse 1 ounce berries or flowers/pint water, drink 3 cups/day; 10-30 drops tincture or wine 3 times/day; 6-12 gm in formula

Hawthorn is highly recognized in the West as a strong cardiac tonic, treating both high and low blood pressure, rapid or arhythmic heartbeat, inflammation of the heart muscle, angina pectoris, arteriosclerosis and valvular heart diseases. It stimulates circulation, regulates blood flow, blood pressure and heart rate, dilates coronary vessels and strengthens the heart muscle, promoting longevity. It is a specific for all cardiovascular diseases, particularly good for heart problems of old age, cholesterol and nervous palpitations or conditions of the heart. It will further help the type of insomnia which occurs with constant mental thoughts or nervousness. It is considered to be gentle and safe with long-lasting effects.

Chinese medicine uses the berries to remove congestion of accumulated food masses due to overeating or poor digestion. It will also stimulate a poor appetite, release abdominal distention, alleviate heart pain and postpartum pain and aid in the digestion of meat. The green fruit is good for diarrhea and the roasted and charred fruits are good to use both for diarrhea and chronic dysentery-like disorders.

The berries and flowers, which have an affinity for alcohol, may be made into a tincture or herbal wine. All three forms of hawthorn are also taken in tea form. There is a growing consensus that the flowers and leaves are more potent than the berries for the heart. Hawthorn is completely safe for long-term use, with no toxic effect or habituation.

WESTERN HERBS

Indications: heart weakness, aging heart problems, palpitations, angina, high and low blood pressure, arhythmia, insomnia, food stagnation, valvular insufficiency, arteriosclerosis, poor digestion

Projects: tea, tincture, wine, capsule, paste

Lemon Balm

Melissa officinalis; Labiatae

Parts used: leaves

Energy and taste: cool; sour, spicy, pleasant

Active constituents: essential oil with citral, citronellal, geraniol and linalool, bitter principle, acids and tannin

Actions: lungs, liver

Properties: carminative, diaphoretic, calmative, antipyretic, antispasmodic

Dose: infuse 1 ounce/pint water; drink 1 cup every 2 hours until the fever or cold breaks, or 1 cup AM and PM for sedative action; 1/2-6 gm in formula

Other: sometimes known as balm or sweet balm

Lemon balm is very effective for breaking fevers and causing a sweat. For simple colds, cough and fevers it is a perfect herb, especially for children, since it has such a delicious lemony taste and smell. For these conditions, drink several cups of tea, take a hot bath and follow by sweating therapy. The tea and sweating can be continued several times in cases of high fevers and is a sure method for breaking them.

Lemon balm is also calming and relaxing, acting on the nervous system as a gentle herbal tranquilizer. It is excellent for those feeling melancholic, homesick, depressed, nervous or hysterical. It may be combined with chamomile for nervous states and insomnia, or for whining, crying, colicy or teething children. It makes a delightful and refreshing summer drink. In fact, during the 16th and 17th centuries in old England many people drank it daily because they enjoyed it so much. Today it is used in salve form by the Europeans to treat herpes simplex.

Indications: fevers, colds, flus, nervous conditions, insomnia, colic, teething

Projects: tea, syrup, sun tea, sweating

Licorice

Glycyrrhiza glabra; Leguminosae

Parts used: root

Energy and taste: neutral; sweet

Active constituents: glycyrrhizic acid (a triterpene glycoside), flavonoids, starch, sugar (glucose and sucrose), lignin, asparagine, a complex volatile oil and a trace of tannins. Substances in this herb seem to produce physiological reactions of desoxycorticosterone, with associated retention of sodium and water and the excretion of potassium.

Actions: general effects on all organs and the whole body; spleen, lungs

Properties: energy tonic, expectorant, alterative, demulcent, laxative, mild sedative, rejuvenative

Dose: decoct 2-3 slices of whole root/cup; drink 2-3 cups/day; 1-9 gm in formula

Precaution: excessive and long-term use of licorice can cause water retention, hypertension and/or edema and reduction in thyroid and metabolism activity—avoid in hypertension, edema and high blood pressure; causes vomiting in high doses

Other: also known as liquorice

The demulcent property of licorice eases sore throats, remedies gastric and duodenal ulcers and other stomach problems (especially when combined with chamomile), soothes mucous membranes, urinary, respiratory and intestinal passages and treats tuberculosis. It also expels mucus in chest complaints, colds and flus and has mild laxative properties which can safely be taken by children and debilitated people. Licorice root can be smoked for relief of sore throat and hoarseness.

A restoring and rejuvenative herb, licorice is a general tonic for the whole body. It strengthens the

Knowing the Herbs / 69

digestive system and improves energy, especially when honey-roasted, which gives it a warmer energy. This increases its use for poor digestion and assimilation difficulties from coldness and lowered functioning. This form also more strongly builds the blood and the energy in those with palpitation or irregular pulse.

Licorice is also calming and alleviates stress, relaxes muscle pains and creates feelings of peace, contentment and harmony. Because it contains substances similar to the adrenal cortical hormones, such as cortisone, licorice is useful in treating adrenal insufficiency and other glandular problems. It is a safe sweetener for diabetics (although it is 50 times sweeter than sugar) and can be added to any tea for flavor.

Licorice is the most used herb in Chinese medicine for several reasons: it harmonizes the various herbs in a formula so they work together better and increases their strength, it alleviates the harsh stimulating effects of bitter herbs without interfering with their use, and it adds a wonderful sweet taste.

Children especially like the taste of licorice (remember sucking on licorice ropes at a show or fair?), and a root or several slices can be given to children when hiking or traveling since they help quench thirst. They can even be safely given to teething babies to stimulate and relieve pain in their gums. Licorice can also be made into little pills which can then be sucked on to treat the throat and lungs, or just for a treat.

Indications: cough, sore throat, colds, flus, bronchitis, ulcers, low energy, laryngitis, general debility, poor digestion, spasms, thirst, stress, spasms, intoxication, toxicity

Projects: pills, tea, honey-roasted, smoked, syrup, gargle, sun tea, milk, paste, cider

Lobelia

Lobelia inflata; Lobeliaceae

Part used: above-ground portion
Energy and taste: neutral; bitter

Active constituents: alkaloids (lobeline is most important one), pyridine and other alkaloids, resin, gum, chelidonic acid and a pungent volatile oil

Actions: liver, lungs, heart, small intestine

Properties: antispasmodic, expectorant, stimulant, emetic, alterative, diuretic

Dose: acute conditions—infuse 1/2 ounce/pint water, drink 1/2-1 cup 3 times/day; 1 "00" capsule, 1-2 times/day; 15 drops of tincture, 2-3 times/day; 6-15 gm in formula

Precautions: overdose can cause nausea and vomiting

Lobelia is a wonderful antispasmodic which relaxes the muscles and nerves. It is useful for asthma and bronchial spasms, whooping and other spasmodic coughs, muscle spasms and twitches, any pains and lockjaw. It can even lessen the strength of contractions during natural childbirth. Lobeline, contained within lobelia, is similar to nicotine, and lobelia is used in commercial smoking preparations to counteract the desire for tobacco. One could include it in a homemade herbal preparation for this, adding comfrey, coltsfoot and mullein.

For muscle spasms, boils and ulcers lobelia may be externally applied in baths, fomentations, poultices and liniments. It can be added to enemas for fevers and infections and to ease spasms and cramps. A few drops of tincture placed in the ear relieves earaches. This herb is most frequently used in combination with other herbs for its relaxing, antispasmodic and pain-relieving properties. When making the tincture, you can use apple cider vinegar to extract its alkaloids.

Indications: spasms and twitches, muscles tension, asthma, bronchitis, pneumonia, hiccough, whooping cough, relaxing respiratory passages, stop smoking, emetic, cough

Projects: tea, tincture, smoking, syrup, liniment, bath, fomentation, capsule, enema, poultice

WESTERN HERBS

Marshmallow

Althea officinalis; Malvaceae

Parts used: root
Energy and taste: cool; sweet, mildly bitter
Active constituents: starch, mucilage, pectin, oil, sugar, asparagin, phosphate of lime, glutinous matter, cellulose
Actions: general effects on the whole body; intestines, lungs, stomach, kidneys, bladder
Properties: nutritive tonic, alterative, diuretic, demulcent, emollient, lithotriptic, anti-inflammatory, vulnerary, laxative, expectorant, galactagogue
Dose: decoct 1 ounce/pint water; drink 3 cups/day; 6-15 gm in formula

Marshmallow is the best source of easily digested vegetable mucilage which lubricates the body, protecting it against irritation and dryness. For this reason it is considered a tonic to strengthen the fluids and substance of the body. This is useful in treating wasting and thirsting diseases such as tuberculosis and diabetes. Its anti-inflammatory action is also beneficial in dry cough, dryness and inflammation of the lungs, sore and irritated joints, gastritis, and ulcers.

Marshmallow also soothes the urinary system and is usually combined with other diuretic herbs to treat kidney and bladder inflammations, difficult or painful urination and kidney stones or gravel. It stops bleeding in the urine, stool or nose, and vomiting or spitting of blood. It can be used with other laxative herbs for constipation due to dryness or lack of roughage and heals irritations associated with diarrhea and dysentery.

Externally it is used as a poultice for inflammations and infections such as wounds, burns, boils, ulcers, abscesses, bruises, gangrene and blood poisoning. The tea can be gargled for sore or irritated throat. In Ayurvedic (East Indian) medicine, it is used as a rejuvenative tonic by decocting it in milk and adding a small amount of ginger. In this way it helps strengthen the body, thus prolonging a healthy life.

Marshmallow is often added to formulas as a good soothing and harmonizing herb with its additional powerful healing properties. In lung formulas it benefits all lung complaints and combines well with diuretic herbs for urinary problems. It also promotes the formation of mother's milk.

Indications: tuberculosis, cough, diabetes, dryness and inflammation of the lungs, kidney stones and inflammation, bladder infections, whooping cough, internal bleeding, malnutrition, wounds, burns, skin eruptions, ulcers, gastritis, increases mother's milk
Projects: tea, syrup, poultice, pill, powder, milk, salve, gargle, capsule, wash

Milk Thistle

Silybum marianum; Compositae

Part used: seeds and above-ground portions
Energy and taste: cool; bitter, sweet
Active constituents: flavolignans collectively known as silymarin
Actions: liver, spleen
Properties: hepatoprotective, hepatic tonic, bitter tonic, demulcent, antidepressant, galactogogue, demulcent
Dose: 10-40 drops tincture or liquid extract 3 times/day; do not use the seeds in tea form as they are not water soluble—they may be eaten as desired, however

Milk thistle protects the liver and regenerates it, even against one of the strongest liver toxins known, the death cap mushroom (*Amanita phalloides*). It treats chronic liver cirrhosis, necroses and hepatitis A and B. It also lowers fat deposits in the liver of animals. It also increases mother's milk.

Indications: liver congestion, disease, cirrhosis and toxicity; hepatitis A and B; insufficient lactation
Projects: tea, tincture, extract

WESTERN HERBS

Motherwort

Leonorus cardiaca; Labiatae

Part used: above-ground portion
Energy and taste: slightly cold; bitter, spicy
Active constituents: bitter principle and bitter glycosides, leonurin, alkaloids, tannin, essential oil, resin, organic acids
Actions: blood stagnation, circulation; liver, heart
Properties: emmenagogue, astringent, carminative, cardiac tonic, diuretic, antispasmodic, antirheumatic
Dose: infuse 1 ounce/pint water, drink 3 cups/day; 2 "00" capsules 3 times/day; 10-30 drops tincture, 3 times/day; 10-30 gm in formula
Precautions: not to be taken during pregnancy

Motherwort is a strong blood and uterine stimulant which treats menstrual disorders such as delayed, stopped or painful menses and pain in the pelvic and lumbar region. A fomentation can be placed over the abdomen and the tea taken for these. It also is a cardiac tonic and eases angina pectoris, cardiac edema, palpitations and other heart conditions. It combines well with hawthorn for all heart problems. As a sedative, nervine and antispasmodic it alleviates cramps, gas, hysteria, nervousness, convulsions and insomnia.

The Chinese use it for PMS pain, postpartum pain with clots, abdominal masses, infertility due to deficient blood, irregular menses and to reduce swellings and promote urination, especially when there's blood in the urine. They often combine it with dong quai as a menstrual regulator. In ancient China it was called *I mu* and used by the courtesans to prevent pregnancy.

Indications: all menstrual disorders, postpartum pain, abdominal masses, infertility, swellings, nervousness, cardiac tonic, palpitations, cramps, gas, insomnia, heart problems, tachycardia
Projects: tea, tincture, capsule, fomentation

Mugwort

Artemisia vulgaris; Compositae

Part used: leaves
Energy and taste: warm; bitter, spicy
Active constituents: essential oil, vulgarin, flavonoids
Actions: circulation, blood stagnation; spleen, liver, kidney
Properties: emmenagogue, hemostatic, antispasmodic, bitter tonic, nervine, diaphoretic, diuretic
Dose: infuse 1 ounce/pint water, drink 1/2 cup, 2-3 times/day; 2 "00" capsules 3 times/day; 10-30 drops tincture 3 times/day; 3-9 gm in formula
Precautions: pregnancy

Mugwort circulates the blood, especially through the lower abdomen and uterus, aiding menstrual difficulties and cramps, leukorrhea and abdominal pains due to coldness. It also calms a restless fetus and arrests threatened miscarriage. Mugwort stops nosebleeds and excessive menstrual bleeding. The Chinese use it to treat infertility due to cold in the womb.

As a bitter tonic, it treats stomach disorders, improves digestion and cures and prevents parasites and worms (although wormwood, another Artemesia species member, is stronger for this). The Native Americans use it for colds, flus, bronchitis, fevers and sweating therapy. Mugwort is also a nervine and can be smoked, filling the lungs three to six times, to help nervousness and insomnia. Externally, it can be applied as a liniment or wash to relieve itching, fungus and other skin infections, or as a douche for vaginal yeast infections.

Mugwort has several other interesting uses. The Native Americans called it "The Great Sage" and used it like incense in smudging rituals (a process of burning the mugwort and using its smoke—see the chapter *Home Therapies*) to purify the spiritual and physical environment. It has also long been used in dream pillows by sewing its dried leaves into a pil-

WESTERN HERBS

low-sack and sleeping on or near it. This helps intensify dreams and promotes dream recall. (A caution in this: it could cause bad dreams in one who needs detoxification!) Mugwort is also the prime ingredient in the Chinese moxibustion (see the chapter *Home Therapies*), valued for its quick and high-burning qualities and deeply penetrating heat. Burning moxibustion over a painful area increases blood circulation, gives relief from pain and aids injuries and bruises.

Indications: menstrual and abdominal pain, excessive menstrual bleeding, nosebleeds and spitting blood—all from coldness; preventative to miscarriage, calms the fetus, parasites and worms, colds, flu, insomnia, nervousness, pain, dreams, rituals

Projects: tea, douche, wash, liniment, tincture, smoking, moxibustion, smudging, dream pillow, sweating, bitters

Mullein

Verbascum thapsus; Scrophulariaceae

Parts used: leaves and flowers

Energy and taste: cool; bitter, astringent

Active constituents: saponins, mucilage, flavonoids, aucubin, traces of essential oil

Actions: lungs, stomach, glands, lymph

Properties: leaves—expectorant, astringent, diuretic, vulnerary, demulcent, emollient, antispasmodic; flowers—nervine, antispasmodic, sedative

Dose: infuse 1 ounce leaves/pint water; drink 3 cups/day; 10-30 drops tincture 3 times/day; 3-9 gm formula; oil—put 5-10 drops in ear every hour until earache is gone

Mullein is an excellent lung herb, useful for asthma, pneumonia, spasmodic coughs, colds, flu, bronchitis, hoarseness and whooping cough. It expels mucus, cleansing the bronchioles and lymphatics. Mullein specifically aids mumps, earaches and glandular swellings. For all these conditions it can be taken as a tea, or the dried leaves can be smoked, which also soothes the throat and is a good substitute for tobacco.

Mullein also stops bleeding from the lungs and bowels. A poultice of mullein leaves can be locally applied to help hemorrhoids, inflammations, wounds and toothache as well. It is said that figs wrapped in mullein leaves will not putrefy.

Mullein flowers have strong nervine, analgesic and anti-inflammatory properties. Oil made from the flowers is an important remedy for earaches and suppurative inflammations of the inner ear. It also helps heal discharges from the ear, frost bite, bruises, hemorrhoids and eczema of the external ear and canal. The oil is excellent for mucous membrane inflammations and hemorrhoids.

Indications: leaves—coughs, whooping cough, asthma, pneumonia, colds, flu, bronchitis, mumps, earaches, stop smoking, lung or bowel bleeding, diarrhea, hemorrhoids, toothache, bruises; flowers—earaches, eczema, bruises, hemorrhoids

Projects: oil, tea, poultice, smoking, gargle

Nettle

Urtica spp.; Urticaceae

Part used: leaves, seeds

Energy and taste: cool; slightly bitter, bland

Active constituents: formic acid, the stinging element, is dissipated by cooking or drying; also contains silicon, potassium, tannin, glucoquinines, high amounts of chlorophyll and Vitamins A and C

Actions: bladder, kidneys, lungs, blood

Properties: astringent, hemostatic, diuretic, galactagogue, expectorant, tonic, nutritive

Dose: infuse 1 ounce/pint water, drink 3 cups/day; 2 "00" capsules, 3 times/day; 9-30 gm in formula

Nettle is commonly called stinging nettle—a name which it definitely lives up to. The tiny prickles on the underside of the leaves and stem sting intensely and seemingly indefinitely when touched, unless poulticed quickly with another plant such as yellow dock

WESTERN HERBS

or plantain leaves. Yet, it is this same stinging quality which has made it an effective, though painful, therapy for arthritis where the person rolls the arthritic area in a nettles patch purposely, causing the intense stinging. It has been said that this process cures arthritis.

Alternatively, one may brush the area with the leaves, a less intense therapy, as a rubefacient to reduce local pains. Use caution if you decide to try it: massive exposure to nettle plants has caused severe symptoms of shock in animals. If you don't need or desire arthritis therapy, then be sure to wear gloves when picking the leaves! Made into a tea or cooked, the prickles "wilt," and then the leaves can safely be eaten as a delicious and nutritious green, especially in spring.

Nettle tea is taken warm for mucus conditions of the lungs, including asthma and excessive mucus discharge from the colon. It also helps skin complaints such as eczema and skin eruptions and stops bleeding and hemorrhage. Taken cool, the tea is a diuretic useful for urinary problems such as stopped urine, gravel and inflammatory conditions of the kidneys and bladder. As a daily tea (three times a day), its high mineral content makes it a tonic for raising low energy and overcoming fatigue.

Indications: arthritis, rheumatism, asthma, eczema, skin eruptions, hemorrhage, low energy, stopped urine, gravel, kidney and bladder infections

Projects: tea, potherb, fresh stinging plant, tincture

Oregon Grape

Mahonia repens, Berberis aquifolium; Berberidaceae

Part used: root
Energy and taste: cold; bitter
Active constituents: the alkaloid berberine
Actions: liver, stomach, colon
Properties: cholagogue, alterative, laxative
Dose: decoct 1 ounce/pint water, drink 2-3 cups/day; 10-30 drops tincture 3 times/day; 2 "00" capsules 3 times/day
Other: the Pacific Northwestern counterpart of barberry, which grows in the Northeast

Oregon grape root is a gentle liver and bile stimulant which improves the function of the liver and purifies blood toxins. It is used for all liver diseases including hepatitis, jaundice, gallstones, skin diseases, cancers, tumors and arthritis. For acute liver problems it combines well with an equal part of dandelion and a quarter part of fennel; drink at least 3 cups daily. Its bile-stimulating action also creates a laxative effect.

Indications: hepatitis, jaundice, gallstones, constipation, skin diseases, cancer, tumors, arthritis
Projects: tea, capsule, tincture, bitters

Parsley

Petroselinum spp.; Umbelliferae

Part used: leaves, root
Energy and taste: warm; spicy
Active constituents: root—contains essential oil, the flavonoid apiin, mucilage, sugar; leaves—have similar but weaker constituents, Vitamins A and C, calcium, iron
Actions: lung, stomach, bladder, liver, uterus
Properties: diuretic, carminative, stimulant, emmenagogue (especially the seeds), expectorant
Dose: infuse leaves and decoct root—1 ounce/pint water, drink 3 cups/day; 3-9 gm in formula
Precaution: pregnancy; acute infections and inflammations

Best known as a culinary herb, parsley is an effective diuretic useful for fluid retention, frequent urination, bedwetting and bladder infections. It helps digestion and gas and eliminates intestinal worms. The root is also diuretic, but more effective for removing stones, including gallstones, if they are not too large.

Parsley tea has an emmenagogic action, promoting menses and dispelling premenstrual water retention from the abdomen, legs and breast. The leaf inserted into and retained in the vagina can bring on delayed menses. Parsley is rich in vitamins, iron and minerals and so is a valuable food. Therefore, when it

WESTERN HERBS

is so often used as a garnish, eat it! Drinking the fresh juice daily (2 tsp) strengthens the kidneys and uterus.

Indications: edema, frequent urination, bedwetting, bladder and kidney infections, indigestion, gas, intestinal worms, stones, delayed menses, menstrual water retention and swollen breasts

Projects: tea, food, bolus, juice

Peppermint

Mentha piperita; Labiatae

Part used: leaves

Energy and taste: cool; spicy, bitter

Active constituents: volatile oils such as menthol and menthone, flavonoids, tannins, Vitamin E

Actions: lungs, liver

Properties: diaphoretic, aromatic, carminative, calmative, mild alterative

Dose: infuse 1 ounce/pint water, drink 3 cups/day; 2 "00" capsules 3 times/day; 1/2-6 gm in formula

One of the oldest medicinal herbs, peppermint is a cooling diaphoretic useful for colds, flus and fevers from heated conditions. It also helps indigestion, gas and colic and counteracts nausea and vomiting. The Chinese use it to clear the head and eyes, and for sore throat, headache, measles and pressure in the chest. Peppermint oil can be applied externally to the forehead to relieve headache and taken internally to treat colds. A few drops may also be added to boiling water and inhaled for bronchitis or general lung and nose congestion.

Mint is used as a flavoring agent in many forms. Children love to pick its leaves and chew on them, and it makes a wonderful cooling summer beverage. The volatile oils in peppermint are strong, however, and prolonged use, especially by infants or young children, can cause a rash or welts.

Indications: colds, flus, fevers, headache, indigestion, gas, colic, nausea

Projects: tea, oil, syrup, sun tea, potpourri, sachet

Plantain

Plantago major; p. lanceolata; Plantaginaceae

Parts used: leaves, seeds

Energy and taste: cool; mildly bitter, bland

Active constituents: mucilage and a heteroside, aucuboside that hydrolyzes into aucubine and sugar, flavonoids, tannin, oleanolic acid

Actions: clears heat; general effects on all organs, especially urinary and gallbladders and small intestines

Properties: vulnerary, astringent, diuretic, emollient, antiseptic, expectorant, refrigerant

Dose: infuse 1 heaping tsp/pint water; drink 1-2 cups every 2 hours until symptoms subside, then 1 cup 2-3 times/day for about 3 days after all symptoms are gone; 5-10 gm in formula

Plantain is another "weed" which grows on lawns and other undesired places that has many medicinal uses. Two commonly used species are *Plantago major*, with very wide leaves (called Broadleaf Plantain), and *Plantago lanceolata*, with very thin lance-like leaves (called Ribwort). Both are valuable healing herbs, with the broadleaf variety having stronger diuretic properties. Its cooling diuretic properties make plantain especially beneficial for kidney and urinary bladder infections and water retention. Its astringent property helps hemorrhoids, diarrhea, constipation and excessive menstrual discharge.

Externally, plantain is a seemingly miraculous poultice for stopping the pain of bee stings, spider and snake bites and other insect wounds. It will draw out the stinger and poisons from these bites and can bring out deeply imbedded splinters if left in place for a day or two. Plantain also heals wounds, burns, scrapes and cuts. It has a soothing effect felt within minutes after applying to the skin and so is one of the best remedies for chronic skin problems. The leaves can also be eaten as a food.

Plantain seeds are similar to psyllium seeds. As such they are helpful for constipation, especially when made into a "seed tea." To do this, soak 1/2 ounce of

WESTERN HERBS

the seeds, preferably overnight, in a cup of water. Drink it down, seeds and all. Native Americans use the seeds as food. In fact, they call plantain "Englishman's foot" because it was brought over by the early European settlers. Its seeds stuck to their feet and scattered throughout this country wherever they walked.

Indications: urinary infections, insect bites and stings, wounds, burns, scrapes, hemorrhoids, infections and inflammations, ulcers, diarrhea, excessive menstrual discharge

Projects: salve, seed tea, poultice, tea, potherb, syrup

Prickly Ash

Zanthoxylum americanum; Rutaceae

Part used: bark

Energy and taste: warm; spicy

Active constituents: coumarins, alkaloids (including berberine), 3-4% volatile oils, resin, tannin

Actions: blood circulation; spleen, stomach, kidney

Properties: stimulant, analgesic, alterative, anthelmintic, astringent, antiseptic

Dose: infuse 1 ounce/3 pints water, drink in frequent small doses, totaling 2 cups/day; take 1 "00" capsule 3 times/day; 10-20 drops tincture 3 times/day; 2-5 gm in formula

Precautions: pregnancy; acute and heated conditions

As a strong stimulant, prickly ash promotes peripheral blood circulation, warms the body, relieves cold extremities and joint pain, aids indigestion caused by coldness and stops diarrhea and vomiting. In addition, it is a blood purifier, useful in treating rheumatism, arthritis, swellings, injuries and wounds that are slow to heal. For these it may be taken internally as well as rubbed on externally in an oil or liniment.

Prickly ash is very warming to the stomach, alleviating stomach aches, colic and cramps. It is also useful for weak digestion. It is excellent added to formulas as a stimulant for acute or chronic ailments. Externally, it is applied as a poultice to help dry up

and heal wounds. Like bayberry, the powder can be used for the teeth, or the bark chewed for relief of toothaches.

Indications: cold hands and feet, joint pain, indigestion, diarrhea, rheumatism, arthritis, swellings, injuries, wounds, colic, cramps, wounds, toothaches, vomiting

Projects: tea, capsule, powder, oil, liniment, poultice, gargle, cider

Raspberry

Rubus idaeus; Rosaceae

Part used: leaves, fruit

Energy and taste: neutral; leaves—bitter; fruit—sweet, sour, astringent

Active constituents: leaves—1-2% organic acids, of which 90% is citric acid; Vitamin C, pectins and sugar; fruit—citrus, malic, and salicylic acids; sugars, fragarin, Vitamin C and niacin

Actions: leaves—spleen, liver, kidney, uterus; fruit—liver, kidney

Properties: leaves—hemostatic, astringent, mild alterative, uterine tonic in pregnancy, parturient; fruit—blood and nutritive tonic, refrigerant

Dose: leaves—infuse 1 ounce/pint water, drink 3 cups/day; take 2 "00" capsules 3 times/day; 10-30 drops tincture 3 times/day; 6-15 gm in formula; fruit—9-15 gm

Raspberry leaves have long been used to strengthen and tonify the uterine muscles for helping with pregnancy and childbirth. Taken freely throughout the entire pregnancy, either as a tea or in capsules, it definitely eases the process and pains of childbirth. It also relieves nausea and prevents hemorrhage. For the menstrual cycle, it relieves cramps, and combined with other herbs such as squawvine and uva ursi, treats vaginal discharge and irregular and excessive menstruation. Like blackberry leaves, raspberry treats diarrhea and dysentery and is a general hemostatic for bleeding.

WESTERN HERBS

The fruit and juice build blood and treat anemia. They also cool the blood and regulate menses. The Chinese use raspberries for frequent urination (day or night), impotence, spermatorrhea and premature ejaculation.

Indications: leaves—pregnancy, childbirth, menstrual cramps and cycle regulation, hemorrhoids, diarrhea, dysentery, bleeding; fruit—anemia, regulate menses, frequent urination, impotence, spermatorrhea, premature ejaculation

Projects: tea, capsule, food, juice, tincture

Red Clover

Trifolium pratense; Leguminosae

Parts used: flowers
Energy and taste: cool; sweet, salty
Active constituents: isoflavones and other flavonoids, volatile oil, coumarins, resins
Actions: liver, heart, lungs, blood
Properties: alterative, antispasmodic, expectorant, antitumor
Dose: infuse 1 ounce/pint water, drink 3-6 cups/ day; 10-30 drops tincture 3 times/day; 6-15 gm in formula
Precaution: contains coumarins, so do not use if the blood does not clot easily

A good blood purifier and mild blood thinner, red clover is gentle in action and therefore good for general and long-term consumption, including by children and the elderly. It cleanses the blood and lymph, clears the skin, lowers fevers and heals inflammatory conditions such as arthritis and gout. Externally as a fomentation, wash or poultice, it aids sores that do not heal, dry and scaly skin, eczema and psoriasis.

Red clover can be applied externally to cancerous growths, or taken internally for tumors and cancers, in which case it should be taken in large amounts. It is more effective for this when combined with chaparral, echinacea and other antitumor herbs. Because it is a mild herb, it is better for those who are weak; for more acute and infectious conditions, other alteratives would give a stronger action.

Indications: skin breakouts, arthritis, gout, skin sores, blood toxicity, fever, eczema, psoriasis, cancer, tumors
Projects: tea, fomentation, poultice, tincture, wash

Sarsaparilla

Smilax officinalis; Liliaceae

Parts used: root
Energy and taste: neutral; sweet, mildly spicy
Active constituents: saponins, glycosides, steroids (sitosterol, stigmasterol, sarsasaoigenin), traces of essential oil, resin, starch
Actions: clears heat and toxins; liver, stomach, kidneys, blood, skin, circulation
Properties: alterative, diuretic, diaphoretic, tonic
Dose: decoct 1 ounce/1 pint water, drink 3 cups/day; 2 "00" capsules 3 times/day; 10-30 drops tincture; 6-15 gm in formula
Precaution: contains estrogen-like compounds; do not use if there are estrogen-sensitive tumors

Sarsaparilla is an excellent blood purifier, useful for skin disorders caused by blood impurities, herpes, skin parasites, psoriasis, gout and rheumatism. It may be taken as a tea or applied as a wash or fomentation for all these conditions. It is excellent for chronic liver disorders, leukorrhea and venereal diseases such as gonorrhea and syphilis, for which it was introduced into Britain in the 17th century. It combines well with other alteratives, especially yellow dock, sassafras, burdock, dandelion and red clover.

A hot decoction promotes profuse sweating, helping colds, fevers and mucus problems, and powerfully expels gas from the stomach and intestines. Sarsaparilla contains estrogen-like substances which make it valuable in glandular balance formulas. It has traditionally been used in root beer and other soft drinks.

Indications: skin diseases, herpes, psoriasis, arthritis, rheumatism, gout, venereal diseases, nervous disorders, epilepsy
Projects: tea, wash, beverage, capsule, fomentation

WESTERN HERBS

Scullcap

Scutellaria lateriflora; Labiatae

Parts used: above-ground portion
Energy and taste: cool; bitter
Active constituents: volatile oil, scutellarin (a flavonoid glycoside), iridoids, tannin, waxes, calcium
Actions: clears heat; heart, liver, gallbladder, large intestines, nerves
Properties: nervine, antispasmodic, sedative
Dose: infuse 1 tsp/cup or 1/2-1 ounce/pint water, drink 3 cups/day; 2 "00" capsules 3 times/day or 4 before bed; 10-30 drops tincture; 3-9 gm formula
Precaution: much of what is sold as scullcap in this country is germander (Teucrium); be sure to ask for the genuine herb

As a nervine high in calcium, potassium and magnesium, scullcap strengthens and quiets the entire nervous system while being essentially nontoxic. It clears restlessness, irritability of the nervous system and insomnia in those with excess or deficient heat. It also gives immediate relief in all chronic and acute nervous conditions and debility including nervous tension, excitability, hysteria, convulsions, epilepsy, nervous twitching and spasms, hypertension, nervous headache, PMS tension and neuralgia. For those with nervous conditions from coldness, valerian is a better choice.

Scullcap is one of the best herbs to break addictions and ease drug and alcoholic withdrawal symptoms and for this should be taken in half cupful doses every hour or two, tapering off as the symptoms subside. It can be combined with other nervines or antispasmodics, such as passion flower or valerian, for a broader action. With chamomile it is a safe daily nervine.

Scullcap is a good brain tonic, calming the mind and aiding meditation. This is interesting since the flower itself looks like a helmet to cover the skull. It also reduces hot emotions like anger, hatred, jealousy and irritability, as well as decreases excessive desires. It promotes clarity, detachment and a calm awareness. Chinese medicine uses it for headaches, irritability, red eyes, a bitter taste in the mouth, thirst and to calm a fetus that is restless from heat.

Indications: restlessness, irritability, insomnia, nervous conditions, epilepsy, headache, drug and alcohol withdrawal, PMS, twitching and spasms
Projects: tea, tincture, capsule

Shepherd's Purse

Capsella bursa-pastoris; Cruciferae

Part used: above-ground portions
Energy and taste: neutral; spicy, sweet
Active constituents: flavonoids, acids
Actions: liver, stomach
Properties: astringent, hemostatic, alterative, diuretic
Dose: infuse 1 ounce fresh herb/pint water, drink 3 cups/day; 1 dropperful of tincture every hour or two to stop bleeding; 5-15 gm in formula
Other: use fresh, or tincture fresh

Shepherd's purse is one of the most effective herbs to stop bleeding of all sorts. It helps stop hemorrhages of the stomach, intestines, lungs, uterus and other internal bleeding. It is also used for excessive menstrual and postpartum bleeding. It is a diuretic and so aids genito-urinary problems, bladder infection bleeding and difficult urination. The herb may be applied topically as a poultice to stop nose bleeds or bleeding hemorrhoids. The tincture is a quick-acting and effective way to take the herb. It must be made from the fresh herb to extract its potent properties.

Indications: hemorrhaging, bladder infection, difficult urination, internal or external bleeding, nosebleeds, bleeding hemorrhoids
Projects: tea, tincture, poultice, juice

WESTERN HERBS

Siberian Ginseng

Eleutherococcus senticosus; Araliaceae

Part used: bark of the root

Energy and taste: warm; sweet, acrid

Active constituents: eleutherosides, essential oil, resin, starch, Vitamin A

Actions: adrenals, spleen-pancreas

Properties: adaptogenic energy tonic, antirheumatic, antispasmodic

Dose: decoct 1 ounce/pint water, drink 3 cups/day; tincture or extract—10-30 drops 1-3 times/day; 3-15 gm in formula; for athletes to increase stamina, take 10-20 gm/day

Siberian ginseng is popularly available as a less expensive ginseng with similar tonifying powers. It increases energy, vitality and endurance. Tests on factory workers and athletes resulted in better workload capacities, faster running times and quicker recovery rates after exertion. Siberian ginseng was thoroughly studied by Dr. I.I. Brekhman and other Russian researchers.

The Chinese variety, Acanthopanax, has a warm energy and spicy taste and acts on the liver and kidneys. It is not used as a tonifying ginseng, but to stimulate blood circulation and eliminate damp heat in the joints for rheumatism, poor circulation, coldness, swelling of the legs, edema and difficult urination. It is frequently given to the elderly in wine form.

Indications: low energy, vitality and endurance, rheumatism, poor circulation, edema, coldness, difficult urination, swelling of the legs

Projects: tea, tincture, wine

Slippery Elm

Ulmus fulva; Ulmaceae

Part used: inner bark

Energy and taste: neutral; sweet

Active constituents: mucilage, polysaccharide, tannins, starches, two polyuronides, calcium

Actions: nerves, stomach, lungs

Properties: nutritive tonic, demulcent, expectorant, emollient, mild astringent, vulnerary, mild emmenagogue

Dose: decoct 1 ounce cut root/pint water; 2 "00" capsules 3 times/day; 9-30 gm of powder

Precautions: pregnancy

Slippery Elm is a highly nutritive and soothing food useful for digestive difficulties, stomach and intestinal ulcers, colitis, wasting diseases, sore and dry throats, coughs, bleeding from the lungs and bronchitis. It may be taken in tea or capsule form or made into a gruel by slowly mixing cool water into the powdered herb until a thick porridge consistency is achieved. Flavored with a little honey or a dash of cinnamon or ginger, this gruel is excellent to take for convalescence and when there is difficulty in keeping food down, even in infants. I have seen those who continuously throw up all food be able to eat and digest this gruel, which settles their stomachs and gives them much needed nutrition.

Slippery elm may be freely eaten except by those with a lot of weight, heaviness or dampness, for then it causes more congestion. If combined with small amounts of spices such as cinnamon, cloves or ginger, or sweetened with honey, it will not congest as much. It may also be decocted in milk as a nutritive tonic, for weight gain and to treat ulcers and hyperacidity. Its tonic properties can be further supplemented for this by preparing it with a tea of ginseng instead of water.

It is the same high content of mucilage that makes slippery elm soothing and drawing for skin disorders. A paste (made by decocting the powder in water until a paste consistency is achieved) may be applied to suppurating sores and bed sores, wounds, gangrene, burns, tumors, boils, damaged tissues and inflamed and infected areas. I successfully applied the powder to cure and prevent my baby's diaper rash. It also

WESTERN HERBS

works well for skin disorders when combined with echinacea, golden seal and comfrey powders.

Indications: indigestion, nausea, ulcers, colitis, sore throat, cough, bronchitis, lung bleeding, hyperacidity, sores, wounds, burns, tumors, boils, rash

Projects: tea, paste, gruel, milk, powder, pill, capsule, salve

Squawvine

Mitchella repens; Rubiaceae

Part used: whole herb

Energy and taste: cool; bitter

Active constituents: resin, wax, mucilage, dextrin, saponins

Actions: uterus, liver

Properties: stimulates uterine contractions; emmenagogue, astringent, alterative, parturient

Dose: infuse 1/pint water, drink 3 cups/day; 10-30 drops tincture; 2 "00" capsules, 3 times/day

Other: also known as partridge berry

Squawvine astringes excessive menstrual bleeding, brings on delayed menses and helps painful or scanty menses. It is also beneficial in preparing the womb for childbirth. Combine with two parts raspberry leaves and one part black cohosh root and take two weeks before delivery to ease birthing. It effectively helps clear and dry the secretions of leukorrhea.

Indications: excessive menstrual bleeding, irregular menses, childbirth, leukorrhea

Projects: tea, tincture, capsule

St. John's Wort

Hypericum perforatum; Hypericaceae

Part used: above-ground portions; unopened flower bud is best

Energy and taste: cool; bitter

Active constituents: essential oil, resin, tannin, alkaloid and a dye (hypericine—a glycoside that is a red pigment), myric acid

Actions: liver, kidney, spleen, stomach

Properties: alterative, antispasmodic, anti-inflammatory, antidepressant, astringent, vulnerary, antiviral

Dose: infuse 1-2 tsp/cup water, drink 1-2 cups regularly morning and night; 2 "00" capsules 3 times/day; 5-10 drops tincture; oil, 1 tsp 2-3 times daily; 3-9 gm in formula

Precaution: when taken internally for long periods of time, it is thought to create sun sensitivity and burning (which it does in livestock, though it has never been proven in humans)

St. John's wort owes its name to the fact that it begins to flower around St. John's tide, the summer solstice, and some herbalists particularly like to pick it on St. John's day. This pretty yellow flowering plant has several beneficial uses. Internally it is a pain-relieving sedative used in treating anxiety, nervous tension and neuralgia. It is also antidepressant and can be used in the treatment of chronic depressive illness, anxiety and restlessness, lightening the mood and inducing a certain euphoria. Although it must be taken for several months before its full effects can be realized, its benefits can be felt within a few weeks. It is also used in AIDS as an antiviral.

The oil treats wounds, burns, ulcers and nerve pain associated with sciatica, rheumatism and varicose veins. It is a specific for the treatment of diseases directly affecting the spine. Homeopathic St. John's wort, called Hypericum, is specific for all types of nerve pain.

Indications: anxiety, nervous tension, neuralgia, nerve pain, sciatica, burns, wounds, depression

Projects: tea, tincture, oil, poultice, wash, salve, bath, liniment, first aid, homeopathic

WESTERN HERBS

Turmeric

Curcuma longa; Zingiberaceae

Parts used: tuber and rhizome

Energy and taste: tuber—cool; rhizome—warm; both—spicy, bitter

Active constituents: rhizome—curcuminoids, volatile oil, protein, sugars, fixed oil

Actions: tuber—heart, liver, lung; rhizome—spleen, stomach, liver

Properties: emmenagogue, carminative, stimulant, alterative, vulnerary, cholagogue, analgesic, antiseptic, astringent

Dose: decoct 1 tbsp/cup water or use 3-9 gm; drink 3 cups/day; mix 1 tsp/cup water, drink 2 cups/day

Precautions: pregnancy, acute jaundice and hepatitis, hyperacidity, ulcers or irritable stomach; stagnation of blood

While mostly known as a spice in Indian cooking, turmeric is used in both Chinese and Ayurvedic medicines for several purposes. The rhizome's warm energy regulates the blood, promotes menstruation and eases cramps, especially in amenorrhea or dysmenorrhea due to coldness congealing the blood. It also helps reduce uterine tumors. Further, it is anti-inflammatory, purifies the blood and stimulates formation of new blood tissue. As such, it is a wonderful herb for women who have PMS and related menstrual problems and as a restorative after blood loss from childbirth.

Turmeric also strengthens digestion, improves intestinal flora, aids in digestion of protein and moves gastric or abdominal congestion and its related pain. It detoxifies and decongests the liver, dissolves gallstones, and may be combined with barberry or Oregon grape root for releasing congestion in the liver as effectively as Chinese bupleurum. Its action on the liver helps flexibility of the tendons and is, therefore, useful for stretching in exercise. The blood-moving and anti-inflammatory properties of turmeric make it useful for wounds, bruises and other traumas or injuries, both externally and internally.

Both the tuber and rhizome stimulate blood circulation, yet because one is cool and the other warm, they do have some different uses. The tuber cools the blood, thus aiding anxiety, agitation, seizures, mental derangement, hemorrhages and jaundice and is used topically for traumatic injuries and sores. The rhizome promotes menstruation, alleviates chest and abdominal pain, amenorrhea and dysmenorrhea due to cold, pain and swelling from trauma and gastric and abdominal pain.

Indications: poor circulation, amenorrhea, dysmenorrhea, indigestion, skin disorders, anemia, wounds, bruises

Projects: powder, tea, spice, milk, poultice, paste, dye, first aid, bitters

Uva Ursi

Arctostaphylos uva ursi; Ericaceae

Part used: leaves

Energy and taste: cool; bitter, astringent

Active constituents: glycoside (arbutin), iridoids, flavonoids, tannins, ursolic acid, phenolic acids, uvalol, resin, and a yellow principle resembling quercetin

Actions: kidneys, urinary tract, heart, small intestine, liver

Properties: diuretic, astringent, antiseptic

Dose: infuse 1 ounce/pint water, drink cool, 3 cups a day; 10-30 drops tincture 3 times/day; 3-6 gm in formula

Precautions: pregnancy

Other: also known as bearberry

Uva ursi is a strong diuretic and urinary antiseptic useful for bladder and kidney infections. When

WESTERN HERBS

combined with marshmallow root, it helps eliminate stones from those organs. It also strengthens and tones the urinary passages and treats blood in the urine. For its diuretic effect it should only be infused in cool or room temperature water. Hot water alters its diuretic properties.

The Native Americans use uva ursi after birthing to help shrink the uterus quickly and to prevent infections. For this, drink the tea and bathe in it. Alternatively, use the tincture for preventing postpartum hemorrhage and shrinking the uterus as they did in many European hospitals. By the same token, it should be avoided during pregnancy.

Indications: bladder and kidney infections, stones, blood in the urine, postpartum hemorrhage and shrinking of uterus

Projects: tea, tincture, bath

Valerian

Valeriana officinalis; Valerianaceae

Part used: root
Energy and taste: warm; bitter, spicy
Active constituents: alkaloids, iridoid compounds, acids, tannin, gum, essential oil
Actions: liver, heart, nerves
Properties: nervine, antispasmodic, carminative, stimulant, anodyne
Dose: infuse 1 ounce/pint water, drink 3 cups/day; 2 "00" capsules 3 times/day and 4 before bed; 1 tsp tincture/1/2 cup water taken as needed or 10-30 drops frequently; 3-9 gm in formula
Precaution: can cause cardiac palpitations in sensitive individuals

Valerian is one of the best herbs for individuals with a cold, nervous condition. It is tranquilizing, calming and sedating, thus relieving pain, cramps, spasms and nervous disorders such as nervous excitement, sleeplessness and palpitations. It is grounding while alleviating dizziness, neurasthenia, fainting,

nervous headache, menopause nervousness, emotional disturbances and hysteria.

Because it is heating, it can have opposite effects on people who have a heated condition. This is a clear example of the need to choose herbs according to their energies rather than properties. For those with heat conditions, scullcap is a better choice. Valerian is often combined in formula for its antispasmodic property, and its actions can be better directed for a specific purpose by doing so. It is best when used fresh.

Indications: nervousness, insomnia, pain, cramps, spasms, palpitations, dizziness, emotional disturbances, headache, menopause

Projects: tea, tincture, capsule

Wild Cherry

Prunus virginiana, P. serotina; Rosaceae

Part used: bark
Energy and taste: warm; acrid, astringent; slightly toxic
Active constituents: prunasin (a cyanogenetic glycoside), p-coumaric acid, scopoletin, tannins, sugars
Actions: spleen, lung
Properties: antitussive, sedative, astringent, carminative
Dose: infuse 1 ounce/pint cool water, drink 3 cups/day; 2 "00" capsules 3 times/day; 10-15 drops tincture; 3-9 gm in formula

Wild cherry bark has been used for centuries in cough syrups as an expectorant to alleviate irritable and persistent coughs and asthma and to calm the respiratory nerves. It is useful in the treatment of bronchitis, mucus, consumption, nervous cough and whooping cough.

It is also a valuable remedy for nervousness and weakness of the stomach with accompanying irritations such as ulcers, gastritis, colitis, diarrhea and dysentery. It is beneficial when combined with digestive tonics, such as licorice, ginseng, citrus peel and

WESTERN HERBS

anise, in rice wine. Taking it with licorice lessens any potential toxicity. The cold infusion is best as this retains most of its properties.

Indications: coughs, whooping cough, asthma, bronchitis, indigestion, diarrhea, gastritis, ulcers

Projects: tea, syrup, tincture, wine

Yarrow

Achillea spp.; Compositae

Parts used: above-ground portions

Energy and taste: neutral; bitter, spicy

Active constituents: volatile oil, lactones, rutin, tannins, coumarins, saponins, sterols, alkanes, fatty acids, alkaloids, salicylic acid, succinic acid

Actions: general effects on the whole body; lungs, liver

Properties: diaphoretic, astringent, hemostatic, antibacterial, stimulant, carminative, antispasmodic

Dose: infuse 1 ounce herb/cup water, drink 1/2 to 1 cup tea every hour or two until cold or fever breaks or bleeding stops; 3-9 gm in formula

Yarrow has been used by many cultures and for thousands of years. Originally yarrow stalks were used for divining the *I Ching*, an ancient Chinese book describing the laws of change and cycles. In Nordic countries the plant was used in place of hops in beer production. In Germany in the 16th century the seeds were put in wine barrels as a preservative. Yarrow flowers are either yellow, white or a dark pink. The white or pink plants are used as medicine, while the yellow are only ornamental.

Its Latin name, *Achillea*, comes from the Greek hero, Achilles, who put yarrow directly on his soldiers' wounds to stop them from bleeding. Achilles further recommended putting yarrow juice in the eye to take away redness. The Native Americans use it for wounds, too. They also roll up the leaves and put them in the nostrils for nosebleed. Interestingly, yarrow does contain a substance which hastens blood clotting from injury, which explains its common name of Nosebleed.

Yarrow's astringent, antiseptic and hemostatic actions make it an invaluable remedy for the healing of burns, cuts, bruises, hemorrhages, inflammations and other wounds, hemorrhoids and leukorrhea. It can be applied directly to wounds to stop bleeding and is used in a bolus or salve for bleeding piles. It relieves cramps and helps stop excess menstrual bleeding and internal hemorrhage when taken internally.

Yarrow also causes the body to sweat. It is perfect for fevers and for helping the first signs of colds, flus and fevers. It is good for chicken pox and measles—it helps eruptions to come out faster, although for some speeding up the healing process may be uncomfortable.

Indications: hemorrhage, nosebleeds, hemorrhoids, bruises, wounds, excessive menstrual bleeding, menstrual cramps, colds, flus, fever, chicken pox, measles, leucorrhea

Projects: tea, salve, bolus, poultice, juice, tincture, dream pillow; for this place the pillow under the head before going to sleep and repeat the following old saying—

"Thou pretty herb of Venus' tree,
Thy true name it is yarrow;
Now who my bosom friend must be,
Pray tell thou me to-morrow."

Yellow Dock

Rumex crispus; Polygonaceae

Part used: root

Energy and taste: cool; bitter

Active constituents: hydroanthraquinone, bras-sidinic acid, oxalic acid, rumicin, calcium oxalate, tannin, calcium, phosphorus, iron, Vitamins A, C and some B

Actions: liver, colon, blood

Properties: alterative, cholagogue, astringent, aperient, blood tonic, skin, circulatory

Dose: decoct 1 ounce/pint water, drink 1/2 cup, 2-3 times/day (it's very bitter!); 1-2 "00" capsules, 1-3

WESTERN HERBS

times/day; 10-30 drops tincture; 1 tbsp syrup, 2-3 times/day; 3-9 gm in formula

Yellow dock is an astringent blood purifier. It is used to treat chronic and acute skin diseases such as skin eruptions, psoriasis, itching welts and eczema since it cools and detoxifies the blood. Very high in iron, it helps build the blood especially when combined with blackstrap molasses. It is very specific for anemia and can be used for this during pregnancy.

Since it detoxifies the liver, yellow dock is beneficial for jaundice, and since it stimulates bile secretion, it causes a laxative action, relieving constipation without causing griping or pain. Externally it is applied to stop bleeding of wounds, hemorrhoids and swellings.

Indications: skin diseases, psoriasis, urticaria, eczema, jaundice, constipation, wounds, anemia

Projects: tea, tincture, capsule, syrup with blackstrap molasses, poultice

CHINESE HERBS

Chinese herbs are extremely useful to us in the West as they include many tonics which are, as yet, rarely found in Western herbalism. Tonic herbs build strength, prevent disease from occurring, balance the body's energy, strengthen the disease-recovery process and nourish the blood and substance of the body.

Western herbal usage is predominantly eliminative in nature since our culture comes from a tradition of excess meat-eating and the use of rich foods. Therefore, few Western tonic herbs have been identified. Because deficiencies in the body need to be handled from a building rather than eliminative approach, Chinese herbs with their thousands of years of use and understanding are perfect for this. Since more and more Western herbalists are beginning to understand this, Chinese herbs are becoming increasingly easy to find in herbal stores throughout the United States, and even in other Western countries. Many are even being grown here, and some day soon we should have readily available organically grown Chinese herbs.

Tonic herbs need to be taken over a long period of time to help strengthen from any deficiencies. For this they are usually taken as a tea, or even better, in soup form. Typically the Chinese prepare a tonic herb soup once a week for maintenance and preventative measures. To learn how to properly make herbal soups, refer to the chapter on *Herbal Preparations*.

Although most of the Chinese herbs included here are tonics of either the blood, fluids, energy, warmth or tonics for specific organs, other Chinese herbs are included which are useful to know for their specific and valuable applications. Under Dose, the grams for tea decoctions are given as this is the traditional Chinese way of preparing herbs. The herbs may be powdered for capsules or tinctured if desired, in which case the standard dose of 2 "00" capsules or 10-30 drops tincture three times daily is given. Under the Chinese names for the herbs, the first is Mandarin (Pinyin) and the second is Cantonese.

Aconite

Aconitum carmichaeli; Ranunculaceae
Chinese: *fu zi, fu jee*

Part used: specially prepared root
Energy and taste: very hot; spicy, sweet; toxic
Active constituents: aconitine, one of the fastest acting and deadliest alkaloids known
Actions: warms inside of body and dispels cold; heart, spleen, kidney
Properties: stimulant, cardiac tonic, analgesic
Dose: In minute homeopathic dosage; decoction of 3-9 gm of specially prepared aconite; 5-10 drops tincture 3 times/day
Precaution: conditions of heat, constipation, pregnancy, high fever, high blood pressure, hypertension; symptoms of poisoning are—numbness of extremities starting at the fingers, followed by dizziness, perspiration, nausea, palpitations, body spasm and decreasing blood pressure; if poisoned, take a thick tea of dry ginger and licorice; only use the Chinese-prepared aconite
Other: also known as monkshood because its flower looks like a monk's hood

Aconite is the hottest herb used in Chinese medicine. It is a powerful internal stimulant which warms the inside of the body and raises the metabolism in cold conditions. As such it relieves severe pain, gas, fluid retention, coldness, numbness, arthritis, sciatica, frequent and nighttime urination, lower back pain, diarrhea, chest and abdominal pain, nervous disorders, general debilitation, poor metabolism, cardiac weakness, chills, kidney infections, impotence and infertility.

It is strictly for use only by those with coldness or for cold conditions of the body. It is almost always combined with other herbs in formula, such as ginseng, cinnamon bark, ginger and atractylodes. Such a formula warms the body, stimulates circulation, aids appetite and digestion and increases energy.

Externally, aconite can be used as a fomentation or wash for sprains, injuries, bruises, neuralgia, arthritis and rheumatism, all caused by coldness. It is also frequently used in homeopathic form at the first signs of acute disease every 15 minutes until symptoms show improvement, and also in times of extreme fear and shock. The homeopathic dose should be about 6X to 30X potency.

Aconite is the most poisonous European plant and in the past was smeared on arrows and spears. Yet today, most of its toxic properties are neutralized by the Chinese method of preparation which takes several months. Therefore, **only the properly prepared Chinese aconite should be used.** If aconite tea causes a numbing sensation in the mouth, this is an indication that its toxicity has not been neutralized and that it should not be used.

Indications: coldness, pain, frequent urination, lower back pain, general debility, lowered metabolism, neuralgia, arthritis, sciatica, nervous disorders

Projects: homeopathic in tincture or pill form; tea, liniment, fomentation, tincture

Astragalus

Astragalus membranaceus; Leguminosae
Chinese: *huang chi; bak kay*

Part used: root
Energy and taste: warm; sweet
Active constituents: 2'4'-dihydroxy-5,6- dimethoxy-isoflavane, choline, betaine, kumatakenin, sucrose, glucoronic acid, B-sitosterol
Actions: spleen, lung
Properties: energy tonic, diuretic, stops sweating
Dose: 6-15 gm in decoction
Precautions: acute heat attacks (like heat stroke), early stages of flus when sweating is desired, acute asthma
Other: the root is long, flat and yellowish-white and looks a bit like a large tongue depressor

Astragalus strengthens the energy and builds resistance to colds, flus, weakness and disease. For those who easily and frequently catch cold and often feel tired, this is the perfect herb as it treats chronically weak lungs with shortness of breath and low energy. It further lifts prolapsed organs, stops spontaneous sweating, eliminates swellings, including a puffy face, and treats collapse of energy, exhaustion, edema due to lack of energy circulation and kidney and bladder infections that do not respond to diuretics.

Astragalus also strengthens digestion, improves metabolism, increases appetite and treats malnutrition and diarrhea. Every sort of wasting or exhaustion disease is benefited by it. It helps heal chronic sores and ulcerations that have formed pus but have not drained or healed well. Astragalus lessens chemotherapy and radiation side effects and inhibits the spreading of tumors. This herb is often included in soups, herbal or vegetable, or cooked in with grains. Taken this way on a weekly basis it helps the whole family get through the winter without a single cold.

Indications: colds, flus, exhaustion, poor digestion and metabolism, low appetite, weakness, shortness of breath, prolapsed organs, spontaneous sweating, tumors

Projects: tea, soup, wine, milk, congee

Atractylodes

Atractylodes alba, A. macrocephalae; Compositae
Chinese: *bai zhu; bak sut*

Part used: rhizome
Energy and taste: warm; bitter, sweet
Active constituents: essential oil comprised of atractylon ($C_{14} H_{18} O$) and atractylol ($15 H_{26} O$)
Actions: spleen, stomach
Properties: energy tonic, diuretic, carminative
Dose: 3-12 gm in decoction
Precaution: dehydration, stomach heat (such as ulcers, burning sensations in the stomach, gum bleeding and bad breath)

CHINESE HERBS

Atractylodes is one of the major herbs used to strengthen the spleen and stomach, thus alleviating poor digestion, lowered appetite, tiredness, lack of strength, vomiting and diarrhea. It helps alleviate fluid retention, edema and stagnant water in the stomach. It also stops spontaneous sweating caused by low energy, and fever and chills without sweating. It can be used in pregnancy for vomiting and a restless fetus. Atractylodes is frequently combined with astragalus, licorice, codonopsis, wild yam and ginseng in tea or soup form.

Indications: poor appetite, tiredness, diarrhea, edema, spontaneous sweating, fluid retention, fever and chills

Projects: tea, soup, wine, congee

Bupleurum

Bupleurum falcatum; Umbelliferae
Chinese: *chai hu; chai wu*

Part used: root

Energy and taste: cool; spicy, bitter

Active constituents: furfurol, sterol, bupleurumol

Actions: liver, pericardium, gallbladder

Properties: antipyretic, diaphoretic, carminative, alterative

Dose: 3-15 gm in decoction

Precautions: fever or headaches due to anemia, if there are signs of heat rising: splitting headache, red eyes and face, bitter taste in the mouth and hypertension; do not use long term as it can cause dizziness

Other: also known as Hare's Ear Root

Note: some people have anger and irritability after taking it for a few days; if this happens, stop for several days and then restart with a lower dose

Bupleurum treats both external acute conditions as well as internal chronic ones. It is one of the best liver herbs and improves liver function, relieves chest and flank pain and congestion, dizziness and menstrual difficulties. It stabilizes emotions, regulates moodiness and eases PMS. Its strong ascending action picks up the body's energy, lifting the vitality, prolapsed organs, hemorrhoids and sagging spirits.

For external conditions bupleurum relieves alternating chills and fever along with a bitter taste in the mouth, flank pain, irritability, vomiting and a sensation of constriction in the chest. Because it harmonizes both external and internal problems, it is good when an acute condition lingers and becomes chronic.

Indications: colds, fever, chest and flank pain, dizziness, menstrual difficulties, PMS, emotion instability, prolapsed organs, hemorrhoids

Projects: tea

Chrysanthemum

Chrysanthemum morifolium; Compositae
Chinese: *ju hua; gook fah*

Part used: flowers

Energy and taste: cool; sweet, slightly bitter

Active constituents: essential oil, adenine, choline and stachydrine

Actions: clears heat; lungs, liver

Properties: antipyretic, carminative, antispasmodic, alterative, tonic

Dose: 3-9 gm in infusion

Precautions: do not use if there is dizzyness; do not take during menstruation

Other: generally the yellow-flowered chrysanthemums are preferred

Chrysanthemum is valuable in treating fevers, headache, colds, flu and pneumonia. It is used to clear heat from the liver which heals red eyes, blurred vision, dizziness, boils and hypertension symptoms. It can be used as an eye wash for sore or swollen eyes. It calms anger and irritability. The Chinese drink it as a summer beverage for its cooling and refreshing taste and rejuvenative properties. The wild chrysanthemum, which is white, is colder in energy.

Indications: fever, headache, colds, flu, pneumonia, red eyes, blurred vision, dizziness, boils, hypertension

Projects: tea, beverage, wash

CHINESE HERBS

Citrus

Citrus reticulata; Rutaceae
Chinese: *chen pi; chen pay*

Part used: aged dried peel of the ripe tangerine (the strongest acting), or of the orange or mandarin orange
Energy and taste: warm; spicy, bitter
Active constituents: essential oils (including limonen, linalool, perpineol), hesperidin, carotene, cryptosanthin, Vitamins B-1 and C
Actions: spleen, stomach, lungs
Properties: carminative, stimulant, expectorant, antitussive, antiemetic, tonic
Dose: 3-9 gm in decoction

Tangerine peel moves stagnant energy in the abdomen and strengthens the digestive functions. It alleviates indigestion, gas, watery diarrhea, vomiting, abdominal swelling, bloating, lack of appetite and nausea. The inner part of the fruit is cold and creates mucus whereas the peel is warming and eliminates it, both from the lungs and the digestive system. Thus, it is always good to eat a bit of the peel whenever eating this citrus. (In fact, Ayurveda says eating a bit of the peel from any fruit will counteract its potentially imbalancing properties.)

Indications: indigestion, gas, bloating, lack of appetite, nausea, diarrhea, vomiting, cough, mucus in lungs, strengthens digestion
Projects: tea, soup, tincture, bitters, cider, congee, chai

Codonopsis

Codonopsis pilosulae; Campanulaceae
Chinese: *dang shen; dong sum*

Part used: root
Energy and taste: slightly warm; sweet
Active constituents: saponin, starch, sugar
Actions: spleen, lung
Properties: energy tonic, demulcent, expectorant
Dose: 6-20 gm in decoction

Codonopsis is used similarly to ginseng but is milder in energy and actions and so is safe to use for long-term treatment, in all climates and by both sexes. It increases vital energy, strengthens digestion and assimilation, helps diabetes and treats hyperacidity. It is given in all diseases associated with weakness, debility, tiredness, lack of strength, poor appetite and anemia. It also helps diarrhea, vomiting, gas and bloatedness and chronic cough and shortness of breath. When combined with astragalus, it helps build resistance to disease. It is very useful for teething babies to "chew" on as it is hard, can be held like a stick and is sweet-tasting.

Indications: low energy and vitality, tiredness, weakness, poor appetite, poor digestion, diarrhea, vomiting, gas, bloatedness, chronic cough, shortness of breath
Projects: tea, soup, wine, congee

Cornus

Cornus officinalis; Cornaceae
Chinese: *shan zhu yu; san yu yok*

Part used: fruit
Energy and taste: slightly warm; sour
Actions: liver, kidneys
Properties: astringent, tonic
Dose: 3-9 gm in decoction

The astringency of cornus berries contains the "essence" in a weak body, retaining fluids which tend to leak out. It treats symptoms of excessive urination and sweating, incontinence, night sweats, seminal emission and excessive menstrual bleeding. It also benefits a weak lower back and knees, impotence, reduction in hearing acuity and dizziness. Cornus is the berry of a Chinese species of the Dogwood tree.

Indications: excessive urination, sweating or menstrual bleeding, incontinence, night sweats, seminal emission, impotence
Projects: tea, soup, tincture, congee, wine

CHINESE HERBS

Cyperus

Cyperus spp.; Cyperaceae
Chinese: *xiang fu; heung fu*

Part used: rhizome
Energy and taste: slightly warm; spicy, slightly bitter, sweet
Active constituents: 0.5% essential oils comprised of cyperol, cyperene, cyperone, pinene and sesquiterpenes
Actions: liver
Properties: carminative, antispasmodic, emmenagogue
Dose: 3-9 gm in decoction
Precaution: use cautiously if there is high blood pressure, as cyperus is prepared in salt
Other: also known as sedge

Cyperus regulates energy in the abdomen. Thus, it aids pain and distention in the abdomen and chest, digestive problems, gas, bloating, food stagnation, irregular menses, cramps and painful menstruation due to emotional causes. It also dispels depression and moodiness. If used for a prolonged period over several months, it can be drying and so should be combined with lycii berries in those with anemia.
Indications: digestive problems, irregular or painful menstruation, depression
Projects: tea

Dioscorea

Dioscorea batata, D. japonica; Dioscoreaceae
Chinese: *shan yao; wai san*

Part used: the tuberous root
Energy and taste: neutral; sweet
Active constituents: 16% starch, mucilage, amylase, albuminoid matter, fat, sugar, amino acids including arginine, leucine, tyrosine and glutamine
Actions: lung, kidney, spleen
Properties: energy tonic, nutritive, demulcent
Dose: 6-15 gm in decoction
Precautions: any excess conditions
Other: this is the Chinese wild yam

Dioscorea strengthens the energy and digestion, helping tiredness, poor appetite, diarrhea, spontaneous sweating and diabetes. It also helps weakness of the lungs and kidneys, chronic cough, frequent urination, spermatorrhea, leukorrhea and emotional instability.
Indications: poor digestion and appetite, fatigue, diarrhea, diabetes, cough, frequent urination, leukorrhea, spermatorrhea
Projects: tea, soup, wine, congee

Dong Quai

Angelica sinensis; Umbelliferae
Chinese: *dang gui; dong kway*

Part used: root, whole or sliced
Energy and taste: warm; sweet, spicy, bitter
Active constituents: 40% sucrose, 0.2%-0.3% essential oil made up of carvacrol, safrol, isosafrol, alcohols, sesquiterpenes, cadinene, n-dodecanol, n-tetradecanol, n-butylphalid; also a non-blycosidal, non-alkaloid and water-soluble crystalline material with B-12 and carotene
Actions: heart, liver, spleen
Properties: blood tonic, emmenagogue, sedative, analgesic, laxative
Dose: 3-15 gm in decoction
Precautions: pregnancy; excessive menstrual flow; nosebleeds; sore throat; due to its coumerins, those whose blood doesn't clot easily should avoid it; it also contains estrogen-like compounds and so should not be used when there are estrogen-sensitive tumors or fibroids
Other: also known as Tang kuei

CHINESE HERBS

Note: usually the entire root is prescribed as the tail, body and head have slightly varying functions (the head tonifies the most, the tail moves the blood more strongly while the body is equally tonifying and invigorating)

Dong quai is the supreme woman's herb for tonifying the blood and regulating the menstrual cycle. It is used for most all gynecological complaints, promoting blood circulation, stimulating the uterus and stopping pain. As such, it is also used for abdominal pain and traumatic injuries. It is invaluable for anemia, a pale face, blurred vision and palpitations. Although usually given to women, it is valuable for men with these signs of anemia. Dong quai is good in menopause and also promotes feelings of compassion. Since it moistens the intestines, it helps constipation due to dryness of the bowels.

Indications: all gynecological complaints, anemia, blurred vision, palpitations, menopause, constipation, injuries

Projects: tea, soup, wine, congee

Ephedra

Ephedra spp.; Ephedraceae
Chinese: *ma huang: ma wong*

Part used: above-ground portion
Energy and taste: warm; spicy, bitter
Active constituents: ephedrine alkaloids
Actions: lung, bladder
Properties: diaphoretic, stimulant, diuretic, expectorant, astringent
Dose: 2-6 gm decoction of Chinese; 4-12 gm of Western
Precautions: contraindicated in false heat conditions, symptoms of hypertension, adrenal exhaustion and any other deficiency; heart palpitations, edema
Other: the Western ephedra is often called Mormon Tea, Brigham tea or joint fur

Chinese ephedra is a strong stimulant with an action-like adrenaline. It is a powerful bronchodilator and valuable for asthma, bronchitis, wheezing, cough and difficulty in breathing. It causes sweating and is helpful in relieving colds, flus and fever without sweating. It also has a diuretic effect.

The American ephedra has similar effects but is far less stimulating and so milder-acting. As a diuretic it is more useful for treating water retention. Either variety should not be taken by weak or frail people or those with deficiencies, as ephedra will only cause further depletion in those cases.

Indications: asthma, bronchitis, cough, fever, colds, flus, water retention
Projects: tea

Fu Ling

Poria cocos; Polyporaceae
Chinese: *fu ling; fuk ling*

Part used: whole fungus (mushroom); it is usually found adhering to the roots of pine trees
Energy and taste: neutral; sweet
Active constituents: tetracyclic triterpenic acid (eburicolic acid, pachymic acid), polysaccharide (pachyman), ergosterol, choline, fat, glucose, lipase, protease
Actions: heart, lung, spleen, stomach, kidney
Properties: diuretic, sedative, tonic
Dose: 6-18 gm in decoction
Precautions: frequent copious urine from coldness
Other: also known as Hoelen

Fu ling is a valuable North American mushroom, called Tuckahoe or Indian Bread, that has fallen out of general use here. Its mildness makes it one of the best diuretics for difficult urination or excessive dampness. It may be used safely by children, the elderly and the deficient. It also calms the mind and emotions, tonifies digestion and relieves anxiety, palpitation and tachycardia from dampness.

Indications: difficult urination, excessive dampness, poor digestion, anxiety, palpitations, moodiness

Projects: tea, soup, congee

Gardenia

Gardenia jasminoides; Rubiaceae
Chinese: *zhi zi; san jee jee*

Part used: the fruit
Energy and taste: cold; bitter
Active constituents: gardenin, crocin, chlorogenin, tannin, mannitol
Actions: clears heat; liver, lung, stomach, heart
Properties: alterative, antipyretic, hemostatic
Dose: 6-12 gm in decoction
Precautions: loose stools, coldness with deficiency

Gardenia is called the "happiness herb" because it clears excess heat in the upper, middle and lower parts of the body which causes restlessness, irritability, anger, fever, hepatitis, jaundice, hypertension, ulcers, urinary tract infections, inflammation of burns, red eyes, mouth sores, bitter taste in the mouth and insomnia. It is also used externally to reduce swellings from trauma. When partially charred, it stops blood in the vomit, stool, urine or nose.

Indications: irritability, fever, hepatitis, jaundice, hypertension, infections and inflammations, red eyes, mouth sores, insomnia

Projects: tea

Ginseng

Panax ginseng; Araliaceae
Chinese: *ren shen; yun sum*

Part used: aged root
Energy and taste: warm; sweet, slightly bitter
Active constituents: triterpenic saponosides (known as ginsenosides), traces of essential oils, trace amounts of germanium (which may be partially responsible for its remarkable action)

Actions: spleen, lungs, heart
Properties: energy tonic, rejuvenative, demulcent, stimulant
Dose: 3-9 gm (up to 30 gm for shock) in decoction
Precautions: false or excess heat conditions, high blood pressure

There are many types of ginseng and this can seem confusing. They all have in common the ability to strengthen the body and its energy, yet otherwise have different specific uses. American ginseng, Siberian ginseng and Tienchi ginseng are discussed separately. Siberian ginseng is mentioned here for clarity: the Chinese are only beginning to recognize that it possesses mild ginseng-like properties.

Korean ginseng is Panax ginseng grown in Korea, from where most of the world's market of ginseng comes. It is treated by steaming, which gives it a red color. They claim it makes the ginseng warmer in energy and increases its blood circulation properties. The white Chinese ginseng is untreated Panax ginseng. Avoid purchasing any powdered form of ginseng unless from a reputable source or company. It is easily adulterated.

Ginseng revitalizes the body and mind, strengthening weakness, low energy and vitality, shock, collapse due to loss of blood, chronic febrile disease, heart weakness, debility, convalescence and weakness in old age. It promotes weight and tissue growth in the body and increases wisdom, longevity and resistance to disease.

Ginseng particularly benefits the digestive process and the lungs, treating lethargy, lack of appetite, abdominal and chest distention, chronic diarrhea, prolapse of the stomach, uterus or rectum, shortness of breath, profuse sweating, wheezing, tuberculosis and palpitations with anxiety, insomnia, forgetfulness and restlessness. Traditionally it is taken at age 40 and over by men, although women take it, too.

Indications: debility, weakness, tiredness, poor appetite and digestion, emaciation, shortness of breath, profuse sweating, palpitations, shock

Projects: tea, soup, wine, congee

CHINESE HERBS

Honeysuckle

Lonicera japonica; Caprifoliaceae
Chinese: *jin yin hua; gum nan fah*

Part used: flowers
Energy and taste: cold; sweet
Actions: clears heat; lung, stomach
Properties: alterative, febrifuge, antibiotic, diuretic, refrigerant, diaphoretic
Dose: 9-16 gm in infusion
Precautions: watery diarrhea from coldness
Other: this is the commonly known ornamental flower

Honeysuckle is valuable for treating infections, inflammations, fevers, viruses, staph and strep infections and other conditions needing an antibiotic. It is also useful in colds and flus, sore throat, headache, conjunctivitis, hot painful eyes, boils and dysentery. It reduces swellings of various types, especially of the breast, throat or eyes, and clears inflammations of the intestines, urinary tract and reproductive organs.

Indications: inflammations and infections, fever, viruses, headache, sore throat, colds, flus, conjunctivitis, swellings
Projects: tea

Ho Shou Wu

Polygonum multiflorum; Polygonaceae
Chinese: *he shou wu; ho sao wu*

Part used: root
Energy and taste: slightly warm; bitter, sweet
Actions: liver, kidney
Properties: blood tonic, astringent
Dose: 9-15 gm in decoction
Precautions: weak digestion with fluid retention or congestion

Ho shou wu is often called *fo ti* in America (a marketing name) and is said to have mysterious prop-erties. When taken for a year, the 50 year old root preserves the black color of the hair, and the 150 year old root causes new teeth to grow in the elderly, whereas the 300 year old root gives earthly immortality. This herb obviously has restorative and reviving powers to the body!

As a blood, liver and kidney tonic, ho shou wu treats dizziness, blurred vision, prematurely gray hair, weak lower back and knees, insomnia, infertility, impotence, premature senility, withered skin, wrinkles, nocturnal emission, spermatorrhea and leukorrhea. It builds blood and sperm, strengthens muscles, tendons, ligaments and bones and counters the effects of aging. I have seen it restore gray hair to black, although it needs to be taken continuously for this. Like dong quai, it moistens the intestines and helps constipation from dryness.

Indications: premature aging signs, dizziness, blurred vision, infertility, impotence, spermatorrhea, leukorrhea, anemia
Projects: tea, wine, soup, congee

Jujube

Zizyphus sativa; Rhamnaceae
Chinese: *da zao; dai jo*

Part used: fruit
Energy and taste: warm; sweet
Active constituents: mucilage, sugar, fat, zizyphic acid
Actions: spleen, stomach
Properties: energy tonic, expectorant, nutritive, mild sedative
Dose: 3-12 gm or 3-10 dates in decoction
Precautions: dampness with bloating and stomach distention; when there are intestinal parasites

These delicious large red dates strengthen the digestion and calm the emotions. They are used for weakness, low energy, nervous exhaustion, insomnia, poor appetite, digestion and memory, diarrhea from coldness and weight gain. They also help stabi-

CHINESE HERBS

lize the emotions when feeling irritable, sad or crying for no reason. They are added like licorice to sweeten and harmonize the other herbs in a formula. After cooking the dates in a tea or soup, it is best to eat them for their full medicinal value.

Indications: weakness, low energy, insomnia, poor digestion and appetite, diarrhea, weight gain, moodiness

Projects: tea, soup, wine, congee

Lycii

Lycium chinensis and spp.; Solanaceae
Chinese: *gou qi zi; gay jee*

Part used: fruit
Energy and taste: neutral; sweet
Active constituents: carotene, Vitamins A and C, thiamene, riboflavin, B-sitosterol, linoleic acid
Actions: kidney, liver
Properties: blood and nutritive tonic, hemostatic, antipyretic
Dose: 5-15 gm in decoction
Precautions: excess heat conditions, weak digestion with a tendency to bloatedness and watery diarrhea
Other: also known as Wolfberry in America

This small, red, sweet-tasting berry strengthens the blood, treating anemia, dizziness, poor eyesight, night blindness, blurred vision, tuberculosis and thirst. It also alleviates sore back, knees and legs and helps impotence, seminal and nocturnal emission, leukorrhea and reproductive secretions. It is very high in beta-carotene.

Indications: anemia, dizziness, night blindness, blurred vision, tuberculosis, impotence, seminal and nocturnal emission, leukorrhea

Projects: tea, soup, wine, congee

Peony

Paeonia lactiflorae; Ranunculaceae
Chinese: *bai shao; bak chuk*

Part used: root
Energy and taste: cold; bitter, sour
Active constituents: 5% asparagin and benzoic acids, paeoniflorin, paeonol, paeonin, triterpenoids, sistosterol
Actions: liver, spleen
Properties: blood and nutritive tonic, emmenagogue, antispasmodic, astringent
Dose: 6-16 gm in decoction
Precaution: watery diarrhea from coldness
Other: also known as white peony (versus a red peony which has other properties)

Peony nourishes the blood. It is useful for anemia, night sweats, dizziness, spontaneous sweating, menstrual irregularities, amenorrhea, cramps, leukorrhea and uterine bleeding. As an antispasmodic it relaxes and calms emotional nervous conditions, muscle spasms, epilepsy, depression and PMS difficulties. In formulas it relaxes tension, which enhances the effects of the other herbs and affects the deep blood circulation of the body. Peony also eases liver congestion symptoms of flank, chest or abdominal pain and spasms in the hands and feet.

Indications: anemia, night sweats, dizziness, menstrual irregularities, depression, cramps, spasms, leukorrhea, nervous conditions

Projects: tea, soup, wine, congee

Pueraria

Puerariae lobata; Leguminosae
Chinese: *ge gen; gwat gun*

Part used: root
Energy and taste: cool; sweet, spicy

CHINESE HERBS

Active constituents: a large amount of starch

Actions: spleen, stomach, intestines

Properties: diaphoretic, antispasmodic, digestant, demulcent, tonic

Dose: 3-12 gm in decoction

Other: also known as kuzu or kudzu root

Pueraria, or kuzu root, is useful for colds, flus (stomach and lung types), fever, headache, thirst, sore throat, early stage of measles, colitis and diarrhea. For colds and flu it works well when mixed with a bit of licorice, cinnamon, ginger and tamari-soya sauce. It is particularly effective in relieving stiff necks, muscular tension—especially of the throat, neck and shoulder—and minor aches and pains since it neutralizes acidity in the body. As it is mildly tonic and replenishes body fluids, it is of benefit in diabetes and hypoglycemia.

Kuzu root is sold as a high-quality starch thickener for sauces, particularly used in macrobiotic and Japanese cooking. As a sauce it works well with some flavoring added and also helps introduce starch assimilation in those who cannot digest grains very well. To use as a sauce, first dissolve it in cold water and then add to the simmering dish. If you add it directly to the hot food, it lumps up.

Indications: colds, flus, fever, headache, diarrhea, measles, muscle aches and pains, tight neck and shoulders

Projects: tea, soup, sauces

Rehmannia

Rehmannia glutinosa; Scrophulariaceae
Chinese-raw: *sheng di huang; sang day*
Cooked: *shu di huang; so day huang*

Part used: the root, either raw or prepared

Energy and taste: raw—cold; sweet-bitter; cooked—slightly warm; sweet

Active constituents: cooked—glycosides, saponins, arginine, b-sitosterol, mannitol stigmasterol, campesterol rehmannin, catalpol, glucose, tannin, resins, coloring matter and a substance similar to myrtillin

Actions: liver, kidney, heart

Properties: raw—clears heat, especially from the blood; cooked—blood and nutritive tonic, hemostatic, demulcent, laxative, alterative

Dose: 9-30 gm in decoction; it is highly water-soluble and does not tincture well

Precautions: raw and cooked—poor digestion with watery stools and abdominal bloating; overuse can cause loose stools; raw—also should not be used in pregnancy with anemia

Other: also known as Chinese foxglove; the root is prepared by cooking in wine

Raw rehmannia clears heat from the body and blood. It is used for high fever, thirst, a scarlet-colored tongue, mouth and tongue sores, irritability, insomnia, malar flush, low grade fevers, dry mouth, constipation and chronic throat pain.

Cooked rehmannia strengthens the blood, treating symptoms of a pale face, dizziness, palpitations and insomnia. It also aids gynecological problems including irregular menstruation, infertility, uterine bleeding and postpartum bleeding. It strengthens the substance of the kidneys, alleviating night sweats, nocturnal emissions and thirst. It strengthens the bones and tendons and is a tonic during pregnancy.

Indications: raw—high fever, thirst, mouth and tongue sores, irritability, insomnia, low grade fever, dry mouth, constipation, chronic throat pain; cooked—anemia, dizziness, palpitations, insomnia, gynecological problems, night sweats, nocturnal emissions

Projects: tea, congee, soup

Reishi

Ganoderma spp., especially lucidum; Polyporaceae
Chinese: *ling zhi*

Part used: whole mushroom

Energy and taste: neutral; bitter

CHINESE HERBS

Active constituents: polysaccharides, lanostans, coumarin, ergosterol, triterpenes, adenosine, uridine, uracil, small amounts of germanium, organic acids, resins

Actions: heart, liver, lungs; entire body

Properties: rejuvenative, antibacterial, antiviral, antitumor, immune tonic

Dose: decoct 1 ounce/pint water over low heat down to 1/3 the amount started with; drink 1 cup 3 times/day; 40 drops tincture 3 times/day; 3-6 gm for less serious conditions, 9-15 for more serious diseases

Precaution: mold sensitive individuals may have allergic reaction; in this case lower dose and take with meals

Note: Reishi is the Japanese name; it comes in many colors, but the red is best

Reishi mushroom has been a rare and secret plant revered by the ancient Taoists. It has been thought to potentially be the elixir of life because it vivifies the entire system and is said to restore life. No wonder it has been treasured more than gold! Fortunately, it is now becoming available in Western markets.

Reishi is a supreme immune tonic. Because of its neutral energy, it is fine for anyone to take. It treats immune disorders including AIDS as it raises the T cell levels (an index of AIDS and immune disorders). It is also specific for Chronic Fatigue Syndrome. It inhibits bacteria and viruses, treats cancer and tumors and its adaptogenic quality protects the body against stress. It treats heart disease, reduces cholesterel and lowers high blood pressure.

This incredible mushroom also alleviates allergies, bronchitis, food sensitivities, chronic pneumonia, rheumatism, insomnia, hepatitis and treats other liver diseases as well as regenerates the liver. It is anti-oxidant against free radicals and protects against the effects of radiation. It calms the body down while revitalizing it at the same time, increasing inner stamina and strength.

Indications: chronic fatigue, AIDS, cancer, tumors, heart disease, cholesterol, high blood pressure, allergies, bronchitis, pneumonia, rheumatism, insomnia, hepatitis, stress, liver diseases, weakness

Projects: tea, tincture, tablet

Schisandra

Schisandra sinensis; Schisandraceae
Chinese: *wu wei zi; ng way jee*

Part used: fruit

Energy and taste: warm; sweet, sour; it really contains all five tastes, which is the meaning of its Chinese name

Active constituents: sesquicarene, schisandrin, schisoandrol, citral, stigmasterol, Vitamins C and E

Actions: kidney, lung, heart

Properties: astringent, tonic, sedative

Dose: 3-9 gm in decoction

Precautions: any heat conditions; early stages of cough or rashes

Other: this herb is also spelled schizandra

As a tonic astringent, schisandra strengthens the tissues, eliminates secretions and helps retain the energy. It treats cough, wheezing, lung weakness, asthma, night sweats, prolonged diarrhea, nocturnal emission, leukorrhea and involuntary sweating. It is also calming and aids forgetfulness and insomnia. Schisandra regulates the blood sugar and has been found to aid in hepatitis. It contains mild adaptogens which regulate various body functions and increase the ability to handle stress.

Indications: cough, wheezing, asthma, night sweats, diarrhea, nocturnal emission, leukorrhea, sweating, forgetfulness, insomnia, hepatitis, blood sugar problems, stress

Projects: tea, soup, wine, milk, congee

Tienchi

Panax pseudoginseng; Araliaceae
Chinese: *tien qi or san qi; som chuk*

Part used: root

Energy and taste: slightly warm; sweet, slightly bitter

Active constituents: arasopanin A and B

Actions: liver, stomach, large intestine

CHINESE HERBS

Properties: tonic, hemostatic, emmenagogue
Dose: 3-9 gm in decoction
Precautions: pregnancy; deficient blood

Because of its ginseng-like strengthening qualities for the energy, tienchi is called a pseudo ginseng. Yet it is primarily an herb to stop bleeding and hemorrhage for blood in the vomit, nose, urine or stool. It is useful for traumas, injuries, wounds and cuts as it also reduces swelling, alleviates pain and dissolves blood clots. In fact, any trauma from falls, fractures, contusions or sprains benefits from it since it quickly promotes the circulation of blood and stops bleeding. For these it can be taken internally or put externally on the wound in powder or liniment form. In its packaged form found in Chinese pharmacies, it is known as *"Yunan Bai Yao."*

Indications: hemorrhage; blood in vomit, nose, urine or stool; traumas, injuries, wounds

Projects: tea, soup, liniment

Zizyphus

Zizyphus spinosa; Rhamnaceae
Chinese: *suan zao ren; shune cho yun*

Part used: seeds
Energy and taste: neutral; sweet, sour
Active constituents: betulin, betulic acid, jujoboside, jujobogenin, ebelin lactone, other saponins, Vitamin C
Actions: heart, spleen, liver, gallbladder
Properties: nervine, sedative, tonic, astringent
Dose: 10-20 gm in decoction
Precautions: it loosens the stools, so avoid if there is severe diarrhea; excess heat

Zizyphus seeds help calm the mind and emotions, treating insomnia, irritability, palpitations, anxiety and nervous exhaustion. It also reduces spontaneous sweating or night sweats, amnesia and poor memory. This moistening, nurturing and strengthening herb helps lack of energy and blood and is safe for children and the weak or elderly.

Indications: insomnia, palpitations, anxiety, nervous exhaustion, sweating, night sweats, poor memory

Projects: tea, soup, wine

HERBS AND THEIR ENERGY

Western Herb	Warm	Neutral	Cool	Western Herb	Warm	Neutral	Cool
Aloe			x	Goldenseal			x
American Ginseng			x	Hawthorn	x		
Angelica	x			Lemon Balm			x
Barberry			x	Licorice		x	
Bayberry	x			Lobelia		x	
Blackberry		x		Marshmallow			x
Black Cohosh			x	Milk Thistle			x
Black Haw			x	Motherwort			x
Black Pepper	x			Mugwort	x		
Borage			x	Mullein			x
Burdock			x	Nettle			x
Calendula		x		Oregon Grape			x
Cardamom	x			Parsley	x		
Cascara Sagrada			x	Peppermint			x
Cayenne	x			Plantain			x
Chamomile		x		Prickly Ash	x		
Chaparral			x	Raspberry		x	
Chaste berry		x		Red Clover			x
Chickweed			x	Sarsaparilla		x	
Cinnamon	x			Scullcap			x
Coltsfoot			x	Shepherd's Purse		x	
Comfrey			x	Siberian Ginseng	x		
Dandelion			x	Slippery Elm		x	
Echinacea			x	Squawvine			x
Elecampane	x			St. John's wort			x
Eyebright			x	Turmeric, rhizome	x		
Fennel	x			Turmeric, tuber			x
Fenugreek	x			Uva Ursi			x
Feverfew			x	Valerian	x		
Garlic	x			Wild Cherry Bark	x		
Gentian			x	Yarrow		x	
Ginger	x			Yellow Dock			x
Ginkgo		x					

Chinese Herb	Warm	Neutral	Cool	Chinese Herb	Warm	Neutral	Cool
Aconite	x			Gardenia			x
Astragalus	x			Ginseng	x		
Atractylodes	x			Honeysuckle			x
Bupleurum			x	Ho shou wu	x		
Chrysanthemum			x	Jujube Dates	x		
Citrus	x			Lycii		x	
Codonopsis	x			Peony			x
Cornus	x			Pueraria			x
Cyperus	x			Rehmannia, cooked	x		
Dioscorea		x		Rehmannia, raw			x
Dong Quai	x			Reishi		x	
Ephedra	x			Schizandra	x		
Fu Ling		x		Tienchi	x		
				Zizyphus		x	

II.
How to Regain &
Maintain Health

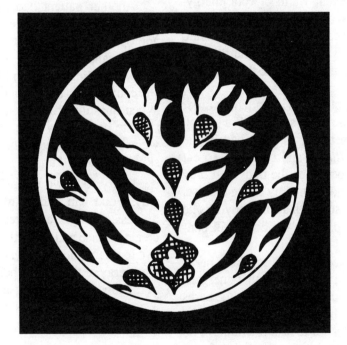

The Energy of Food

In *The Energy of Herbs* we learned that all herbs have a warm, neutral or cool energy. Like herbs, every type of food has an inherent warm or cool energy. The warming or cooling energy of food affects the body by creating more heat or coldness in it. While Western cultures are used to thinking of nutrition as food groups, Eastern cultures recognize the energy of food regardless of the group it is in.

Learning the energy of food is important in order to regain and maintain the body's health. If a person has a lot of heat in the body, as described in the chapter *The Energy of Illness* and continues to eat warming and heating foods, then the body will only become warmer inside and eventually create disease. The same is true for a person with a cold body. If s/he eats a lot of cooling foods, then the body will continue to get colder.

As a result, even when a person is taking herbs for healing, if s/he is eating in a way that energetically opposes what the body needs and what the herbs are intended to do, then the herbal treatment will be less effective, will take longer to heal or will have no effect at all. For this reason, it is extremely important to learn about and understand the energy of food.

As an example, one patient had low energy and frequent colds. He was given warming and building herbs and a balanced diet to eat. Yet, in two weeks time little progress was made. When questioned about the diet, he admitted to consuming fruit and juices, believing they were healthy and important foods to eat. Yet, these same foods were continually causing his poor digestion, mucus, lowered immunity and tiredness. When he eliminated these foods, within a week he felt stronger and had better digestion and more energy.

Another patient had skin problems, frequently breaking out on her face and shoulders. Again an appropriate energetic diet was given along with heat-clearing and detoxifying herbs. Within a few weeks she was feeling better and her face had cleared, but she continued to break out on her back and shoulders. When questioned further it was discovered that she still ate her weekly dose of chocolate chip cookies, white sugar included. When these were stopped, her skin fully cleared up.

Every food we eat affects our bodies in some way. Food can add warmth, coldness, dampness, dryness, strength and weakness, maintain balance, create disease and so forth. Because most people eat two to three times a day, then two to three times a day the energy of the body is being affected by the energy of the food ingested. You are what you eat is not such a strange adage from this perspective.

A Balanced Diet

A balanced diet is one which uses foods energetically. It incorporates more foods with a neutral to warm and neutral to cool energy, a little less food with warm or cool energies and sparing use of foods with hot and cold energies. If these energies are placed on a continuum, it is easier to visualize how they affect us.

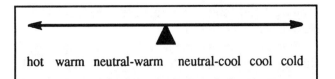

hot   warm   neutral-warm   neutral-cool   cool   cold

Consider this continuum as a child's seesaw and imagine a person sitting at each of the hot and cold ends, one in the air and the other on the ground. Now if the person on the ground suddenly gets off, the one in the air slams to the ground quickly and strongly. Likewise, when eating at the extreme ends of hot and cold foods, the disease "crash" is likely to be sudden, more intense and harder to cure.

Now imagine both people sitting a little distance away from the center point. If one gets off, the other only lightly taps the ground. Eating closer to the balanced energy point creates less disease potential. Any minor ailments which occur can be more easily taken care of.

When eating according to the energy of foods, we want to include more foods close to the balance point and fewer foods away from it. In terms of percentages, an energetically balanced diet includes 50-60% of neutral-warm and neutral-cool foods, 30-40% of somewhat warm and cool foods and 10% warm, cool, hot and cold foods. Translated into specific foods this means that an energetically balanced diet includes 50-60% grains and legumes, 30-40% vegetables, mostly cooked, and 10% meat, dairy, fruit and juices. When viewed from this perspective, we can see how so many of us eat in an energetically imbalanced way, perhaps having the 10% category make up 90% or more of our diets.

We can determine ourselves how food makes us feel by noticing its effects in us after we eat it. These effects can be evident immediately, such as the spiciness of hot peppers, or it may take three days or more, such as the effects of cold-energied ice cream. Most foods affect us within three days to a month. An excess amount of one type of food builds over time until we feel the effects of that food more readily. Ultimately, we become so sensitive to certain foods that we become "allergic" to them.

Another way of looking at the warm-cool energy of food is in terms of acid-alkaline. In general, foods that are cool or cold tend to make the body alkaline.

Foods that are warm or hot tend to make the body acidic. The acid-alkaline determination is not the Ph of the food itself, but the residue ash which forms when that food is oxidized.[1]

The taste of each food also indicates its warming, cooling or neutral energy. Foods which are bitter, like endive or spinach, tend to cool us down and eliminate toxins. Sour foods, like sauerkraut, are refreshing and cool, and small amounts aid digestion. Spicy foods are stimulating and heating. They move blood and energy. Salty foods, like seaweed and miso, are cool and softening because they hold fluids in the body. Full sweet foods, or complex carbohydrates which break down slowly, are warm to neutral in energy. These complex carbohydrates help nourish bones, muscles and blood.

The energy of a food is its natural inherent energy regardless of how it is eaten or prepared. It can be modified somewhat by eating it raw (more cooling) or cooking it (more warming). Overall, adding heat, pressure, cooking time and spices makes a food less cooling and more warming. Adding coldness, water, refrigeration or freezing and eating raw and unspiced makes food less warming and more cooling.

Yet, despite preparations, a cool food can never be warm and vice versa. For example, an apple which has a cool energy can be baked with walnuts and cinnamon to make it less cool in energy instead. Likewise, eating warm shrimp in a raw state gives it a less warm energy since the shrimp isn't cooked.

Empty-Full

Along with warming and cooling energies, foods have a quality of being either empty or full. Empty and full refer to the effects that a food has on the body and not its nutritional contents. Like energy, empty-full is on a continuum so that a food is not absolutely empty or full, but is slightly or strongly empty or full. This is an important concept to grasp in terms of food because it gives us a broader and deeper understanding of how food affects the body.

Relative to each other, fruit and juices are empty, vegetables are neutral to somewhat empty, meat and dairy are full and grains and legumes are neutral to

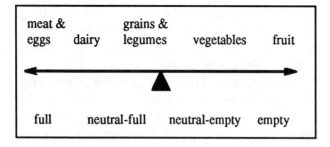

full. From this it appears that protein-rich foods are full and more water-containing foods are empty.

Prolonged eating of mostly empty foods creates elimination in the body. This can affect the energy, blood, strength and working capacity of the organs, and it ultimately results in some sort of deficiency. People who predominantly eat empty foods often feel tired, unfocused and depleted.

For instance, fruit and juices are empty foods, although they range from warm to cold in energy. They generally lower the body temperature and metabolism by creating elimination. A little periodically eliminates toxins and moistens dryness. Yet, if eaten too frequently or predominantly, they can create poor digestion, gas, possible low back pains, dampness, lowered immunity and resistance and feelings of being ungrounded and unfocused.

On the other hand, prolonged eating of mostly full foods creates too much "building" or strengthening of the body. This usually leads to congestion and stagnation of the energy, blood and organ functions. It ultimately results in some type of excess condition, either heat, dampness or both. People who predomi-

nantly eat full foods often feel congested, stuck, explosive and hypertensive.

For example, red meat and dairy are full foods, although they are neutral to warming in energy. Small quantities eaten occasionally strengthen the blood and energy and build strength and endurance. However, red meat or dairy every day or even several times a day ultimately creates too much congestion, resulting in a red neck and face, irritability, a loud voice, aggressive behavior, constipation and toxicity in the blood and organs.

Putting empty-full together with warming and cooling energies helps us look at food in a different way. For instance, some foods may be warm in energy but also empty, such as the spice cayenne. It is hot, but it doesn't build or strengthen. Instead, it is stimulating and dispersing and in excess can cause elimination. On the other hand, some foods may be cool in energy but also full, such as barley. It expands the intestines and so helps stop diarrhea. It also strengthens the digestion and the substance of the body. Likewise, American ginseng is a cool herb, but it strengthens the substance of the body and gives energy.

Overall, it is a question of balance. It is best to eat a diet comprised predominantly of foods with a neutral-warm and neutral-cool energy and neutral-full, and neutral-empty quality. Eating large amounts of the more extreme foods, those that are hot, cold, full and/or empty, creates imbalance and disease. Now let's look at each of these food groups individually to understand their energetic uses better.

GRAINS, LEGUMES, NUTS & SEEDS				
Energy				
Hot	**Warm**	**Neutral**	**Cool**	**Cold**
———	sweet rice black bean pine nuts sesame seeds walnut chestnut	aduki bean peanut kidney bean corn string bean peas rice rye yellow soybean black soybean sunflower seeds almond	barley wheat mung bean tofu buckwheat millet soybean	———

Grains, Legumes, Nuts and Seeds

Grains, legumes, nuts and seeds are predominantly neutral-warm and neutral-cool in energy. They are neutral to full in quality. Grains give complex carbohydrates to the body which break down slowly and provide long-lasting energy and strength. Beans, nuts and seeds provide a protein balance to grains, and should be eaten regularly by those who don't eat meat. For those who do, they can be used as a periodic protein substitute to alleviate the potential of creating too much congestion and toxins from eating meat all the time.

Some people need more protein than others. Protein gives strength, endurance, immunity, resistance and heat to the body. But in excess, it creates toxins, congestion, irritability and too much heat. Each person needs to determine his/her own level and needs. Don't go by an intellectual idea or theory but experiment with how you feel when you don't eat enough or eat too much. Find what amount helps you feel good, strong, energetic and flexible. Bear in mind that your protein needs change from day to day and week to week according to what is going on in your life. In general, physical work requires more carbohydrates to sustain it, while mental work needs more protein.

Grains and beans should comprise about 50-60% of every meal in various forms. Bread is not a substitute for grains. One meal with bread in a sandwich is fine, but beyond that, whole grain cereals, pilafs and pasta should be used.

Vegetables

Vegetables range from slightly neutral-warming to neutral-cooling. They are neutral to empty in quality. In general, compact vegetables which take a long time to grow and mature into the fall and winter are slightly cooling in energy. Vegetables which grow quickly, expand easily, have a high water content and occur mostly in summer are more cooling in energy. Cooking vegetables makes them a little less cool, but their inherent energy is still cooling to the body. Eating them raw partakes of their full cooling energy.

Vegetables are an important addition to any type of diet; in fact, most people don't eat enough of them. They should comprise about 20-40% of each entire meal. Greens and sea vegetables should be included in abundance. They aid in the digestion of grains and give important vitamins and minerals. Raw vegetables are colder in energy and take strong digestive power to break them down, whereas slightly cooked ones are much easier to digest and so more of their nutrients are assimilated.

A large controversy exists around raw versus cooked foods. Raw food proponents believe that cooking vegetables kills their live vital energy and renders them useless to health in the body. Frankly, I have seen just as many sick raw vegetarians as I have meat eaters, and generally it is more difficult to bring them to health.

Raw and cold food in excess does several things: it thins the blood, it cools the body down and it slows the metabolism, almost snuffing out the digestive

VEGETABLES				
Energy				
Hot	Warm	Neutral	Cool	Cold
————	onion garlic winter squash mustard leaf kale	carrot celery beet potato pumpkin sweet potato yam shitaki mushroom cabbage	watercress lettuce cucumber radish eggplant celery spinach asparagus button mushroom alfalfa sprouts summer squash broccoli	tomato bamboo shoots seaweed snow pea

FRUITS & JUICES

		Energy		
Hot	**Warm**	**Neutral**	**Cool**	**Cold**
————	cherry coconut milk guava peach raspberry date kumquat	fig grape olive papaya pineapple plum apricot coconut meat	orange apple mango tangerine mandarin orange pear strawberry loquat lemon	banana grapefruit persimmon watermelon star fruit (carambola) cantaloupe

fires in some cases. Aches and pains, stiffness, anemia, arthritis, gas, bloatedness, lethargy and other problems can result. Raw foods in an already cold diet of fruits, juices, salads and no meat quells the metabolic ability of the body to break the food down and assimilate it. If this break down and assimilation cannot occur, or happens poorly, then the vitality of raw foods is totally lost.

In addition, the body needs little hydrochloric acid to digest vegetables. When only eating vegetables the body tends to produce small amounts of hydrochloric acid. Over time this situation decreases the digestive ability of the body since other foods need more hydrochloric acid to break down. Overall, the body may be able to assimilate and get more out of cooked rather than raw vegetables.

On the other hand, vegetables should never be over-cooked or mushy. Overcooking destroys important nutrients. Cooked and still slightly crunchy, vegetables are less cold and digest and assimilate well. A little bit of raw food is beneficial, and meat eaters can healthily include salads, fruits and juices to help counteract their warmer diet.

Fruit

Fruit and juice have a neutral-warm, neutral-cool or cold energy. Their predominant emptiness (there are a few exceptions) creates elimination and dampness in the body. In excess and over time, however, they cause lowered strength, resistance and immunity, resulting in loose stools, diarrhea, frequent and recurring colds and flus, poor digestion, mucus, chronic asthma and other lung problems, low back pain, sciatica, impotence, infertility, nasal drip or runny noses and other such problems.

Used correctly, meat eaters can benefit from these foods, especially for fasting purposes. In the summer and when fruit is in season, a little is important for all of us, yet even then if eaten to excess, it can cause abnormal dampness in the body, injuring digestion and causing water retention. Vegetarians should eat these foods more sparingly, especially fruit juices, and perhaps bake or stew their fruit, adding cinnamon and walnuts to make it less cool. Vegetable juices are less empty than fruit juices.

DAIRY

		Energy		
Hot	**Warm**	**Neutral**	**Cool**	**Cold**
————	butter	cow's milk cheese yogurt	————	————

Dairy

Dairy products can add valuable protein to the diet, especially for vegetarians. Yet most dairy products are full in quality and therefore can be very congesting to the energy: they create mucus, with stagnation and poor digestion resulting. Therefore, these highly concentrated foods should be eaten in moderation.

For a body that is dry and underweight, a little milk can actually moisten and build. For this, use raw milk, warm it up and add a little cinnamon or ginger. It can then be followed by a half teaspoon of honey to counteract the mucus-producing aspects of milk.

For those who have a lot of mucus in general, are overweight, have dampness, are prone to cysts, have chronic coughs or runny noses or experience such obvious problems as asthma or allergies, dairy will only aggravate these conditions. Often children's asthma, coughs, runny noses, diarrhea or constipation will disappear by simply eliminating dairy and juices from the diet.

Meat

Meat ranges from neutral-warm to neutral-cool and some cold in energy, yet it is full in quality. Meat is a powerful food-medicine and should be treated as such. At the most 2-4 ounces per day, preferably organic, is building, strengthening and warming to the body. More than this creates stagnation over time, resulting in toxins and congestion with their accompanying problems.

For people who have eaten a lot of meat, it may be best to eliminate meat from the diet for awhile until the body becomes balanced. If you are going to eat meat, it should always be cooked and eaten with a little raw ginger root. Ginger aids in the assimilation and detoxification of meat in the body.

The issue of whether to eat meat or not is a personal one. I have seen people who eat it three times a day eliminate it from their diets and become healthier and stronger than ever. I have also seen ten year vegetarians begin to eat a little meat and become healthier and stronger than ever.

In general, vegetarians need to eat a more limited diet since, without meat, most other foods are neutral-cooling. If a balanced diet is followed consisting mainly of grains, beans, cooked vegetables, some dairy items, a little fruit in season and an adequate protein level, then balance can be maintained. This does not allow for many empty foods to be included in the diet such as fruits, salads, juices and other raw uncooked foods. Warming and building herbs can be included to help provide warmth, resistance and immunity.

Likewise, for those who desire to eat meat, some empty foods can be incorporated more abundantly to help balance the fullness of meat and create elimination of possible toxins. However, as meat is a strong food, for the body to stay in balance it should be limited to 2-4 ounces per day. This is a vast reduction from the Western tradition of 4-8 ounces of meat almost three times a day. If eaten this frequently and in this quantity, toxins and congestion result, such as hypertension, heart attacks, cancer, arthritis, strokes, constipation, aggressiveness, irritability, red face and neck, rheumatism, stiff neck and shoulders and gout.

MEAT				
Energy				
Hot	**Warm**	**Neutral**	**Cool**	**Cold**
lamb	chicken fresh ham mussel shrimp anchovy	herring oyster beef goose duck tuna eggs sardine pork whitefish carp	———	clam crab

EXTREME FOODS				
Energy				
Hot	Warm	Neutral	Cool	Cold
————	coffee tobacco vinegar wine brown sugar malt and maltose molasses	honey white sugar	beer	salt tea sugar cane

Extreme Foods

There are several other foods worth discussing here, including sugar, salt, alcohol, caffeine and tobacco. All of these are extreme foods. Eating one usually sets up a craving for the other and creates an endless cycle. For example, after eating sugar for awhile, the body craves salt and vice versa. Yet this type of "balance" is extreme, like the seesaw described earlier.

Refined sugar cane is a cold food that is empty. It leeches important vitamins and minerals from the body, such as calcium. It is also well known as a leading cause for a diseased body. Heavy meat eaters often crave sugar because its emptiness offsets the fullness of meat. Sugar also causes salt cravings, and the heavy eating of salty foods conversely causes sugar cravings. Whole sugars such as maple sugar, honey, barley and rice malts and raw sugar cane are much better for the body, though they should be used sparingly as they are empty.

Alcohol, caffeine and tobacco all cause heat and irritation in the body. In meat eaters this creates excessive amounts of heat. In vegetarians, alcohol, caffeine and tobacco can provide heat which the body craves if provided with a very cooling diet. This quite often makes it much more difficult, if not impossible, for vegetarians to quit smoking cigarettes and drinking coffee without a diet change, even more so than meat eaters. In addition, alcohol, because of its sugar content, creates the problems sugar does in the body. This is why it goes so well with a meat diet: its emptiness helps offset the fullness of meat.

Caffeine taps into the energy stores of the adrenals, the fire aspect of the Kidneys. In time this leads to adrenal exhaustion. Drinking coffee to push through tiredness ultimately leads to an exhaustion which is very difficult to replenish. It may take years for this to show up, suddenly taking you by "surprise."

Tobacco restricts the circulation, promoting excessive coldness in the extremities. It also robs the cells of their much-needed oxygen supply, which causes a weakening of their functions throughout the whole body. It then injures the blood.

Water is worth mentioning here because it, too, can cause disease in the body when taken improperly. Most meat eaters tend to drink lots of iced water to eliminate some of the fullness and acidity they feel inside. Yet iced water is one of the largest contributors to a weakened digestion causing gas, bloatedness and lethargy after eating. Imagine throwing iced water on a fire and the resulting steam and eventual dead fire if enough is used. The same occurs in the stomach where the digestive fires are very much needed. Likewise, excessive drinking of carbonated water causes symptoms of gas, bloatedness, hiccough, poor digestion, dizziness, spaciness and lethargy.

Quantity is another issue. Eight glasses of water a day is fine for meat eaters. This much is needed to flush the heat, toxicity, acids and irritations of the meat from the body. However, for those who eat little or no meat at all, too much water causes dampness in the digestive system, quelling the fire and causing the kidneys to constantly work unnecessarily. If eating little or no meat, 4 glasses a day of room temperature or hot water or herb tea is adequate. Cold water is aggravating to all bodies, and even more so to vegetarians. This goes for cold juices, too!

Food Therapy

Food can be used therapeutically to heal disease by following its inner warming or cooling nature. A body that has too much heat can be balanced by eating more cooling foods and less heating ones. A body that has too much coldness can be balanced by eating more warming foods and less cooling ones. Because all people's bodies are different, everyone requires different types of foods to stay in balance, and even this may vary from season to season and year to year. Therefore, there is no such thing as one type of diet that is healthy for all people. Instead, each person should learn what his/her current body needs are and eat the right foods for those personal conditions.

If dealing with a disease or imbalance in the body, it is important to tailor the diet accordingly along with taking the proper herbs. This is known as food therapy, and will not only enhance the healing process, but usually speeds it up. In contrast, eating improper foods can actually drain the body's healing energies.

To use food therapeutically, first determine if your condition is one of coldness, heat, dampness, dryness, excess or deficiency as outlined in the chapter *The Energy of Illness*. Then create your food plan accordingly. For instance, if experiencing constipation, irritability, frequent sweating and always feeling warm, then eliminate those foods with a hot energy, eat a few with a warm energy and focus more on neutral, cool and a small amount of cold-energy foods.

Likewise, for someone experiencing frequent cold and flus, lowered immunity, runny nose, tiredness, weakness and feelings of chill and cold, eliminate all cold foods, eat some cool foods, but only in cooked form, and focus more on neutral, warm and some hot-energy foods. If the plan is to maintain existing good health or if one is recovering from an illness, then follow the balanced diet outlined under the section, *A Balanced Diet*.

Here are a few basic guidelines. If there is too much coldness in the body, only cooked food and warming foods should be eaten. If there is too much heat, more fruits and juices should be ingested and little or no meat eaten. If there's dampness, use more drying foods such as grains. If there's too much dryness, add moistening foods like milk, coconut and some unsaturated fats and oils.

Whole Foods

It is important here to distinguish between whole healthy foods and disease-causing foods. Whole foods are those which come to us in their purest form from nature with the least possible interference. This means they are preferably organic and without chemicals, additives or preservatives. They are also unrefined and in their whole natural state. Brown rice, maple syrup and earth salt are examples of whole foods. Refined white rice, white sugar and table salt are examples of processed, disease-causing foods. The following chart suggests many healthy foods to eat and unhealthy foods to avoid.

WHOLE FOODS	
Healthy	**Unhealthy**
whole grains	white sugar
beans	white flour
vegetables, especially organic	white bread
sea vegetables	"junk foods"
seeds, nuts	additives
greens	preservatives
a little sea salt as needed	refined salt
a little honey, maple syrup or grain syrup as needed	artificial colorings
fruit in season, baked, if needed	chemicals in foods
salads in season	soda pop
a little bit of meat as needed (optional)	any sweets with white sugar in them
small amounts of dairy	tobacco, caffeine

Food should never be cooked in aluminum pots and pans. Aluminum is toxic and contaminates the food. Gas or wood heat is best for cooking. Electric heat is fine for strong bodies, but I have seen it interfere with the healing process in those with weakness and deficiency. Thus, for those with lowered immunity and severe or degenerative diseases, gas or wood is better.

A microwave should preferably not be used. It heats food differently by creating friction between the food molecules. Food heats from the inside out rather than from the outside in as with other heating methods. Because of this, food can cook unevenly and often tastes strange. In my opinion, a microwave alters foods enough so they are different than nature created them. Therefore, it is best to avoid microwaves.

Get in the habit of reading labels and shopping selectively. There are plenty of healthy alternatives available. Eating whole foods according to a balanced energetic diet is eating to maintain strength and health and prevent disease.

Food Energetics

The following chart lists a number of commonly used foods, their energies, flavors, organs and therapeutic applications according to the Traditional Chinese concept of food and nutrition. For specific applications and recipes, refer to the Natural Healing and Food Therapy section of the *Bibliography*.

---

[1] The macrobiotic delineation of foods according to a Yang-Yin continuum fairly well matches the acid-alkaline differentiation. Foods categorized as Yang tend to be acid-forming and those classified as Yin tend to be alkaline-forming.

FOOD ENERGETICS

Name	Energy/Taste	Elements	Therapeutic Conditions
Aduki bean	neutral; sweet, sour	heart, small intestines	edema, beriberi, mumps, jaundice, diarrhea, discharge of blood from anus, reduces weight Avoid: dryness or emaciation
Almond	neutral; sweet	lungs, spleen-pancreas	relieves cough, resolves phlegm, lubricates lungs
Apple	cool; sweet, sour	spleen-pancreas	lubricates, clears heat counteracts depression, moistens; low blood sugar, indigestion, morning sickness, chronic enteritis
Asparagus	cool; sweet, bitter	lungs, kidneys	clears heat, dries dampness, lubricates dryness; cough, mucus discharge, swelling, various kinds of skin eruptions, shortage of mother's milk, diabetes, TB, wasting heat diseases
Banana	cold; sweet	spleen, stomach	lubricates, clears heat, counteracts toxins; constipation, bleeding piles, hemorrhoids, alcoholism
Barley	cool; sweet, salty	spleen, stomach	regulates stomach, promotes urination, clears heat, lubricates dryness, expands intestines; edema, dysuria, indigestion, burns
Beef	neutral; sweet	spleen, stomach, colon	tonifies energy and blood, strengthens tendons and bones, tonifies stomach and spleen; emaciation, edema, diabetes, weak knees and low back pain with emaciation; various parts are good for responding organs

FOOD ENERGETICS

Name	Energy/Taste	Elements	Therapeutic Conditions
Beet	neutral; sweet	spleen	nourishes fluids; rheumatic pains, congested chest, poor energy circulation
Black Pepper	hot; pungent	lungs, spleen, stomach, large intestines	warms the body, carminative, removes stagnation and coldness, dries mucus; vomiting of clear liquid, diarrhea from coldness, food poisoning, locally on toothache, weak nerves; not good for false heat signs or wasting heat
Black Sesame Seeds	neutral; sweet	kidneys, liver	liver and kidney tonic, lubricates; treats vertigo, constipation, grey hair, weak knees, rheumatism, dry skin, shortage of mother's milk; black sesame seeds are better for the kidney-adrenal, and the yellow for the spleen-pancreas
Black Soya Bean	neutral; sweet	spleen, kidneys	promotes blood circulation and urination, detoxifies, nourishes kidney and liver blood; lower back pain and knee pains, infertility, seminal emission, blurred vision, difficult urine, edema, jaundice, rheumatism, muscular cramps, lockjaw, drug poisoning
Buckwheat	cool[2]; sweet	colon, stomach, spleen	clears heat; eliminates swelling, boils, chronic diarrhea, dysentery, skin lesions and eruptions Avoid: vertigo, indigestion
Butter	warm; sweet	spleen, stomach	promotes blood circulation, expels coldness; scabies, skin eruptions, body odor
Cabbage	neutral; sweet	spleen, stomach	promotes urination, beneficial to kidneys and brain after long consumption; constipation, thirst due to intoxication, ulcers, depression, coughs and colds, hot flashes Avoid: lack of energy, poor digestion, nausea
Carrot	neutral; sweet	lung, spleen	diuretic and digestive; improves eyes, removes swellings and tumors, indigestion, cough, dysentery, difficult urination, skin eruptions, chronic diarrhea and dysentery
Cayenne	hot; pungent	spleen, heart	warms, moves blood, disperses congestion, expels cold; poor appetite, cold abdominal pains, diarrhea, vomiting Avoid: false heat signs, wasting diseases, excess heat or cough

[2] The buckwheat found in China is cool in energy, but the variety in the United States seems to be warming.

FOOD ENERGETICS

Name	Energy/Taste	Elements	Therapeutic Conditions
Celery	cool; bitter, sweet	stomach, liver, kidney	clears heat, promotes urine; hypertension, headache, dizziness, discharge of blood in urine, conjunctivitis
Cheese	neutral; sour, sweet	liver, lungs, spleen	tonifies energy, moistens, quenches thirst; fever, dryness, constipation, skin eruptions, itchy skin Avoid: weak digestion or mucus conditions
Cherry	warm; sweet	heart, spleen	moves blood circulation, expels cold and damp; rheumatism, arthritis, lumbago, paralysis, numbness, frostbite
Chicken	warm; sweet	spleen, stomach	tonifies energy, warms; underweight, diarrhea, edema, poor appetite, vaginal bleeding and discharge, lack of mother's milk, general weakness, frequent urination, weakness after childbirth, diarrhea, dysentery, diabetes, edema. Avoid: excess conditions, external diseases
Corn	neutral; sweet	stomach, colon	regulates digestive organs; weak heart, difficult urination, sexual weakness.
Cucumber	cool; sweet	stomach, spleen, colon	detoxifies, clears heat, promotes urination, quenches thirst; sore throat, pink eyes, inflammation, burns
Date (red)	warm; sweet	spleen, stomach	tonifies energy and blood; weak stomach, palpitations, nervousness, hysteria from weakness.
Duck	neutral; sweet, salty	lungs, kidneys	tonifies energy and blood, lubricates dryness, treats swelling and edema, hot sensations, cough Avoid: weak spleen, stagnant energy, symptoms of hemorrhage
Eggplant	cool; sweet	colon, spleen, stomach	clears heat, removes stagnant blood, relieves pain, swelling; dysentery, bleeding discharges from anus, urine and dysentery, boils, skin ulcers and mastitis, prevents strokes
Fig	neutral; sweet	colon, stomach, spleen	detoxifies, stomach tonic; heals swelling, constipation, hemorrhoids, sore throat, diarrhea, dysentery

FOOD ENERGETICS			
Name	**Energy/Taste**	**Elements**	**Therapeutic Conditions**
Garlic	warm; pungent	lungs, stomach, spleen	warms, expels cold, promotes energy circulation, destroys worms and kills parasites, antiviral, anti-bacterial; arthritis, cold abdominal pain, edema, diarrhea, dysentery, whooping cough
Ginger (dried)	hot; pungent	lungs, stomach	warms, carminative, expels cold, benefits digestion, relieves cramps; colds, coughs, cold limbs, diarrhea, vomiting, nausea, mucus, rheumatism, cold abdominal pain
Gluten, wheat (seitan)	cool; sweet	stomach, spleen, liver	tonifies energy, clears heat, reduces fever, sedates hypertension, quenches thirst
Grapes	neutral; sweet, sour	lungs, spleen, kidneys	red variety is very tonifying to energy and blood, strengthens bones and tendons, promotes urine, harmonizes stomach, relieves anger and irritability; blood and energy deficiency, cough, palpitations, night sweat, rheumatism, difficult urination, edema Avoid: excessive consumption can decrease appetite, cause blurred vision
Honey	neutral; sweet	lungs, spleen, colon	tonifies energy and blood, lubricates dryness, relieves pain; dry cough, constipation, stomachache, sinusitis, mouth cankers, burns, neurasthenia, hypertension, TB, heart disease, liver disease Avoid: phlegm and dampness, diarrhea, stomach congestion
Kidney Bean	neutral; sweet	spleen, kidney	promotes urination, clears heat, diuretic, reduces swelling; edema
Lamb	hot; sweet	spleen, kidneys	tonifies energy, warms and expels coldness, removes blood stagnation; indigestion, fatigue, emaciation, coldness, lumbago, general weakness, underweight, abdominal pain, cold sensations post partum, sore loins; strengthens sexual power and penis erection Avoid: cold external diseases
Lemon	cool; sour	liver	produces fluid, considered good for pregnancy; cough with mucus discharge, diabetes, indigestion, laryngitis, reduces fat

FOOD ENERGETICS

Name	Energy/Taste	Elements	Therapeutic Conditions
Lettuce	cool; sweet	colon, stomach	clears heat, drys damp, promotes urination and milk secretion, calming, inhibits bleeding Avoid: eye disease; overconsumption can cause dizziness and blurred vision
Lotus Root	cool; sweet	stomach, spleen, heart	cools blood, strengthens appetite, tones spleen, produces muscles; thirst, dryness, weakness, bleeding, anorexia and diarrhea
Lotus Seed	neutral; sweet	spleen, heart, kidneys	nourishes heart, tonifies heart and kidney-adrenals; premature ejaculation, frequent urination, dream-disturbed sleep
Loquat	neutral; sour, sweet	spleen, liver, lungs	lubricates dryness and lungs, quenches thirst; cough, constipation, laryngitis
Mango	cold; sweet, sour	stomach	quenches thirst, strengthens stomach, relieves vomiting, promotes urination; cough, indigestion, bleeding from gums Avoid: common cold, indigestion, during convalescence; overconsumption can cause itching or skin eruptions
Milk	neutral; sweet	lungs, stomach, heart	tonifies blood, produces fluids, lubricates dryness and intestines, tonifies deficiencies; indigestion (take scalded and warm), upset stomach, difficulty swallowing, diabetes, constipation Avoid: for weak spleen-stomach with mucus tendencies
Millet[3]	cool; sweet, salty	stomach, spleen, kidneys	tonifies energy, clears heat, benefits kidneys, lubricates; indigestion, counteracts toxins, diabetes, vomiting and diarrhea; Avoid: undigested food in stools, poor digestion
Mung Bean	cool; sweet	stomach, heart	promotes urination, clears heat, detoxifies, relieves hypertension, summer heat; diarrhea, dysentery, diabetes, boils, edema, burns, lead and drug poisoning; sprouts are good for alcoholism
Mushroom (common button)	cool; sweet	lungs, colon, stomach, spleen	clears heat, calms spirit, reduces tumors; edema, mucus discharge, vomiting, diarrhea Avoid: cold stomach, skin problems or allergies

[3] Millet found in China is cool in energy. The variety found in the United States seems warming.

FOOD ENERGETICS			
Name	**Energy/Taste**	**Elements**	**Therapeutic Conditions**
Mustard Greens	warm; pungent	lungs	carminative, regulates energy, removes stagnation, expels cold, dries mucus; cough, mucous discharge, chest congestion Avoid: skin eruptions, eye disease, hemorrhoids, anal hemorrhage, heat conditions, bleeding, pink eye
Olive	neutral; sweet, sour	lungs, stomach	clears lungs; sore throat, coughing blood, alcoholism, diarrhea
Onion	warm; pungent	lungs, stomach	diuretic, expectorant; external applications for trichomonas vaginitis and ulcers; common cold, headache, constipation, cold abdominal pain, dysuria, dysentery, mastitis, nasal congestion, facial edema
Oyster	neutral; sweet, salty	kidney, liver	tonifies blood, hormone tonic; stress, insomnia, nervousness
Papaya	neutral; sweet	spleen, heart	promotes digestion, destroys intestinal worms; stomachache, dysentery, difficult bowel movements, rheumatism
Peach	warm; sour, sweet	spleen	promotes blood circulation, removes energy stagnation, expels cold, lubricates; dry cough, hernial pain, excessive perspiration, indigestion; excess can produce internal heat
Peanut	neutral; sweet	lung, spleen	lubricates lungs, good for stomachache; dry cough, upset stomach, promotes mother's milk
Peas	neutral; sweet	stomach, spleen	diuretic, induces bowel movements; spasms, counteracts skin eruptions
Pear	cool; sweet, sour	lungs, stomach	produces fluids, lubricates dryness, eliminates mucus; cough with mucus, constipation, alcoholism, indigestion, difficulty when swallowing, difficult urination
Plum	neutral; sweet, sour	kidneys, liver	promotes urination and digestion, promotes fluids; liver disease, diabetes, fatigue; excess can cause bloating and gas
Pork	neutral; salty, sweet	kidney, liver	lubricates dryness; diabetes, weakness, emaciation, dry cough, constipation Avoid: mucus with heat (yellowish discharges), or congestion

FOOD ENERGETICS

Name	Energy/Taste	Elements	Therapeutic Conditions
Potato	neutral; sweet	spleen, stomach	heals inflammation, tonifies energy and the spleen; lack of energy, mumps, burns
Radish (seed)	cool; sweet, pungent	lungs, stomach	detoxifies, promotes digestion, eliminates hot mucus discharge, expels cold; abdominal swelling due to indigestion, laryngitis due to continual cough with mucus discharge, vomiting of blood, nosebleed, dysentery, headache, bloating, hoarseness, diabetes, occipital headache, epistaxis, dysentery, trichomonas vaginitis Avoid: when there's a lack of coldness
Raspberry	neutral; sweet, sour	liver, kidneys	checks frequent urination, sharpens vision; impotence, dizziness, spermatorrhea, polyuria, enuresis, deficiency fatigue, blurred vision Avoid: painful or difficult urine
Rice	neutral; sweet	stomach, spleen	tonifies energy and spleen, harmonizes stomach, relieves depression, quenches thirst; diarrhea, morning sickness, thirst
Rye	neutral; bitter	heart	dries dampness, diuretic; post partum hemorrhage, migraine; can be toxic
Salt	cold; salty	colon, small intestine, stomach, kidneys	detoxifies, lubricates dryness, causes vomiting, cools blood; abdominal swelling and pain, difficult bowel movement, dysuria, pyorrhea, sore throat, toothache, corneal opacity, skin eruptions, constipation, bleeding from the gums, cataract Avoid: edema
Seaweed	cold; salty	kidneys, stomach	lubricates dryness, softens hardness (lumps and tumors), eliminates mucus, promotes water passage; goiter, abdominal swelling and obstruction, edema and beriberi
Sesame Oil	cool; sweet	stomach	detoxifies, lubricates dryness, promotes bowel movements, produces muscles; dry constipation, abdominal pain caused by indigestion, roundworms, skin eruptions, ulcers, tinea, scabies, dry and cracked skin Avoid: diarrhea with lack of energy

FOOD ENERGETICS

Name	Energy/Taste	Elements	Therapeutic Conditions
Shitake Mushroom	neutral; sweet	stomach	tonifies blood, benefits the stomach, anti-inflammatory; cholesterol, hypertension, common cold, chickenpox, cancer, kidney problems, gallstones, hemorrhoids, lack of vitamin D, softening of the bones, cataract, oxena, pyorrhea, ulcers, neuralgia, anemia, measles Avoid: during convalescence of chickenpox, childbirth or general illness
Spinach	cool; sweet	colon, small intestine	lubricates dryness, arrests bleeding, clears heat, tonifies the blood; nosebleed, discharge of blood from anus, thirst in diabetes, constipation, alcoholism, scurvy, hemorrhoids Avoid: spermatorrhea
Squash (winter)	warm; sweet	stomach, spleen	heals inflammation, relieves pain, expels cold; pulmonary abscess, roundworms Avoid: dampness or energy congestion
Strawberry	warm; sweet, sour	liver, kidneys	removes blood stagnation, expels cold; polyuria, vertigo and motion sickness
Sweet Potato	neutral; sweet	spleen, kidneys	tonifies energy and spleen, removes blood stagnation, expels coldness, produces fluid, induces bowel movements, jaundice, emaciation, skin eruptions, stomach and kidney weakness, premature ejaculation Avoid: energy and food congestion
Swiss Chard	cool; sweet	colon, lungs, stomach	clears heat, detoxifies, hemostatic; delayed eruptions of measles, dysentery, amenorrhea and carbuncle
Tangerine	cool; spicy, sweet	lungs, kidneys, stomach	promotes energy circulation, strengthens spleen, relieves coughing; chest congestion, vomiting, hiccupping, stimulates appetite, quenches thirst, diabetes Avoid: cough and sputum from external coldness
Tofu	cool; sweet	lungs, colon, stomach	detoxifies, clears heat, sedates Yang, produces fluid, lubricates dryness; conjunctivitis, chronic amoebic dysentery, diabetes, sulphur poisoning, alcoholism Avoid: spermatorrhea

FOOD ENERGETICS

Name	Energy/Taste	Elements	Therapeutic Conditions
Tomato	cold; sweet, sour	stomach, liver	clears heat, produces fluid, quenches thirst, strengthens stomach, promotes digestion; thirst and anorexia
Vinegar	warm; sour, bitter	stomach, liver	disperses coagulations, detoxifies, arrests bleeding, dries dampness, induces perspiration, expels cold, hemostatic, vermifuge; post partum syncope, genital itching, abdominal swelling and obstruction, jaundice, food poisoning Avoid: poor digestion with undigested food in the stools and lack of energy, muscular atrophy, rheumatism, tendon trauma, and beginning of a common cold
Walnut	warm; sweet	lungs, kidneys	tonifies kidney, lubricates intestines, checks seminal emission, expels colds, solidifies sperm, warms lungs, calms; asthma, cough, lumbago, impotence, spermatorrhea, frequent urination, dry stools, kidney and bladder stones, constipation Avoid: false heat signs or mucus with heat
Water Chestnut	cold; sweet	lungs, stomach	clears heat, relieves fever and indigestion, promotes urination, disperses accumulations; hypertension, diabetes, jaundice, conjunctivitis, measles, dysentery with bloody stools, smoker's sore throat Avoid: anemia, coldness or weakness
Watercress	cool; pungent	lungs, stomach	removes blood stagnation, clears heat, benefits water; jaundice, edema, urinary strain, leukorrhea, mumps, oliguria Avoid: poor digestion with low energy or frequent urination
Watermelon	cold; sweet	stomach, heart, bladder	promotes urination, lubricates intestines, clears heat stroke, relieves mental depression, quenches thirst, diuretic; oliguria, sore throat, canker sores, diminished urination Avoid: excess dampness, anemia, frequent urination or coldness
Wheat	cool; sweet	spleen, heart, kidney	heart and kidney tonic, clears heat, calms, quenches thirst

SHOPPING LIST FOR HEALTHY FOODS

Grains

Brown rice—long grain for the summer and short grain for the winter season (about 3 or 4 pounds)

Basmati rice—a good flavor and offers tasty variety (about 2 or 3 pounds)

Whole rolled oats—oatmeal for breakfasts (1 or 2 pounds)

Nine-grain cereal or something similar for breakfasts

Barley (1 pound)

Millet (1 pound)

Mochi—mugwort variety is best to start with

Beans

Japanese aduki or azuki beans—the darker red the better (2 or 3 pounds)

Black beans (2 or 3 pounds)

Green mung beans (2 or 3 pounds)

Lentils (1 or 2 pounds)

Split peas (1 or 2 pounds)

High-Protein Bean Substitutes

Tofu (1 or 2 pounds)

Tempeh (1 or 2 pounds)

Seitan—wheat gluten (1 or 2 pounds)

Miso paste—one dark variety for soups and a light variety for sauces

High-Protein Nut and Seed Butters

Tahini or sesame butter

Sunflower seeds, walnuts, almonds, pecans, etc., to be used as a garnish and protein supplement

Vegetables

More frequently used:

broccoli, cabbage, brussel sprouts, Chinese cabbage, bok choy, carrots, turnips, onions, garlic, mushrooms (especially shitake mushrooms), beets, kholrabi, winter squash, yams or sweet potatoes, plantains, collards, kale, dark leafy greens

Less frequently used or used in warm climates:

leaf lettuce (not iceberg), cucumbers, tomatoes, potatoes, peppers, green peppers

Sea Vegetables

Kombu seaweed, wakame—used in soups with beans

Dulse—high in iodine and used for seasoning and garnish

Nori—used for sushi rolls

Arame, Hiziki—good with vegetables or grains

Kelp powder or tablets—similar to kombu but can be taken in tablet form until one gets used to cooking with it or it can be sprinkled on as a seasoning

Fruits

Year-round use dried raisins, apricots and figs as a sweetening with cereal grains if desired. When well, eat small amounts of seasonal fruits. Baked apples, pears and prunes can be eaten year-round. Remember, fruit serves the important function of adjusting our blood to the season in which we are living (usually thinning it in warm weather). Thus, overeating raw fruits and juices can severely imbalance the immune system.

Juices

Juices are even more extreme than fruit. They should be taken only in small amounts during the warm season or periodically in warmer climates. Meat eaters can fast on a single fruit juice for 1 to 3 days maximum to effect a cleansing. Generally, for vegetarians, it is better to do a short fast with vegetable broth.

Dairy

Yogurt during warm weather (not more than one or two tablespoons a day)

A little goat's milk if tolerated

A little raw, unpasteurized cow's milk

Raw, unsalted butter to make ghee

Use cheese sparingly

Flesh Foods

Specify organically raised if at all possible

Fish and fowl can be eaten once or twice weekly, especially in cooler weather

Cooking Oils

Sesame or olive oils

Ghee (clarified butter)—Make it yourself by heating a pound of raw unsalted butter in a skillet over a medium flame. When it melts, allow the white milk solids to separate out and keep the pure golden oil which is the unsaturated fats. This is the best cooking oil and will keep a long time, even unrefrigerated, without going rancid. It imparts great health benefits as well as flavor to simple foods.

Condiments

Soy sauce (aged)

Umeboshi plums

Seaweed sprinkles,

Healthy sauces and similar alternatives

Gomashio (sesame salt)

Nuts and seeds

FOOD THERAPY

IMBALANCE[1]	ENERGETIC DIET TO FOLLOW[2]				
	warm	neutral			cool
Coldness cold hands and feet, clear urine, loose stools or diarrhea, gas, bloatedness and/or lethargy after eating, lack of appetite, pale, soft voice and manner, clear runny discharges	10% Eat red and white meat more frequently, 3-7 days/week, 2-4 oz./time	3%-5% Some dairy items	50%-60% grains & legumes	30% cooked vegetables	Eat all cooked food Avoid: fruit, juices, sweets, salads, raw food
Heat frequent sweating, feelings of heat, loud voice, heavy breathing, constipation, burning feelings, skin eruptions, boils, red face, scanty and/or yellow urine, yellow or red discharges, thirst	2%-4% Eat no red meat Eat white meat infrequently, 1-2 times/week, 2-4 oz./time	No dairy items	40%-50% grains & legumes	30% raw & cooked vegetables	20% salads, fruits, juices
Dampness *with cold*: clear frequent urine, swollen, puffy, edemic, watery diarrhea or stools, mucusy, labored breathing, thick white mucus and discharges	10% Eat some red and white meat, 3-7 days/week, 2-4 oz./time	No dairy items	60%-70% grains & legumes	20% all cooked vegetables	Eat all cooked food Avoid: raw foods, salads, juices, fruit, sweets
with heat: thirst but no desire to drink, yellow hot stools and diarrhea, copious thick yellow pussy discharges, mucusy, labored and painful breathing	2%-4% Eat no red meat, some white meat, 2-3 times/week, 2-4 oz./time	No dairy items	60%-70% grains & legumes	30% all cooked vegetables	5% Some salads okay Avoid: juice, fruit, sweets
Dryness dry stools, cough, tongue, mouth, skin and lips, unusually thirsty, cracked or chapped lips, skin, some heat signs	2%-4% Eat no red meat, some white meat infrequently, 1-3 times/week, 2-4 oz./time	2% Some dairy items	40%-50% grains & legumes	30% cooked vegetables, soups	20% Some salads, fruit, juices okay
Deficiency signs include lowered immunity, chronic recurring ailments, weakness, no odors, tiredness	10% Eat red and white meat more frequently, 3-7 times/week, 2-4 oz./time	3%-5% Some dairy items	50%-60% grains & legumes	30% cooked vegetables	Eat all cooked food Avoid: fruit, juices, sweets, salads, raw food
Excess signs include acute severe conditions, buoyant spirits, aggressive, loud, strong	*With cold*: 10% Eat red and white meat more frequently, 3-7 days/week, 2-4 oz./time *With heat*: 2%-4% Eat white meat 1-2 times/week, 2-4 oz./time	No dairy items	40%-60% grains & legumes	20%-30% cooked vegetables	*With cold*: avoid raw foods, salads, fruits, juices, sweets *With heat*: some salads, fruits, juices okay

[1] There need to be 3 or more signs in the category for it to apply

[2] The percentages indicate the amount of food in that category to be eaten in proportion to that entire meal. Note: This is a general outline and is not intended to be all-inclusive.

The Process of Health and Healing

We all define health differently. Some feel a little stomach pain and think they are terribly ill. Others have diagnosed ulcers and yet live cheerfully, as if nothing is wrong. Thus, it is difficult to define health other than saying it is feeling good physically, mentally and emotionally. Health is a dynamic process, not a static state. Our bodies, minds and emotions constantly process our changing experiences. How we handle these changes on all levels determines how healthy we really are.

Some of these changes come in the form of external influences, such as cold, heat, wind and dampness. Others occur internally from harmful food, drinks and emotions. Our bodies constantly need to adjust to climatic conditions, some extreme—like sweltering heat or a blustery snowstorm—as well as extreme internal environments caused by excessive meat eating (heat) or prolonged intake of fruits, juices and raw foods (coldness). When our bodies can't cope with these conditions, illness develops.

The Causes of Disease

Ideally, we maintain balance with our diet, habits, emotions and environment. This keeps us well and prevents disease from setting in. You can do this by being aware of the various factors which cause illness and then taking the appropriate measures to balance them as they occur. Factors which cause illness include:

- inappropriate foods or drinks for your personal condition
- climatic conditions
- poor lifestyle habits
- emotional extremes and negative mental patterns

These can be corrected by determining the appropriate diet for your needs, living according to climatic influences, regulating lifestyle habits and moderating emotions. Many of these issues are addressed in other chapters.

Living our lives in balance to prevent sickness does not mean it needs to be bland, boring and without risks. Maintaining balance through simplicity in diet and lifestyle exercises our essential creativity as human beings. We need to recognize and honor our personal limits as extensions of our uniqueness. If we are tempted to explore and venture beyond our boundaries, we must recognize the early signs of trouble and take appropriate compensatory measures.

For instance, if we stay up late at a party and enjoy food indiscretions, then the next several days may require more rest and a stricter diet than normal to counterbalance this. Or if we are feeling on the verge of a cold, then we narrow our diets for awhile to only balancing foods, get more rest and curtail extracurricular activities which require a strong immune system. When the threat of the cold is gone, we can then broaden our dietary and lifestyle choices. In this way we can enjoy the things we desire and still maintain balance.

The Search for Health

In the West most of us have been raised to believe that what we eat, drink, feel, express and do has little effect on our health. We pay them little attention and then wonder why we get frequent colds or flus, have a chronic cough, feel low energy, have high blood pressure or experience recurring bladder infections. Then we get diagnostic tests, take whatever medicines are prescribed and hope for the best. This approach is one of treating the body mechanistically, like a machine which has broken down and needs to be repaired. As a dynamic, complex inter-related whole, the body is quite unlike a machine. Treating it that way is like mistaking the carburetor for the car or a single plant for the garden.

For those of us who are frequently sick, the search for balance needs to take a different approach. The first step is to choose to get better and make the necessary changes in our situation. This is two-way: 1) recognizing that something we are doing and/or ingesting has caused our illness, and 2) actively and personally undertaking appropriate measures in order to get well.

This goes beyond taking medications to patch up symptoms. Often, taking medications can treat the symptoms, but does not eliminate the original, or root, cause of the condition. Instead, many medications disturb the fragile chemistry of the body. Antibiotics, for instance, are now known to destroy and imbalance important beneficial bacteria. This can lead to weakened assimilation, elimination, a lowered immune system and consequently, a variety of disease complexes ranging from chronic fatigue, allergies and multiple food sensitivities to premenstrual syndrome in women and candida yeast overgrowth.

For true healing to occur then, it means treating the root causes of the illness and eliminating or limiting the many ways we make ourselves sick. We can see that disease symptoms are simply the result of not living in harmony with the natural flow—inadequate sleep, poor dietary habits and overuse of harmful substances such as sugar, alcohol, drugs and tobacco. We often look for an external cause on which to blame our discomforts and disease rather than changing our lifestyle and dietary habits. It may be necessary to go to bed earlier each evening, eat better meals or cut back on sugar, alcohol or tobacco to get well. I have seen many people "miraculously" heal an annoying condition by doing these things.

Since so many other factors can play a telling role in our wellness, we may also have to look at some more difficult and complex issues and how they affect our well being. These can include the deadening effects of radiation exposure from sitting too close to a colored t.v. monitor or a microwave, the weakening carcinogenic pollutants that are not only present in our outdoor environment but now identified as being literally built into our homes, the profound effects of our job and our personal relationships. If we see acid rain killing the forests, how can we believe it is not having an effect on us?

However, we often ignore the need to change what we know is making us sick. The threat of death is, in many cases, an insufficient motivator. For instance, despite having chronic fatigue or skin blemishes, we continue to abuse sweets or eat chocolate. For some, even the threat of lung cancer may not be enough reason to quit smoking. This reveals that spiritual and emotional issues are generally the root of most diseases. True change must ultimately be created from the inside of our spiritual and emotional self out to our diet, activities, friends and environment.

Admittedly, such addictions as tobacco, sugar, caffeine, chocolate and alcohol can be very difficult to overcome. Help in some form or other is often necessary to make the transition to a healthy way of life. Many people have found acupuncture, herbs, massage therapy, macrobiotics, hypnotism and counseling to be invaluable tools for eliminating tobacco, alcohol, sugar, chocolate and coffee from their lives.

Whatever illness-causing habits you have may not be easy to change. It is often a choice, however, between changing those habits or experiencing recurring or sustained bouts of sickness. A further threat is that by not correcting such habits, minor complaints will continue to occur and possibly result in a chronic degenerative condition. What seems expedient to ignore in the present may cause more grief, pain and expense in the long run.

Some Factors That Weaken the Body and Predispose it to Illness

- refined foods, such as white flour, white sugar, white rice, white pasta, refined salt
- chemicals and preservatives in food
- extensive use of canned foods
- frequent indulgence in "junk foods"
- polluted air and water
- proximity to major electrical wiring anywhere in the home, or living close to power plants
- excessive noise
- stress-causing situations or conditions
- job stress or incompatibility
- relationship problems
- proximity to color t.v. monitors
- extensive computer use without proper screening of the monitor
- living near toxic waste dumps
- frequent use of antibiotics
- synthetic fibers in clothing and home and office furnishings
- fast-paced life
- carcinogenic pollutants from materials built in the home or office
- side effects of drugs
- mercury amalgam fillings in teeth

Inherited Constitution

People frequently ask me: Why do I get sick after eating just a few cookies when my friend and even my Uncle George seem to be able to freely consume anything they want ranging from frequent indulgence in candy, sodas and alcohol to several cups of coffee every day? This is a complex question which requires much thought.

First, are these people really well? We may have to refer to our definition of health and wellness. Do we agree that having to rely on medication to feel well constitutes health and wellness? Do we consider those all-too-frequent outbursts of anger, depression or compulsive and addictive patterns of behavior to be something apart from our health or the way we feel?

Perhaps for us, the way we feel physically and emotionally after eating even a single fruit-juice-sweetened cookie is unacceptable while Uncle George, after two hamburgers, four beers, two cups of coffee and several pieces of cake, does not consider his acid indigestion, recurring headaches, chronic tiredness or disturbing outbursts of impatience and anger as signs of sickness or even ill health!

The body is being affected, however, and will ultimately manifest illness. Seemingly "healthy" people who suddenly have cancer are examples. Because cancer and other degenerative diseases take quite a while to develop, it is hard for us to connect the disease with the poor habits or life style factors that created it.

Another reason it appears Uncle George can indulge without problems is that he may have a strong constitution. Each of us inherits a unique body which represents our potential for withstanding disease and sustaining the many lessons life provides. Health and disease is part of the evolutionary process: balance is individual for all. We each inherit health imbalances, and some of us help their progress along. Eventually, each of us reaches a point where our body cannot sustain the indulgences of the past. Something must give. For some this occurs later in life; for others, earlier.

While constitution affects our health and longevity, it is not everything. Too often I have seen self-proclaimed and apparently healthy people suddenly die of a stroke or some terminal illness, while seemingly weak and sensitive individuals who need to pay more attention to what they eat or how things affect them live a long, fruitful life. In fact, it is more often the beef-eating, coffee-drinking, beer-swilling and sugar-addicted Uncle Georges who often die suddenly of an "unexpected" stroke or heart attack.

It behooves those of us with strong constitutions to moderate our habits and those of us with weak constitutions to build ourselves so that we pass strength, rather than weakness, on to our children. When we don't, our children or grandchildren get sick earlier in life or develop diseases in childhood, such as immune weakness, asthma or even diabetes. If we understand this, then perhaps we'll be motivated to make the needed changes to heal ourselves and strengthen our bodies.

Desire to be Healed

Many of us need to delve deeply into our whole being to attain true healing. This usually means being honest about our habits and underlying motives. Paradoxically though, many of us are not even sure that we want to get better. Our illness may be providing us with something which we cannot get in any other way. This can be attention, love, a way around doing something we don't want to do, avoidance of people, situations or work, indecision about something or fear of confronting unresolved childhood issues.

We often use illness as an excuse to cover hidden motives. Despite our proclaimed intentions to heal ourselves, we may have hidden reasons for staying sick. For example, we may have learned how to thrive on the sympathy and attention that sickness brings to us from others. It is important to examine whether our sickness is simply an excuse for attention, a poor substitute for some much needed love and affection, or some other need.

When we have hidden reasons for staying sick, we can sabotage our efforts to get well. Rather than taking your herbs three times a day, you forget and take them sporadically. Instead of eliminating fats from your diet, you follow Uncle George who says that a few pieces of bacon couldn't possibly cause any harm. Rather than going to bed by 11 PM, you continually stay up until 1 AM or later, saying that tomorrow night you will definitely start going to bed earlier. All of these are tactics our hidden motives use to keep us sick.

For the healing process to occur then, we need to truly want to get well and willingly make the necessary changes. There are several questions we can ask ourselves which, when answered honestly, can reveal to us if we have hidden motives for staying ill. Some of these are included in the Self Inquiry Questions Chart that follows.

Writing these questions and your answers in a journal can be very helpful and revealing. Refer to the chapter on *Home Therapies* for guidelines on journal writing. It could also be a good exercise to talk about these issues with a close and trusted friend. Or perhaps use a tape recorder and speak your answers out loud when you are alone.

Self Inquiry Questions

Do I *truly* want to get better?

Am I ready to be healed, to be different than I am now?

And am I willing to do the necessary work to make those changes?

Do I try to sabotage my healing process? If so, why?

Why do I continue my harmful habits? What do they give me that I don't get otherwise?

Do I have enough love in my life?

Do I get enough attention in my life?

Am I satisfied emotionally? spiritually? physically? creatively? mentally?

How important am I to me?

Do I feel good about myself and my life?

Do I allow the world to control and dominate me? Or am I involved in my healing?

What unresolved issues am I carrying around from my childhood or any other time of my life?

Do I like my work or my job?

Am I happy with my career?

Are my relationships satisfying?

What is my true heart's desire?

What changes can I make to start following my heart's desire?

What changes can I make to start bringing more satisfaction into my life in the areas that are lacking?

What can I do to assure I follow the changes necessary for improving my health?

What specific help can I seek to make these changes?

"Going Through It"

During the healing process it is important to maintain a positive attitude. Using alternative methods hardly ever results in a quick cure. Alternative healing methods are usually a much slower but deeper healing approach. It is not a quick cure, but a long-lasting change towards balance. Because it is slow, people often loose confidence and trust in the process — they get impatient because they have been taught to expect fast results.

Therefore, it is necessary to remain confident in the face of what may be a minor "setback." Part of healing is elimination, and, for most, this is a necessary step before the stage of rebuilding can take place. Just as it may be difficult to let go of old debilitating patterns of eating, living and, for some, jobs and relationships, so it may be uncomfortable and inconvenient for your body to eliminate patterns of sickness, old thoughts and emotions.

When your body is eliminating in this way, you are now in the midst of what is called a "healing crisis." Specifically, a healing crisis manifests externally as an acute illness such as a cold, fever, diarrhea, minor skin eruptions and other forms of elimination. It can also evoke emotional responses such as vulnerability, fear and anger. It usually comes on quickly and lasts a short time. Afterwards, you often feel better than you did before the healing crisis. A healing crisis is actually a very positive sign of improvement. When such symptoms happen they shouldn't be stopped, but dealt with as part of the entire healing process through herbs and nutrition.

Sometimes the healing crisis manifests as symptoms of an old illness. When this happens, it is called the Law of Cure. This law was observed by Samuel Hahnemann when he founded homeopathy in the 1700's. The Law of Cure is a description of how healing progresses. It states that the body heals the most recent disease experienced first. It then works back through other diseases until the oldest one is healed. Also, symptoms first occur on the surface of the body and move from the top of the body downwards. Thus, the various symptoms which arise reflect the healing stage of the body.

For example, when naturally healing a recurring condition of bronchitis, you may experience a renewal of teenage chronic sore throat for a period of time. Then you might see your childhood eczema return. The eczema may start on the arms and then move down to the legs. If you persevere with natural remedies and appropriate diet, the body gathers strength and energy to complete the healing process. These symptoms eventually disappear, and a healing of your chronic bronchitis can occur. Through this process you are healing the root cause of these conditions. However, if you return to your poor eating and living habits after healing, you will most likely get sick again.

Healing Crisis Characteristics

In order to distinguish a healing crisis from a genuine sickness, there are several guidelines:

1) A healing crisis usually occurs in the midst of much greater improvement. Therefore, examine all factors of what you are experiencing and look for the genuine indications of health, such as increased energy and vitality. When indications of health are also present, then the disease symptom is only part of the healing crisis.

2) A healing crisis is of relatively short duration. The illness comes on and leaves quickly.

3) The particular sickness or emotion being expressed may be occurring for the last time. Usually when an elimination of old physical or emotional symptoms occurs during a healing crisis, there are no further experiences of them.

4) After the healing crisis you often feel better with a new sense of well-being than before it occurred. In a genuine sickness, there is not a sense of feeling different or better.

5) A healing crisis often yields symptoms of an old illness that are suddenly reoccurring from your teenage or childhood years.

6) Healing crisis symptoms usually first move from the inside of the body out so that surface ailments begin appearing such as skin eruptions, colds and flus. The symptoms also usually occur from the head down so that a rash reappearing from childhood might first appear on the face, then move down the body, disappearing as it goes.

In other instances some people experience what they think is a healing crisis when actually they are overdosing themselves with herbs or are having minor allergic reactions to them. This is important to differentiate from a true healing crisis. Overdosing with herbs or having allergic reactions to them usually appears soon after starting the herbs, and the symptoms don't let up after the "crisis" occurs. A healing crisis, on the other hand, can take longer to appear, the problem occurs for a short period amidst general improvement and the symptoms go away after the healing is complete.

When going through the healing process it is most important to be gentle and forgiving of yourself. Don't abandom play and humor. Remember how Norman Cousins literally laughed his cancer away by immersing himself in old comic movies. Note how Dr. Bernie Segal is helping many terminally ill people recover by learning to forgive themselves and to renew their commitment to joy and love. Louise Hay helps terminal AIDS patients live longer and have better lives, with some experiencing miraculous cures, by teaching them to develop positive self-images through the use of affirmations. These positive methods can definitely help make aches and pains easier to live with during recovery.

It is important to remember that natural healing takes time and effort. It is not a quick cure or fix. Yet, it has longer-lasting results as it aims at eliminating the cause of disease rather than just acting as a palliative to its symptoms. Above all, don't berate yourself for being ill. Remember, life is a "terminal condition"; it is not a question of right and wrong, but of growing and learning.

The Role of Herbal Healing

There are several principles to be aware of in using natural therapies. First, treat acute conditions with a few strong herbs. These conditions appear quickly, such as a cold, flu or fever. They need to be treated directly and immediately. If too many herbs are used in a formula, their individual effects are weakened and they cannot quickly treat the illness. Take small amounts of the herbs frequently (every 2 hours or so), possibly in a variety of forms, and take for a short period of time.

On the other hand, treat chronic diseases slowly and gently. You want to give the body's weakened organs the needed support over a longer period of time. If treated too quickly or strongly, this can further deplete the body's reserves or cause it to get weaker. Combine several herbs together in a formula for chronic conditions. In this way the possible strong effects of any one herb are tempered and won't tax the body. Take small amounts of the herbs two or three times a day over a longer period of time.

In treating chronic, seriously acute or degenerative diseases, it is important to take plenty of herbs and use several natural therapies to heal the condition. For example, if you have pneumonia, then it isn't effective to only drink three cups of herb tea a day. Instead, you also need to rest, use onion poultices on the chest twice a day, do a ginger foot bath, take herbal syrup and capsuled herbs every 2-4 hours and drink 4-6 cups of strong herb tea per day. This may be why some people who try herbs don't feel they are effective: they did not take enough herbs or do enough therapies to overcome the disease.

In general, the acute manifestations of excess diseases are easier to cure. Conditions from deficiencies take more time and can be more difficult to heal (refer to the chapter on *Energy of Illness* to understand excess and deficiency). This is because it is easier to eliminate when there is too much of something than it is to build up what has been depleted.

Deficient conditions often involve more complex issues, such as we discussed earlier, involving emotional needs for the illness, or job or relationship issues, for example. On the other hand, excess to extreme ultimately causes a condition of deficiency because at that point the body's healing ability has been depleted. As with deficiencies, healing is then more difficult since it takes more work, time and patience.

Health and Healing Routines

Establishing a healing or health maintenance routine is incredibly supportive and beneficial to the healing process. It also serves as a preventative measure and, over time, may become a way of life. Many cultures have specific living and eating routines or rituals for daily health. For example, some Native American and Andean Inca tribes welcome (and gaze into) the sun upon awakening, the Chinese go to the parks in the morning to do tai chi, or the Indian yogis do netibol (see the chapter on *Home Therapies*) before their morning meditation. Many of us have been cut off from these ancestral, parental, ethnic and cultural roots. Reuniting with all that is of value in our past can be tremendously healing.

You can adopt and create your own daily routine based upon your personal needs and what helps you feel good. For some of us, adapting routines or rituals from other cultural ways of life can sustain us through our various daily changes. As a basic guideline, I suggest you include starting the day with prayer (or meditation), then do some form of exercise (aerobics, yoga or tai chi), plan food for the day and set out and/or prepare the day's herbs. Then, as the day progresses these aspects which are so essential to your healing are already attended to and can be easily incorporated with your other activities.

For instance, I find that if I plan and start my evening meal in the morning, then it takes little time or effort to complete when dinner time arrives. If I don't do this, then in the late afternoon when I am often the busiest juggling home, business, children and answering the door and phone, I don't have time to make a good meal. I am also so hungry that I have little patience to prepare the food I and my family really need. Instead, I fix something quick.

Over time these meals aren't nearly as satisfying or healing as those made with some care, imagination and preparation. Cooking wholesome and nourishing food takes some time and effort. Popping a frozen dinner in the oven or microwave may be quick and easy, but it is usually lacking in the many essential and vital nutrients our bodies need. We eventually feel less energy, strength and ability to cope with the day's demands. This is especially true if we've only had a quick cereal and sandwich previously in the day.

If you are single or have cooked for large families for many years, you may lack incentive to carefully cook meals for yourself. This situation can be improved if you take 1-2 hours two times a week to plan out your upcoming meals. During these times you can also cook a big pot of rice (or other grain), a big pot of beans and a soup stock. These three items can be combined in many ways to prepare quick and delicious meals. Vegetables and perhaps more protein can be easily added.

Our mental state when we cook our food is also important. In some way we eat the thoughts and emotions of the cook. If angry or upset, the cook might hold the salt or spice shaker too long over the food. Of, if distracted, the food may get overcooked. If the cook is sad and lonely, then food may be made too sweet in search for the needed emotional nourishment. Thus, how we feel when cooking our food affects what we eat.

I have discovered that eating a full meal (like dinner) at lunch time or even for breakfast is very health supportive. Vegetables, grains and legumes give us much more energy and strength to handle a busy day than a simple cereal. Each person's needs are different this way. Yet, many have found making this switch to a more complete meal at breakfast and/or lunch makes all the difference in their energy and health.

Similarly, those who experience weak or poor digestion may need to carefully plan their meals throughout the day. Often symptoms of gas, bloating, overweight, abdominal distention, the need to sleep after meals, or insomnia or restless sleep occurs because we ate too late in the evening and went to bed on a full stomach. Over time, not only is our sleep poor, but our digestion becomes further impaired. For good digestion, assimilation and sleep, therefore, it is best to complete the evening meal by 6:00 PM. These benefits are further enhanced if this meal is light.

Since our health and well being is so affected by the food we eat, it may be useful for you to keep a food diary during the healing process. Many people have found this invaluable. You can discover what foods cause you problems and if and when you're over-eating. A food diary can help you see what foods might be missing from your diet and learn what meals work best for you. This journal can also help you examine why and under what conditions you eat certain foods. Then, you can correlate certain foods or meals with how you feel that day and into the next few days. We often don't feel the effects of many foods until 1-3 days later.

To keep a food diary, write down everything you eat on a daily basis. Include how much of each food you eat and when you eat it. Also note how you feel throughout the day. Review the diary after the first week. Then make whatever alterations you see necessary and keep the diary another week. If you follow your insights and advice from doing this, eventually you will learn much about how to heal yourself through food.

How we eat is also important. Our digestion works best when we eat in a calm, slow manner. Eating standing up, in the car or on the run creates nervousness, gas, bloating and ultimately, poor digestion. Praying or meditating briefly before meals is calming to the mind and body and slows us down. Rather than sleeping or working immediately after meals, it is more healthful to sit for 15 minutes or so and then take a walk.

Laughing and singing before and after meals enhances the digestive fire and strengthens its action (see the chapter on *Home Therapies* for guidelines). Sitting with your legs folded under you (as the Japanese sit to eat) aids digestion and alleviates gas and bloatedness. You can eat in this posture, or sit this way after the meal for 15-20 minutes.

It is also best to eat only when hungry. True hunger means the previous meal has been digested. Likewise, avoiding between-meal snacks allows the digestive organs a rest. It also increases your appetite for healthy foods at meal time. If you find snacks are frequently necessary, it could be you are either not eating enough at meal times, or what you are eating is insubstantial for your needs.

It has been scientifically demonstrated that eating less is the best tonic for longevity. Overeating uses more energy to break food down than we ultimately receive from it. As we grow we need less and less food. Yet, we often eat for stimulation and sentimen-

tal reasons rather than for nutrition. Or we overindulge in food when under stress. It is important to determine the difference between a desire for food and a real physical need.

For good digestion, avoid extremes. This includes food that is either too hot or too cold, or food that is overly greasy or dry. Preferably, all food should be fresh rather than frozen or canned. Likewise, it is best to freshly prepare each meal before eating to receive the maximum amount of nutrients. Frequently eating reheated and canned foods causes gas and is devitalizing.

Going to bed by 11 PM each evening is another important health habit to form. In Chinese medicine, the Wood element rules the body between 11 PM to 3 AM. This is the time the Liver is most active in its functions of storing and cleansing the blood. If we are awake and active at this time, the Liver has less energy to perform these tasks. Many of us find we wake up refreshed and lively when we go to sleep by 11 PM. On the other hand, when we go to bed later we don't feel as well when waking up, even if we get the same amount of sleep. It may not be the length of sleeping time that matters, but the quality. This is affected by the time we go to bed.

Where we live and work also affects our health. Our local environment, climate, house and workplace all influence how we feel. For example, some of us have too much dampness in the body with symptoms of asthma, bronchitis, allergies, bloatedness, water retention and lack of taste or no desire to drink. We should not live or work in damp locations such as near the sea, where it rains a lot, or in concrete rooms or buildings underground. All of these create more dampness in the body. Instead, we would feel good in dry, hot, even desert areas, houses above ground in the sun and upper stories of work buildings.

Likewise, those of us who have too much dryness and heat dislike hot locations. We feel better in wet, moist and cool areas such as basements, the sea or places where it snows or rains frequently. We should avoid extremely heated buildings, rooms at the top of buildings where the heat rises, the desert, sunbathing and other hot, dry activities or locations. To live in environments which match your needs may mean moving or making a change in job locations. Even Western medicine often recommends those with severe allergies to go live in desert areas. Usually we don't need to make such radical changes. Just finding a dry home with a sunny exposure may be sufficient.

The seasons also affect how we feel. Living according to their various differences can influence us and our health tremendously. Each season requires different dressing, eating and lifestyle habits to stay in harmony and balance. Because this is important to look at in-depth, it is covered separately in the next chapter, *Living with the Seasons*.

Living with the Seasons

No matter where we live, we are constantly affected by the seasons and their changes. Even in extreme heat or cold climates, there are seasonal differences with distinct qualities and traits. Coping with these changes can be difficult for some of us. For example, the switch from Summer to Fall often causes many of us to get the flu. For others, not adjusting to each season's differences lowers our resistance to disease and later creates sickness. For instance, when we frequently drink juices and eat fruit in the winter, we eventually feel cold, or get a cold, because these foods create coldness and dampness in the body.

The ancient Chinese have long acknowledged the effects of the seasons on health. They associate each season with particular aspects of nature and climate, organs of the body, emotions, foods, activities, energies and ways to dress. By knowing these we can learn each of their unique opportunities and discover how to balance the extremes of each season's energy.

Spring

Spring is the beginning of the year, the time when the earth awakens and new life bursts forth. This season stirs the uprising of vital energy. We begin moving out of Winter's cocoon with renewed life, new possibilities and ideas. It is a time of planting seeds, physically and mentally, and for the year's creative endeavors.

This is the season of the Wood element, the Liver[1] and Gallbladder in Chinese medicine. A healthy Liver is like a young tree sapling growing strong yet flexible and bending. The energy is clear, flowing and solidly rooted. As such, the Liver is responsible for the smooth movement of energy throughout the body which gives grace to our movements and cleans and stores the blood.

When the Liver is aggravated, it is susceptible to irregular movement, called Wind. This causes tension, stiffness, spasms, tics, clumsiness, numbness, headaches, allergies, convulsions, itching and pains which change location. The Liver then becomes congested, which can result in anger, frustration, irritability, stiff neck and shoulders and hypertension.

Therefore, Spring's new growth must be nurtured and allowed to occur slowly according to your own individual energy and needs. If you suddenly change from Winter's quietness to full outward activity, then you can feel ungrounded or uprooted. On the other hand, if you don't allow new ideas or activities to grow or push through rigidity and ineffective emotional or behavioral patterns, then the energy can become stuck. Balance the focus between your inward and outward energies in Spring and pace yourself. Since regulating your habits also keeps the energy flowing smoothly, set routines for eating, sleeping and exercising and keep them with regularity.

Although we feel warmer air in Spring, our body's fires are only beginning to rise from being deep inside during Winter. As the outside temperature rises, so does our internal body heat begin to move toward the surface. Yet there is still a sensitivity to cool air. This is true even though it may be the same temperature as in Fall when you needed fewer clothes and could keep the windows open at night. If your body is sluggish, it doesn't effectively make this change, and Spring fevers and colds can result.

Until our "fires come up" in Spring like sap in a tree, it is best to remain well wrapped up when outdoors, even when the urge is to throw off heavy clothes. Otherwise, we expose ourselves too early to the elements and sickness sets in. This is particularly true of the back of the neck and shoulders where the wind most easily penetrates the protective energy of the body. What we call "colds" and "flu" the Chinese call "wind chill" and "wind heat," or the wind penetrating the body's resistance.

Likewise it is best to continue eating warm foods well into this season. Add more green vegetables, steamed greens and some salads to the diet as these help overcome any sluggishness. Limit raw fruits, or eat them stewed or baked. Avoid heavy rich foods, fats, oils, nuts and dairy as these all congest the Liver. Limit meat-eating to 1-2 times/week to lighten the diet. From this, the body will adjust better to temperature changes.

The Liver is most active between 11 PM-3 AM when it is at the peak of its functions. Directing the Liver's energy into creativity during this time diverts it from its physical function of cleaning and renewing the blood. So resist the urge to be a "night owl" and go to bed by 11 PM.

Cleaning the blood is a way of housecleaning, the traditional ritual in spring time. Herbal "spring tonics" and fasting help cleanse the blood and assist the liver in releasing stored toxins. Herbs which are gently stimulating, pungent, bitter and sour are particularly good for Spring. *Sorrel, dandelion, nettles, watercress* and other young green leaves provided by nature then are a perfect balancing food for the liver. They help strengthen by thinning the blood and releasing toxins. They also help attune the body to Spring's growth and prepare it for summer. *Dandelion, gentian* or *barberry* cleanse the liver, bowels and strengthen digestion.

Summer

Summer is the essence of life, growth, heat and activity. Our energy, like that of the season, is expansive now, flowing outward to act on the plans and seeds sowed in Spring. Our natural inclination is to be outside most of the day, pursuing sports, gardening, yard work, hiking or other outdoor activities. Our energy flourishes and compels us to get things done, to work, socialize and actuate our potentials. This is the season of the Fire element with its organs of the Heart and Small Intestines which are associated with joy, forgiveness and laughter.

If we experience low energy now, it is often because we didn't rest sufficiently during Winter. Or, if we are too active, we can "burn out" and deplete our energy reserves. This stunts our development and growth and robs our body of its needed essence the rest of the year. Summer is the time to protect your energy for the rest of the year, especially for those of us who already have low energy.

In summer our body heat is more on the surface to keep us cool inside. We can become more easily overheated through over-exposure to the sun, heated environments or hot-natured foods. This causes a flare-up of heat in our bodies such as fevers, heat stroke and aggravated high blood pressure. It is important to continue paying attention to the heating and warming qualities of foods and herbs in this season.

Lighter, easier-to-digest foods are appropriate now. Eat cooling foods such as local fruit, juices, salads and raw foods along with the more balanced grains and legumes to guard against overheating. Red meat and excess meat-eating should be kept at a minimum, if at all. Those of us who already have too much heat in our bodies crave cool liquids. Yet we should avoid ice in drinks since it injures (by cooling down) our metabolic "fires" needed for digestion.

Those of us who always feel cold and tired, however, need warmth even in Summer. We then must resist the tendency toward cooler foods and drinks and build our heat, instead. To do this, we should restrict our fruit, juice, salad and raw food intake to small amounts and continue eating meat along with grains and legumes.

Herbs which are cooling, spicy and bitter, such as *red clover, peppermint* and *chrysanthemum*, help keep the body's temperature down. The bitter taste strengthens the Heart and Small Intestines, the organs attributed to Summer. These in turn nourish the blood. The cooling and drying qualities of bitter help by eliminating excess fluid and cholesterol from the blood. Spicy herbs, such as *chillies* and *curries*, open the pores and create perspiration to cool the body off. That is why people living in southern climates eat spicy food—it is ultimately cooling although it tastes hot. Herbs such as *mint* and *lemon balm* also cool the body and make refreshing summer drinks.

Dressing in summer seems easy, the fewer the clothes the better. Yet those of us who are frequently cold should maintain our body heat by covering up on cooler summer days. Being in air conditioning and then going out into the hot air stresses and imbalances our bodies through the temperature extremes. This leads to a weakening of resistance and a greater susceptibility to illness, like the horrible summer colds. Therefore, if air conditioning is a must in your life, try to keep it at a higher temperature to more closely match that of the outdoors. It also helps to wear a sweater when in the air conditioning.

Late Summer

Many climates throughout the world have five definite seasons, and late Summer, or Indian Summer, is usually the fifth. This is the period of ripening and fruition. It is a time of being stable, grounded, balanced, down-to-earth and rooted. These qualities give us full and complete nourishment no matter what the changes of upcoming Fall, or life, bring us. At this time we are fully assimilating our year's experience from the initial planting to its full growth.

The Earth element rules Late Summer along with its organs, the Spleen, the Pancreas and Stomach. Their special function is digestion. These organs nourish the physical body and transform food and fluid into bones, muscles, energy, blood and so forth. Poor digestion can lead to gas, bloatedness, lethargy, low energy and vitality and excessive mucus in the lungs which shows up in the Fall. Obsession, over-concentrating, excessive studying or sitting too much all can injure the digestion.

Dampness or humidity is also attributed to this season as seen in monsoons, hurricanes or late summer rains. It can imbalance the energy, especially for those who are fluid-retentive. For those who are dry or emaciated, it may help. Poor digestion can lead to mucus which may create cough, allergies, poor appetite, bloating and malnutrition.

The sweet taste, attributed to the Earth element, strengthens the digestion. This includes complex carbohydrates, dairy and protein. Adding more of these foods in the diet along with plenty of vegetables and some seasonal fruit is appropriate now. As Fall is around the corner, it is best to begin limiting the intake of juices, salads and raw foods.

Herbs which are sweet and strengthen the Spleen's digestive functions include *ginseng*, *codonopsis*, *dioscorea* and *fu ling*. Other beneficial herbs at this time are *comfrey*, *slippery elm*, *dandelion*, *hawthorn*, *licorice* and *marshmallow* and carminatives such as *citrus peel*, *cardamom* and *ginger*.

Fall

The energy of Fall is one of harvesting the fruits and labors of Spring's planting and planning. It is a pulling in and building up of your energy reserves to be stored for Winter. This is the time to discriminate and separate out what is needed from what isn't. The ability to receive, or take in, and to release the unnecessary is attributed to the Metal element which rules this season. Change and old age represent this, and when we don't release the old or accept changes, we experience grief and sadness.

The Metal organs are the Lung and Colon. The Lungs bring in vital air, which is nourishing, supportive, building and essential to life. The Colon and skin (associated with the Lungs) eliminate what is unnecessary. Therefore, skin eruptions and constipation often show a toxic condition of the body or suggest an overactive life. Asthma, bronchitis, allergies and other lung ailments also result and often kick up at this time of year. Colon purification and mucus elimination from the lungs (letting go!) are beneficial now.

The taste of the Metal element is spicy. Herbs that are spicy stimulate the functions of the body and break through obstructions and congestion. In turn, this eliminates any mucus which the lungs have over-produced. *Peppers, spices, black pepper, cinnamon, citrus peel* and *raw ginger* are all good herbs for Fall. Those who have dryness or feel dizzy, light-headed or ungrounded periodically should take *licorice* with the spices to soften their stimulating effects. Do not eat spices in excess, however, as they could then cause dryness and result in these symptoms. Expectorants and laxatives may also be appropriate, such as *elecampane, coltsfoot* and *cascara sagrada.*

When Fall arrives, the surface heat of our bodies starts slowly moving inward. We can stay warm long in to the Fall, wearing fewer clothes and keeping our windows open. However, if we dress too lightly or if we continue to eat a lot of cooling foods, then we make ourselves vulnerable to the cooling winds that occur in Fall. We also dissipate our heat so that when Winter arrives, the much needed deep internal heat to keep us warm is lessened and we frequently feel cold, instead. Our immunity and vitality also become weakened from this.

Further, Fall winds are cool and, like Spring, can penetrate the back of the neck and shoulders if left uncovered. This creates colds, flus and other similar illnesses. Therefore, on windy and cooler days, coats and even scarves are essential even though one doesn't feel the need for them. Likewise, any window which is open should be located away from the bed so a draft does not blow on the neck or shoulders. Nasal drip and mucus often appear at this time if we don't dress adequately or if we overindulged in damp and cool foods during summer.

Including more warm foods in the diet is appropriate, with emphasis on grains, legumes and cooked vegetables. Root vegetables, lots of steamed greens, winter squash and some seasonal fruit are beneficial. It is better to eliminate juices and raw foods and have salads less frequently as these cooling foods are no longer appropriate for the Fall and cold Winter to come.

Winter

Winter provides us with a time of retreating, of going within ourselves and replenishing our reserves. It is the season of storage and conservation of energy. The Water element rules this season and its organs are the Kidneys, Adrenals and Bladder. These store the deep inherited and vital constitutional energy of the body. This root energy can be protected or wasted in life, but not replenished.

It is especially important in Winter to get plenty of rest and nourish ourselves quietly. Go to bed early and sleep late, stay warm and cozy and do not expend much energy. Conserve and preserve your resources, essence and energy in Winter; it is not a time for extravagance. Winter provides us with the opportunity for inner reflection, assessing the past year, the goals we set and did or did not meet and learning from our experiences.

The Kidney is a unique organ in Chinese medicine. Although its element is water, which is cooling, it also has a fiery aspect. This is linked to the Adrenal, hormonal and reproductive processes. Too much cold can injure the fire quality. Those of us with coldness usually dread Winter. Those of us who expended too much of our energy in Summer or who ate inappropriately then and in the Fall, feel cold in Winter, as if nothing we do can keep us warm.

If our bodies get too cold, depression, fear and even paranoia, the emotions of the Water element, may result. We may also experience low back pain, sciatica, frequent or night time urination, weak knees, impotence, infertility and hearing problems. Therefore, it is especially important to contain the heat in our bodies at this time to protect these fires.

Dressing warmly as appropriate is one way to do this. Moxibustion on the back at waist level also helps replenish lost heat from the body. Another method of retaining heat is to wear a harimake, a type of waist vest or band traditionally worn by the Japanese around the waist to cover the location of the Kidneys and Adrenals. This protects the stored vital energy and essence of the body. (Refer to the chapter on *Home Therapies* for instructions on moxibustion and harimake.)

Pay careful attention to the energy of food and herbs in Winter. The outside cold drives the body's heat deep inside and food and herbs need to be taken to reinforce and support this. Spicy foods, like salsa and curries, seem warm but are used in hot climates to induce perspiration, which takes heat out of the body. Instead, foods and herbs which are internally warming are necessary. All food should be cooked at this time, which is a way of adding heat to the body and keeping our inner fires burning strong.

Soups, including oxtail, bone marrow or lamb and dong quai soups with ginger are especially warming to the body. Plenty of grains, root and leafy green vegetables, aduki and black beans, winter squash, walnuts, some meat and a little baked fruit are health supportive in Winter. Grain teas and other warm drinks are good, too. Cold drinks, ice cream, tropical fruits and raw salads and foods are all cold in nature and so have a cooling effect on the body. These should be avoided in Winter.

Herbs which are internally warming and strengthening are best in this season such as *cinnamon*, *dry ginger*, *fenugreek*, *cornus*, *dioscorea*, *ho shou wu* and *rehmannia*. Many of these herbs can be cooked with food in soup form, an excellent way to increase nutrition and strengthen the body's reserves. (Refer to the chapter on *Herbal Preparations* for directions on making soups.)

Salty is the Water element taste. A little salt and herbs high in mineral salts, such as *seaweed* and *nettles*, can be added to teas, grains and soups to help the Kidney energy. Too much salt, on the other hand, causes water retention and other imbalances of water in the body.

In Winter we tend to become lethargic. If exercise is not kept up our energy can stagnate. This often results in frustration, irritability, anger or depression, known as cabin fever in the cold country. To prevent this from happening, exercise regularly as a balance to Winter's rest.

Likewise, if we keep the temperature too hot indoors, we get tired and sluggish. Then when we go out into the cold, we create stress on the body through exposing ourselves to such extremes. Therefore, keep the heat down indoors to more closely match the temperature outside.

After making this journey through all the seasons we can see how intimately our well-being is connected with nature. Our eating, dressing and lifestyle habits are all affected by the seasons' energies, qualities and traits. When we adjust our life patterns to match these seasonal influences, we promote health and enhance our quality of life.

---

[1] The Chinese organ systems are capitalized throughout the book to differentiate them from the physical organs which are in lower case.

Home Remedies

The use of preparations applied to the surface of the body is an important aspect of home healing. There is an intimate connection between the skin and internal organs and systems. The skin is the largest digestive organ in the body and, as such, quickly and effectively takes into the blood stream and tissues anything which is placed, rubbed or massaged on it.

Therefore, applying herbs to the skin can affect the blood and internal organs, can draw out or drain that which is causing pain or inflammation, or can stimulate and promote the body's own innate healing potential. External applications such as baths, foot soaks, washes and rubs are especially useful and effective for children, the elderly and the infirm.

Of the many uses of herbs, external applications and folk remedies have come down to us from the "beginning." They are extremely valuable and important to the healing process. Taking herbs internally is the first line of defense in treatment, yet external applications can often reach the desired area faster, beginning work there before the herbs arrive internally. Often there is a blockage in the body which stalls herbs taken internally from reaching the necessary location quickly. Applying herbs externally tremendously enhances and speeds up overall treatment.

External applications can be learned and used by anybody. They put the power and responsibility of healing back into each individual's hands. They are usually made out of items already in the home. One can put them into use immediately upon the first signs of a problem, such as a cold or flu, or relieve problems from getting more complicated or advanced.

Until about two generations ago, folk remedies were casually used in the home on a regular basis. My grandmother would hang a bag of asafoetida around my mother's neck when she went to school to prevent her from catching colds, flus or other bugs. Interestingly, asafoetida is an antiseptic, among other things, and so could definitely help in these circumstances.

Coughs, pneumonia, colds, fevers, sprains, burns, cuts, swellings, arthritis and poor circulation, to name just a few conditions, can all benefit from external herbal treatments. However, by themselves external treatments do not usually compose a complete cure. The root cause of the problem always needs to be identified and treated. Usually, changes in diet or lifestyle habits need to be made.

The following are several specific food and herbal remedies. **You will need to refer to the chapter on *Herbal Preparations* for their exact instructions.** Here we learn what each remedy is good for and what it helps heal and prevent.

When recipes provide formulas for herbs the amount of herbs given is usually listed as parts. A part is the ratio of that herb to the quantity of the entire formula. For example, in a formula comprised of 6 parts total, one herb listed as 2 parts means that the herb comprises 2/6 or 1/3 of the entire amount of herbs in that formula. If you want a total of 6 ounces of herbs, therefore, you would use 2 ounces of that herb.

Baths

An herbal bath can be made just for a specific part of the body, such as the hands, hips or feet, or can be a full body bath. Baths are especially useful and effective in treating infants as the baby will assimilate what it needs through the skin without needing to take the herbs internally. Likewise, this is a safe method for treating the elderly.

Ginger Bath

Made from freshly grated *ginger root*, this bath stimulates circulation, alleviates aches and pains, breaks a cold, helps arthritis and warms the body. A ginger bath is also wonderful for flus, gout, bursitis, feeling cold and tiredness. Immerse the entire body in a tub full of hot water with 1/3 of it being ginger tea.

This same bath may be made in smaller quantities and used as a soak for aching, sore, swollen or numb hands, feet or any other body part. A hot ginger foot bath eases sore and aching feet, stimulates the circulation, warms the body and helps energy and mental tiredness.

The ginger foot bath is also useful in causing sweating to break fevers and colds. To do this, sit in a chair with the feet in a tub of ginger tea. Then wrap blankets about the head and body, encompassing the tub of ginger tea. Leave in place 5-10 minutes after a sweat has occurred. Then rinse off, dress in clean clothes and go to bed well-covered.

Calming Bath

Combine equal parts *lavender*, *rose*, *chamomile* and *scullcap*. This bath calms the mind and body, relaxes the muscles and helps cramps and spasms.

Radish Leaves Bath

A hip bath in *radish leaf* water is specific for bladder infections, acute or chronic. It is good for any other genito-reproductive disorders such as endometritis, leukorrhea and menstrual difficulties. In the hip bath, only the pelvis or hips are immersed in the tub with the feet and upper area covered and hanging out of the tub. Daikon radish leaves are best to use since they are more stimulating than most radishes, yet any radish leaves may be used.

Chop up a large handful of radish leaves, add 1 tablespoon grated fresh ginger and tie up in a thin cloth bag. Put under the faucet while letting hot water run over them to fill the tub. Soak the hips for 20 to 30 minutes.

Stimulating Bath

Combine equal parts *bayberry bark*, *ginger*, *prickly ash* and 1/4 part *cayenne pepper*. This bath helps relieve fever and chills, produces a sweat, helps colds and flus and stimulates the circulation.

Bolus

A bolus is a suppository inserted into the rectum to treat hemorrhoids or various cysts, or into the vagina to treat infections, cysts, irritations and tumors.

Toxins, Cysts and Tumors

Useful for drawing out toxins, reducing cysts and tumors in the rectum or vagina. Use equal parts of: *chickweed*, *comfrey root*, *goldenseal root*, *marshmallow root*, *mullein leaves*, *slippery elm*, *squawvine* and *yellow dock*.

Vaginal Infections

This will reduce vaginal infections and with repeated use over time, heal the area. Use equal parts of: *comfrey*, *goldenseal* and *echinacea roots*.

Hemorrhoids

Very specific for hemorrhoid relief, this formula is astringent and soothing. Use equal parts of: *bayberry bark*, *chestnut bark*, *comfrey root*, *slippery elm* and *witch hazel bark*.

Compress/Fomentation

A fomentation, sometimes called a compress, is an herbal fluid wrapped on the body and kept warm. It benefits swellings, pains, colds and flus, stimulates fresh blood circulation and warms the area where placed. Herbs that are too strong to be taken inside the body can be put on the outside, and the body will then slowly absorb the herbs in small amounts.

Ginger Fomentation

Ginger fomentation is excellent for congestion, sprains, cramps, pains, coldness, swellings, colds, flus, coughs, excessive mucus and strained muscles. It is also very effective for drawing out blood toxins and stimulating the circulation. Ginger is a very warming herb which also moves blood, energy, fluids and toxins.

Place over the lower abdomen and perineum during childbirth to help prevent tearing and stop pain; place over the chest for congested lungs, cough, asthma and pneumonia; over the abdomen for pains, spasms, poor digestion, coldness, bladder infections (in a cold person) and menstrual cramps; over the lower back for pain and ache, lowered immunity and energy and poor digestion; over any other part of the body where there is congestion, sprain, cramps or pain.

Charcoal Compress

A charcoal compress is very effective for treating infections and slow-healing wounds. It can be placed over small or large areas, such as an inflamed abdomen. Leave on for 1-2 hours. It should not be put on open wounds, however, as this will cause a tattoo. The charcoal should first be powdered, then moistened and placed between layers of gauze to form the compress. Charcoal tablets may be purchased at any drug store.

Castor Oil Compress

Castor oil compress is made a little differently than other compresses. In a pan, soak with castor oil a piece of felt, cloth or cheesecloth cut to fit the desired area. Heat in the oven till very warm but still touchable. Place over desired area, cover with plastic wrap, then follow compress directions given in the chapter on *Herbal Preparations*. Generally, this compress is left on for several hours or overnight.

Castor oil compress is a fabulous way to rejuvenate scarred and failing tissues and organs. The oil is very close to natural oils in the body and so penetrates the cells easily, healing and rejuvenating them. It detoxifies, heals cysts, growths, warts, treats epilepsy, paralysis and other nervous system disorders, stimulates the body's deep circulation and heals body tissues, detoxifying and healing liver disorders or chronic bladder infections, for example. Apply the compress over the affected area, be it the liver, bladder, kidneys, cyst or other growth. Repeated applications are necessary over time to heal these conditions. Often a pattern is followed of applying the castor oil compress for 4 days in a row and then left off for 3 days. This is repeated for several weeks to months or until the condition is healed.

Congee

Congee is a well-cooked soupy grain or type of fortified porridge. It is a very therapeutic food which is perfect during convalescence from sickness, for treating acute diseases, strengthening the digestion and assimilation ability, general debility and low vitality. A congee is made with a grain, usually rice, water and your personally chosen herbs. It has a long cooking time over low heat which slowly and thoroughly breaks down the grain so that it is extremely easy to digest and assimilate. Thus, the body gets the most nutrients out of it possible, which is perfect for weak digestive power that can't break down or assimilate food well.

Possible Formulas

Poor digestion, gas, bloatedness, lowered energy and immunity: *ginseng, dong quai, codonopsis, red date* and *astragalus*

Cough, asthma, mucus, bronchitis: *apricot kernel, comfrey root*

Fever, detoxification, diarrhea and dysentery: *mung bean* mixed with rice and sautéed cumin, *turmeric* and *coriander*, it becomes Indian Dahl, called *Kicharee*, or the "Food of the Gods"

Edema, gout, retention of urine or frequent urination and other kidney-bladder problems: *aduki bean*, cooked *rehmannia*, *ho shou wu* and *cornus*

Coldness, poor circulation and as a blood rejuvenative after menstruation: *lamb*, *dong quai* and *ginger*

Malnutrition, hypoglycemia, tiredness, diarrhea and weakness: *beef*, *ginseng*, *licorice* and *ginger*

Juice

Potato juice taken internally is beneficial for gastric, stomach and duodenal ulcers. Squeeze through cheese cloth the washed and grated raw potato and collect the juice. Take 1/2 cup three times a day before meals. Red potato is best, next is blue-skinned and less effective are the white and yellow potatoes.

Liniments

Liniments are herbal extracts that are rubbed into the skin for treating strained muscles and ligaments, bruises, arthritis and some inflammations. Liniments usually include stimulating herbs, such as cayenne, to warm the area and increase the circulation, and antispasmodic herbs, such as chamomile, to relax the muscles.

Dit Dat Jiao Liniment

This is called "Kung Fu Medicine" by the Chinese because it is a type of liniment used when someone is injured while practicing martial arts. There are many prized secret variations of this liniment which is used by different practitioners. The following formula is one example:

angelica and *comfrey roots*	6 parts each
cinnamon bark and *valerian root*	4 parts each
hyssop leaves and *safflower*	3 parts each
calendula flowers	3 parts

All-Purpose Liniment

This is a general liniment good for blood circulation, bruises and sore and aching muscles. It may be rubbed into these areas or massaged into the fingers for arthritis. Use:

goldenseal	1 part
myrrh gum	2 parts
cayenne	1/2 part

Milk

Ginger milk is a tasty treat which is also very warming to the body. By first scalding a cup of milk and adding 1/2 teaspoon honey and 1/2 teaspoon powdered ginger, the mucus-producing and congesting properties of milk are mitigated, and the body receives a warming nutritive tonic instead.

Oils

Herbal oils are a method of extracting the active principles of herbs into an oil. They are used on the outside of the body, like liniments. They are good for sore and aching muscles, cuts and stings and are wonderful for massage. My whole family loves to be massaged regularly with herbal oils. Spices, mints and other strong-smelling herbs are especially good to use in oils.

Arthritis Oils

Good for rheumatism, arthritis, sprained and aching muscles and tendons, the following are two possible formulas:

1) Use equal parts: *bay*, *eucalyptus*, *mugwort*, *rosemary*, fresh grated *ginger* and *cayenne*. Add 1 tbsp medical grade *turpentine oil* (turpentine is sap from the fir tree) and 1 tbsp *rosemary oil* for every cup of oil.

2) 1 tbsp *camphor oil*   1 tbsp *clove oil*
   1 tbsp *peppermint oil*   1 tsp *eucalyptus oil*
   1 tsp *rosemary oil*
   1 tbsp juice from fresh grated *ginger*

All-Purpose Oil

Use equal parts: *calendula, chamomile* and *elder flowers* and 1/2 part of *rose* and/or *lavender*. This is good for minor skin irritations, burns and blemishes and as a mild chest and back rub for flus, colds and lung congestion.

Comfrey Oil

This is a very healing and simple oil which can be used as is or as a base for a more complex oil or salve. Comfrey is very healing and soothing to the skin, activating new cell growth and quickly "knitting" skin tissue and bones together. It is very useful for any cuts, abrasions, bites, stings, wounds, breaks or other skin irritations.

Use freshly mashed *comfrey root*, if possible, but dried is also fine. Use fresh roots in a ratio of 1 part root to 3 parts oil. For dried roots use 1 part root to 1 part oil, but soften the root before cooking by soaking it in the oil an hour or two. *Comfrey leaves* may be used, but the root is stronger.

Ear Oil

An ear oil is used to relieve the pain of an aching or inflamed ear while also inserting antibiotic or decongesting properties. Three of the most effective herbs for this are *mullein flowers, garlic* and *echinacea root*. Make a standard oil with one or a combination of these herbs in sesame or olive oil. Then insert 5-10 drops of the warm oil into the ear, having the patient lean the head to the side. Next place a small piece of cotton in the ear to prevent it from spilling out. Repeat this process 5-6 times throughout the day until the symptoms are gone. A hot water bottle next to the ear may further enhance the healing process.

Ginger Sesame Oil

This oil activates the functions of the blood capillaries, circulation and nerve reactions. Use for aches and pains, headaches or pain in the spine or joints by massaging it into the skin. It can also be used for earaches by placing 2 or 3 drops of the oil on cotton, which is then placed in the aching ear for several hours, keeping the head tipped sideways for a while until the oil has penetrated. Leave the cotton and oil in the ear for a few hours.

It is also useful for scalp diseases and dandruff. Rub ginger sesame oil on the scalp and leave it there for at least 8 hours—overnight is good. Then wash with an herbal shampoo. Do this 2-3 times a week.

To make, use a mixture of equal amounts of *sesame oil* and fresh *ginger juice*. To extract the ginger juice, grate the ginger and express the juice by squeezing it through a cheesecloth.

Tree Flower Oil

An herbal first-aid kit in itself, tree flower oil can be used both externally and internally for all acute ailments such as the first signs of colds, cough, flu, headache, pain, bruises, sprains, indigestion and low spirits. Since it is very concentrated, only a drop or two at a time should be used. It consists of a blend of the volatile oils from herbs, made by pressing the herbs to extract their natural oils. They may be obtained already in oil form, usually found in your local herb store.

Try equal parts: *cinnamon, thyme, camphor, cajeput, eucalyptus, marjoram* and *olive oils*. Combine and pour into a bottle for storage and ready use.

Pastes

An herbal paste is also called an electuary or herbal candy because it is mixed with sweeteners and tastes good. In fact, in East Indian Ayurvedic medicine, herbs are often administered powdered and mixed with a little honey as a carrier.

Trikatu

Trikatu is a traditional Ayurvedic (East Indian) formula composed of three spices: *ginger, black pepper* and *pippli* (Indian long pepper). Because pippli is not easy to obtain, *anise seed* may be substituted. Equal parts of the powders are combined and taken with warm milk, or mixed with enough honey to form a paste, and then eaten.

Spicy and stimulating, trikatu is useful to stimulate the body's energy and circulation and to dry wet conditions. It helps dry mucus and so is fabulous for colds, flus, mucus congestion, lung ailments, sore throat, allergies and cough, all from coldness. It helps reduce fat, aids digestion and circulation and warms internally. A specific remedy for clear damp discharges that often occur in cold, damp climates, trikatu should be taken in winter by nearly everyone living in such environments and then suspended during warm summer months.

Umeboshi Plum

Umeboshi plum is a Japanese plum which is pickled in salt. It can be found in oriental groceries, health food or macrobiotic stores either in the form of whole plums or as a paste. It is very sour and salty, and when taped to the navel, will stop motion sickness. Taken internally, it aids digestion, certain types of headaches, nausea, morning sickness, stomach aches and cramps, migraines and acidity.

It also counteracts fatigue and acts as a preventive against dysentery. It is further effective to counteract the intake of sugar or alcohol, as it will balance out the system after ingestion of these substances. In Japan it is traditionally added to bancha tea along with a little tamari soy sauce for hangovers. When traveling I always carry some ume plum paste with me and eat a little after meals to aid digestion and prevent unwanted bugs with attending diarrhea.

Pills

Herbal pills are used for more chronic illnesses and during periods of convalescence. They are used in the same way as gelatin capsules but have the advantage of being prepared entirely with herbs. For strict vegetarians they are advantageous since most capsules are made from animal gelatin. Powdered herbs are used in pills, but do not need to be as finely ground as those for capsules. Any formula which can be taken in tea or powder form may also be taken as pills.

Longevity Pills

Chinese tonic pills for longevity can be made using equal portions of the following herbs: *dong quai, ginseng, ho shou wu (Polygonum multiflorum), licorice, atractylodes (Pai shu)* and *fu ling (Poria cocos)*.

Colds and Flus

Helpful in alleviating colds and flus, this formula is also good to take periodically for their prevention. If taken regularly at the first onset of colds and flus, it can knock them out in their early stages. Use equal parts: *echinacea, golden seal* and *ginger root* powders.

Sore Throats and Cough

This is soothing to the throat and dispels coughs. Use equal parts: *licorice, wild cherry bark* and *comfrey* with *honey* added.

Digestive Aid

These pills stimulate digestion, aid assimilation, dispel gas and calm an upset or nauseous stomach. They can also be helpful for those who cannot stomach any food. Use equal parts: *slippery elm* and *ginger*.

Plasters

A plaster is an herbal mash that is wrapped up in a protective cloth or combined in a thick base material such as slippery elm, oil or Vaseline and then placed on the skin. It is first placed in the cloth or oil because the herbs used in a plaster are stronger and might burn or extremely irritate the skin if they were put directly on it. Mustard and garlic are two common examples.

Plasters are good for muscle spasms, swelling, arthritis, rheumatism, tumors, fevers, mucus congestion in the chest, bronchitis and pneumonia. They can be used in treating enlarged glands and organs (neck, breast, groin, kidney, liver, prostate) and various eruptions (boils, abscesses).

Albi Plaster

Albi is the *taro potato* found growing abundantly in Hawaii. Albi plaster is especially useful in dissolving hardened tumors and lymphatic swellings and cancers, especially breast cancer. If used regularly and consistently enough it will draw out poisonous waste that is stored in the cells and shrink the tumor, cancer or swelling. It can be applied to any part of the body where needed, such as over the eye for eye trouble, behind the ear for ear problems, on the face, throat, arms, legs and so forth.

Ideally the plaster should be changed every four hours, though it may be left on overnight. After this time the poultice becomes saturated with poisons and often will turn black. Repeat applications until the problem is alleviated. For cancer and tumors first apply a ginger compress for 20 minutes, then the albi plaster.

To make, grate taro potato (found in oriental grocery stores or in powdered form in some health food or macrobiotic stores). Then add 1/10 part grated fresh ginger root and 1/5 part flour. If albi cannot be found, regular potatoes may be substituted, though they are not as effective.

Buckwheat Plaster

As a food, *buckwheat* is strengthening and nourishing. Buckwheat plaster, however, is wonderful at drawing fluid out of the body. Mix buckwheat flour with enough water to make a paste and apply as a plaster for local edemas and other swellings. I have seen this work well on knees, ankles and other joints, on the abdomen, breast and arms. It is important to repeat application of the buckwheat plaster throughout the day and for several days to totally eliminate the swelling.

Chlorophyll Plaster

Chlorophyll plaster can be used instead of the albi plaster and will further treat inflammations and infections. Pound any fresh leafy greens and add 1/5 part peppermint leaves and 1/10 part flour. Mix together well. No water is necessary since fresh leaves contain moisture. Apply as a plaster to the afflicted area for a few hours and renew if necessary. *Radish* and *carrot tops*, *swiss chard*, *watercress*, *parsley* and *spinach* are good as a few examples.

Garlic Plaster

It is well known that rubbing the soles of the feet with a clove of *garlic* causes a garlic odor and taste to occur in the mouth within a minute or so. It is such a powerful herb that it quickly passes into the blood stream and moves throughout the entire body.

When placed on the feet, garlic can have a beneficial effect on the lungs. A garlic plaster placed on the soles of the feet is very good for stopping coughs and aiding colds. It is made by mincing several cloves of garlic, mixing them with a little olive oil to cover and then making a plaster out of them.

Mustard Plaster

A *mustard* pack, or plaster, is a well known folk remedy. It is excellent for aches, sprains, spasms, cold areas needing circulation and to cause mucus expectoration. It is made with 1 tablespoon mustard powder, 4 tablespoons whole wheat flour and enough water to form a paste. If the skin is sensitive or if it seems too strong, use an equal amount of egg white instead of the water to prevent blistering. After removing the plaster, the skin may be powdered with flour and the area wrapped with dry cotton.

Mustard plasters are usually placed on the chest to draw out mucus congestion, dispel coldness, aid asthma, eliminate coughs and heal colds and flus. It can also be placed where needed to treat body and joint pains and heal watery, oozing and chronic sores or boils.

Onion Plaster

Onions are a natural antibiotic and so aid infections and inflammations. Made into a plaster and placed over the lungs, they are a tremendous aid to pneumonia, lung infection, bronchial inflammation and asthma and will clear the lungs of mucus congestion and coldness. Slice 3 large onions (preferably organic) and steam or saute in a little water until slightly soft. Follow plaster steps.

Salt Plaster

A *salt* plaster is good for aching or sore muscles and joints. Place heated salt in a bag and apply directly to the sore places of the body. Many find relief from knee pains, arthritis or tennis elbow with this remedy. The salt bag may also be tied to the feet at night and held in the hands to ease arthritis in these areas.

Tofu Plaster

A *tofu* plaster is specific in lowering fevers, helping head wounds, concussion, headache and earache. Because it is very cooling, it should only be applied to the head and neck areas and left on until the fever drops or the ache goes away. Muramoto in *Healing Ourselves* claims 100% effectiveness for cerebral hemorrhage with tofu plaster if applied within 48 hours of the injury.

Wrap 1/4 to 1/2 lb tofu in cheesecloth and squeeze out any remaining liquid. Make the plaster with 1/5 part pastry flour and 1/10 part grated fresh ginger root. Apply as a plaster to desired location.

Poultices

A poultice is an herbal pack applied directly on the skin. It is useful for inflammations, bites, stings, skin eruptions or cancers, pain, infections, pus and wounds, to soften and mature boils and ulcers and to cleanse and heal the skin. A *comfrey* poultice is the most effective remedy I have ever found to get rid of spider bites. It also takes away itching and pain.

Cabbage Poultice

A *cabbage* poultice is detoxifying and stimulates the blood circulation, bringing in a fresh supply of blood to the area applied. Placed over the liver it will break up congestion and detoxify. Placed over the lower abdomen it treats genito-reproductive disorders.

Clean 8 whole cabbage leaves and lightly steam. Then place over the affected area by overlapping them in layers, like laying shingles. Cover with a towel and heat source as in any poultice. If used over the liver, leave on for only 10 minutes the first time and slowly work up to longer as its effects could be too strong until things start moving and the liver starts detoxifying.

Potato Poultice

A *potato* poultice is good for drawing out toxins and fluids from the part of the body where placed. Though not as strongly effective as albi (taro potato), it is easier to obtain. Use the raw grated potato.

Poultice for Painful and Swollen Joints

This is effective in relieving pain and reducing swelling in joints. Combine:

3 parts	*plantain* and *comfrey*
1 part	*marshmallow root* and *lobelia*
1/8 part	*cayenne*

Add enough *honey/wheat germ oil* mixture to form a paste, and apply as a poultice.

Powders

Powders may be used as is and not always put in capsules or rice papers. For instance, powdered echinacea and goldenseal are healing when sprinkled on infections, inflammations and spider bites. I successfully used this combination on my son's umbilicus after the cord was removed to prevent infection, and many friends have found echinacea powder to be equal to comfrey poultices in drawing out the poisons in spider and other insect bites. Powders may also be made of combined herbs for other uses, such as the following:

Composition Powder

This powder was named by Dr. John Christopher (one of the foremost herbalists in this country at the start of the herbal renaissance) and has since been known this way even though the herbs may somewhat vary. The powder is comprised of several very stimulating herbs which activate the circulation, open the pores and cause sweating to occur. As such, it is valuable in preventing and healing colds, flus, sore throats, coughs, bronchitis and other lung and mucus conditions. It is most effective when taken directly as a powder mixed in hot water and sipped slowly. It may also be taken in capsule, pill or tablet form. One composition powder recipe is as follows:

1 part	*ginger, cinnamon, bayberry bark* and *clove*
1/2 part	*cayenne, licorice*
1/4 part	*marshmallow*

Toothpowder

A toothpowder made from your own personalized combination of herbs can be very healing. I have one friend who prevented gum surgery by just brushing her teeth daily with cayenne powder. Because this is extremely stimulating, it may be better to combine the cayenne with other herbs. The following recipe is effective in healing inflamed or bleeding gums, alleviating tooth and gum infections, tightening the gums and whitening the teeth:

Combine equal parts: *myrrh, cinnamon, bayberry bark, horsetail* and *echinacea*. Add 1/2 parts *prickly ash, cayenne* and *baking soda*. *Dentie* and/or *salt* may also be added in 1/2 part amounts if desired. The horsetail is a key herb to use since it is high in silicon which helps in calcium absorption and has a mild scouring effect on the enamel, which whitens the teeth. Cinnamon also whitens and stimulates blood circulation along with cayenne and prickly ash. Bayberry bark stimulates and tightens teeth and gums. Echinacea and myrrh fight infections and inflammations.

Footpowders

Powders may also be used on the feet for fungus or itch or to keep the feet warm. For fungus, combine 1 ounce powdered *black walnut hulls* (a strong antiseptic), 1/2 ounce powdered *calamus root* (a deodorizer) and 1/4 ounce *sage* (an antiseptic and deodorizer). Powder this combination on the feet and toes before putting the socks on for the day.

For stimulating the circulation in the toes and feet, especially when outdoors on a cold day, first put on a thin pair of inner socks, then sprinkle a teaspoon of *cayenne pepper* into a thicker pair of outer socks. Next, put these on over the inner socks. Many people have remarked about how effective this is in keeping their feet warm!

Salves

A salve is a thick herbal oil that can be put on the skin and left there. Used for bites, stings, cuts, sores, scrapes, burns and other skin problems, salves heal the skin quickly. They also reduce pain and eliminate itching almost immediately. Whenever my child gets a cut or scrape, he asks me to put salve on it right away. Then after it has been on a few minutes, he usually forgets the hurt was ever there! Salve works especially well for me, too, on mosquito bites, cuts, sores and much more.

Salves can be made with fresh, dried, whole or powdered herbs. They are easy to use: place your finger in the salve and spread it on the sensitive area. Salves are a good first aid remedy to have on hand or to take on a trip.

Sore Muscles

To help sore, aching muscles, combine equal parts of: *chamomile, carnation, elder, gardenia, lavender, mint, mugwort, mullein flower, rose, rosemary* and *St. John's wort.*

Itching and Rashes

This is a single herb salve made only of fresh *chickweed*. It is even more powerful if you can extract the juice from the fresh chickweed and use along with the fresh chickweed herb.

Healing Salve

This is useful in the treatment of all skin rashes, swellings, wounds, eruptions and bites. Combine:

1 part	*echinacea, yarrow, comfrey* and *calendula*
1/2 part	*plantain leaves, mugwort* and *chickweed*

Syrups

A syrup is used to treat coughs and sore throats, relieve tickling and irritation of the throat, loosen phlegm, facilitate expectoration and heal and soothe the throat and lungs. Syrups work well for these situations because they coat the area and keep the herbs in direct contact with problem areas.

Herbal syrups are usually a delicious way to take herbs. When I have a bottle of herbal cough syrup out on the counter, my little boy often fakes a cough just so he can take some! I think you will find them delicious, too.

Cough and Sore Throat Syrup

This formula aids mucus expectoration, calms coughs and soothes the throat. Use equal parts: *elecampane, wild cherry bark, licorice, comfrey root, coltsfoot* and *lobelia.*

Stubborn Cough Syrup

For especially stubborn coughs or deep lung ailments, combine 1 cup *lemon juice* (fresh squeezed preferable), 5-7 cloves of pressed or minced *garlic,* 1 tbsp grated *ginger* and 1/2 tsp *cayenne* powder. Take in tablespoon doses frequently or as needed. This works very well for coughs, bronchitis, pneumonia and mucus and lung congestion due to coldness.

Onion Syrup

This is very beneficial for mucus congestion, coughs, bronchitis, colds and flus. Blend 1 medium minced *onion* with enough *lemon juice* to cover and 1/8-1/4 cup *honey* or brown sugar. A little *cayenne pepper* may be added if desired.

Teas

Herbs that have a mild flavor and are taken internally are usually made into tea. Herbal teas can be taken medicinally and also as a beverage. I enjoy a cup of herbal tea daily.

Teas are made from fresh or dried herbs, either cut or whole. If you are using a fresh herb, it should first be rubbed between the palms of your hands, or broken up in a mortar and pestle (called "bruising" the herb), to help release its active ingredients. Powdered herbs can be used in a pinch, but they do not taste as good and are gritty in tea form.

Teas should be made in such non-metallic containers as glass, earthenware or enamel pots. Stainless steel is all right to use if the others are not available. Whenever possible, spring or purified water, rather than tap water, should be used.

There are two basic methods of preparing teas: infusion and decoction. An infusion is used with delicate plant parts: flowers and soft leaves. It is also used with herbs that have strong smells and contain volatile oils, such as mint. Decoctions are used with herb parts that are sturdy and need to be broken down: course leaves, stems, roots and barks. Herbs that do not have much smell or volatile oils are also used in this way. Decocting herbs dissipates any volatile oils.

Aduki Bean Tea (Juice)

Aduki beans are very healing for any kidney trouble and symptoms related to kidney problems such as swelling. Decoct 2 1/2 cups aduki beans in 5 cups water for one hour. Strain out juice (the beans may be used as food), and drink 1/2 cup aduki bean juice 1/2 hour before meals for two or more days.

Black Bean Tea (Juice)

Black bean juice is effective for treating laryngitis, hoarseness, lung complaints and convalescence. Decoct 2 1/2 cups black beans in 5 cups water for one hour. Strain out the juice (the beans may be further cooked and eaten as food) and drink 1/2 cup black bean juice 1/2 hour before meals for two or more days.

Chai Tea

Chai is a delicious tea traditionally enjoyed in India. Because it is quite spicy and stimulating, it is good for poor circulation, coldness, low appetite, poor digestion, gas, bloatedness and colds. It is also a wonderful winter beverage as a preventative to these conditions. I know people who make up a big pot of it at a time and drink it as their main winter tea daily. For those with heat signs of any sort, it may be too spicy and so should be avoided.

To make: combine 1 ounce fresh grated *ginger*, 7 *peppercorns*, 1 *cinnamon stick*, 5 *cloves*, 15 *cardamom seeds* and one *orange peel* with 1 pint of water. Cover the pot, heat and simmer for 10 minutes. Add 1/2 cup milk and simmer covered another 10 minutes. Strain and sweeten with honey. It is usually made with black tea in India. However, for those who do not want to ingest the caffeine, make it with herbs alone.

Ginger Tea

Ginger tea is useful for indigestion, gas, flus, colds, sore throats, poor circulation, coughs, lung congestion, low energy and lack of appetite. If used at the first sign of any of these ailments it will generally knock them out of the system. After a condition has developed or ripened, the tea should be ingested several times a day until the problem goes away. Ginger tea is made by grating 2 inches of the fresh

ginger root to yield 1-1/2 ounces grated root and making it into an infusion with 1 pint of water.

Kuzu Root Tea

Kuzu root is widely known as a thickening agent for sauces. Yet it has many medicinal qualities which cure colds, heal weak intestines, neutralize acidity, relieve body pain and relax tight muscles. For these conditions, make a tea by dissolving 1 teaspoon of kuzu in 1 cup cold water (it will lump in warm water). Add one teaspoon of soy sauce. Cook over low heat for 3-5 minutes. Drink 1 cup about an hour before meals and throughout the day on an empty stomach.

Sometimes the kuzu root is added to some bancha tea along with a little umeboshi plum. This tea is good for soothing the digestion, neutralizing acidity, picking up low energy and fatigue, helping ward off intestinal and pulmonary colds and flus and alleviating hangovers (for which it is traditionally used in Japan).

Mung Bean Tea

Mung bean tea is helpful in relieving hypertension and lowering blood pressure. Steep two tablespoons of mung beans in 1 cup boiling water for 20 minutes. Then strain and drink 1 cup 3-5 times a day. The beans can be reused several times for a tea and finally eaten at the end of the day. By then they should be sufficiently cooked.

Scallion-Ginger Tea

For the common cold, make a tea using 2 *scallions* (the white part) and 1 tsp. fresh grated *ginger root* to one cup of water. Drink freely as needed.

Walnut Tea

Walnuts strengthen the blood, overcome debility and tonify the kidneys, liver and brain. They are good for relieving coughs, aiding intestinal smoothness, seminal emission in men, dry and withering skin, white hair, weight loss, forgetfulness, insomnia and neurasthenia.

To make walnut tea add 1 tsp walnut powder (grind chopped walnuts in a nut and seed or coffee grinder) to 1 cup boiling water and drink before meals several times a day. The powder or crushed whole walnuts may be added to soups and foods to benefit the above conditions, also.

Tinctures

In a tincture the medicinal parts of herbs are extracted and preserved by one of the solvents alcohol, vinegar or glycerine. They are useful for bitter tasting herbs, those too strong to drink in teas or for herbs taken over a long period of time. They are good for herbs which do not extract well in water but do better in alcohol.

Antibiotic Tincture

An excellent formula to use as a natural antibiotic, antiseptic, blood purifier and lymphatic cleanser contains equal parts of fresh *garlic*, *echinacea root*, *goldenseal root*, fresh *nasturtium* (whole plant—this may be left out if it cannot be located).

Cyclone Cider

This vinegar tincture is good for sinus infections, colds, flus, mucus congestion and lung complaints. Use equal parts: *onion*, *garlic*, fresh *ginger* and *horseradish roots*, *mustard seeds* and *black pepper corns*. Grate the fresh herbs, combine the seeds and corns, then add 6-8 whole chilies. Make the vinegar tincture, then strain and add 1 part honey or glycerine to 3 parts vinegar extract mixture (heat it first). Take 1 teaspoon to 1 tablespoon every hour.

Additional Remedies

Ashes

Ashes are specific for stopping bleeding and hemorrhage, both internally and externally. They can be sprinkled on the skin or body wound, or taken 1/2 teaspoon per cup of water for internal bleeding or hemorrhage. (For severe or dangerous cases of any sort of bleeding, or bleeding which will not stop in a reasonable time, be sure to consult your family healer.)

Dentie, an ash made from the *calyx of eggplant*, also works well to stop bleeding as do fireplace ashes and the leftover ashes from burning moxibustion (a therapy described in the chapter on *Home Therapies* which burns the herb mugwort). Yet, in a pinch, the ash from burning some strands of human hair will work effectively. To do this, cut off enough hair to yield 1/2 teaspoon of ash, probably a 1" by 3" section. The hair does not need to be that of the person bleeding; anyone's hair will do.

Using ashes to stop bleeding is a valuable cure which has been traditionally known and used by people in China for thousands of years. In fact, one Chinese folk tale includes a monster who stops the wounds on his hands from bleeding by thrusting them into the cool ashes of a fireplace! (Because most fireplace ashes today result from newspaper, they might be toxic and best not used.)

DENTIE. This is an ash made by preserving the *calyx of an eggplant*. One part eggplant calyx and 1/5 part salt are placed in a closed jar and left for several years, then dried and charcoaled. The resulting ash, when used to brush the teeth each evening, will cure any toothache, pyorrhea and other mouth and gum disorders. The ash can also be applied externally, or internally ingested, to stop any kind of bleeding. Since it takes so long to make, you may want to purchase it already prepared from your local health food or macrobiotic supply store.

Charcoal

Charcoal is very effective in eliminating occasional gas and bloating from poor digestion. At times gas can be extremely painful, and it may seem like some other major problem is occurring in the abdomen instead. Ingesting some charcoal at these times alleviates the pain, eliminates the gas and reduces the bloating. This remedy is not suitable for long-term use. If you have gas all the time, the deeper underlying cause needs to be addressed.

Charcoal may be purchased from drug stores in tablet form and chewed when needed. However, for emergency purposes, it is also possible to burn toast until it is black and use the scrapings from it as the charcoal. To take, swallow a tablespoon of the charcoal scrapings with a little warm water.

Egg Oil

This is considered to be an excellent remedy for a weak heart. Roast the yolks of 5 eggs in a frying pan until black. At this stage the oil will emerge. Take one half teaspoon of the oil daily for a long period of time.

Moxibustion Smoke

The burning of certain herbs, usually mugwort, which are then applied to the body is called moxibustion. While described in the chapter on *Home Therapies*, I wanted to mention it here because the specific use of its smoke is beneficial in treating sinus infections and blockages.

For this, one may obtain dried mugwort in an herb store. Light the herb, then blow out the flame and keep the herbs smoking by periodically fanning with your hand. Then close one nostril and inhale the smoke into the open nostril. Next close that nostril and inhale smoke into the other nostril. Continue alternating in this way for about 5 minutes. Repeat two to three more times until the problem is gone.

It is also possible to use the smoke from a moxibustion stick. It is used in the same way as the loose mugwort, but may be a little harder to obtain.

Rice

RAW BROWN RICE. To remove intestinal parasites, eat a tablespoon or two of raw brown rice first thing each morning for a week or two. One may also eat raw brown rice in this way to prevent intestinal parasites while traveling in those countries where they abound. The natives in the Himalayas do this as a matter of course in daily life.

RICE CONGEE. Rice congee is a tonic soup which is very easy to digest and assimilate. It is especially useful for those recovering from disease or surgery, or for those who are weak, tired, have poor digestion or experience gas and bloatedness after eating. It is also useful to help people who can not digest any grains or carbohydrates at all. Rice congee will help them begin doing so.

The congee may be made plain, or a variety of tonic herbs such as *ginseng, dong quai, astragalus, lycii berries, jujube dates* or other Chinese tonic herbs may be added to create a valuable tonic for the whole body. Herbs combined with food in this way are best used in the treatment of all deficiency diseases including weakness, tiredness, low appetite, lowered immunity, depression and poor digestion and assimilation.

To make *rice* congee, combine 1 cup rice with 9 cups water and cook over low heat slowly for about 9 hours, until the rice is broken down and forms a thick soup. If herbs are to be included, add at the beginning and cook down with the rice. Then strain out before eating the congee.

Salt Tonic

SALT. A *salt* tonic is made by adding a pinch of salt to an herbal tea. In this way it acts as a tonic for the urinary tract and as a carrier for the other herbs in the formula, bringing their action to the kidneys. Since the kidneys are the "residence" of the entire body's energy and resistance, it is important to preserve and strengthen their functions.

SESAME SALT (GOMASIO). This is a delicious seasoning for foods which is also a tonic for the heart and body. One teaspoon of this salt can be taken nightly by people suffering from heart weakness. It is also beneficial for heartburn and headache (take as these occur). In those who feel cold, weak and tired, a sprinkling of sesame salt on food daily will help strengthen the body.

Sesame salt does not create thirst, as the oil from the sesame seeds coats the salt, preventing it from causing an excessive attraction for water. The oil helps the salt enter the cells when necessary. Sesame salt can be made using different proportions, from 1:5 to 1:12 (salt to sesame seeds). Try 1:8 to start, and if it is too strong, change the proportion according to your taste and needs.

First roast sea salt in a pan until a faint odor of chlorine rises from salt. Then roast sesame seeds in a pan, continuously stirring, until they have popped for about 10 minutes. Then combine salt and seeds according to your chosen ratio in a suribachi (a nut and seed or coffee grinder will do) and stir constantly with a wooden pestle until most of the seeds have been crushed.

Variations of gomasio are made in other countries. The Arabs eat a mixture of dried powdered thyme and coriander seeds mixed with gomasio. They eat this with olive oil on bread. It is quite delicious and has actually become the gomasio staple in our household. I am told by some people who live in Israel that the people there combine sesame seeds and salt with hyssop for a similar seasoning.

Home remedies are valuable preparations for healing and health maintenance. Along with remedies, there are many wonderful therapies which can also assist in the healing process. These may or may not include herbs. The next chapter gives many valuable home therapies.

Home Therapies

Therapies are modalities we can employ in our homes for healing and preventative health. Quite often it is not enough to just take herbs internally. Rather, therapies are needed as important supplementary healing approaches. These help correct any internal imbalances which cause the illness as well as speed up the healing process.

Many therapies have been used around the world and by various cultures for thousands of years. Some are shared by different cultures although located quite far apart, such as sweating therapy. Others are unique to the culture itself, such as dermal hammer. Some therapies treat the subtle aspects of our beings more directly, affecting states of consciousness, acting as magnets and utilizing the more subtle energies of plant life. While some therapies have direct effects on the body, others are less physically tangible.

Breathing Exercises: The Four Purifications[1]

The Four Purifications are a set of breathing exercises which are extremely beneficial to the body, mind and spirit. Consisting of four different breathing techniques, they calm the body, quiet the mind, energize and rejuvenate the entire body and mind, tone the lungs, blood, circulation, brain, internal organs and heart and give strength to the whole body. Interestingly, in Chinese medicine the lungs are considered responsible in part for giving the body strength. The lungs have always been associated with air and its essential and vital life-giving properties.

These breathing exercises purify the nerve channels in the body, clear and stimulate the digestive system and strengthen the nervous system. Thus, they aid such ailments as nervousness, insomnia, indigestion, lung and breathing problems, poor circulation, low energy and vitality, fatigue, lethargy and poor memory. As such, they are invaluable for helping the body recover from many health problems.

For those who have never done any breathing practices, these four techniques are safe to do. For those already doing their own form of breathing practices, these are a perfect adjunct and starting exercise. Sit quietly with your back straight either in a chair with your feet on the floor or on the floor with your legs crossed. For those who desire, you may concentrate your attention on the space between the eyebrows while doing these exercises.

The four breathing techniques are: alternate nostril breathing, skull shining, fire wash and horse mudra. Do them in the order given. After practicing them for a few months, move on to the intermediate method described at the end, if you so desire.

Alternate Nostril Breathing (*Nadishodhana*)

Begin by gently exhaling all air. Then close the right nostril with the thumb of the right hand and inhale slowly and deeply through the left nostril. When finished, close the left nostril with the ring finger of the right hand, releasing the thumb, and exhale slowly and fully through the right nostril. Next, immediately inhale through the right nostril in a slow and steady

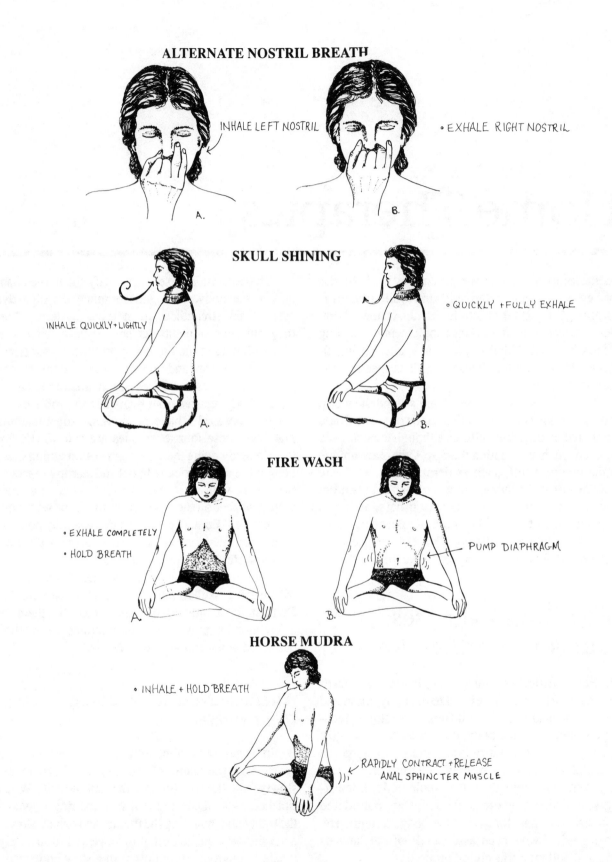

ALTERNATE NOSTRIL BREATH

INHALE LEFT NOSTRIL

∘ EXHALE RIGHT NOSTRIL

A.

B.

SKULL SHINING

INHALE QUICKLY + LIGHTLY

∘ QUICKLY + FULLY EXHALE

A.

B.

FIRE WASH

∘ EXHALE COMPLETELY

∘ HOLD BREATH

PUMP DIAPHRAGM

A.

B.

HORSE MUDRA

∘ INHALE + HOLD BREATH

RAPIDLY CONTRACT + RELEASE
ANAL SPHINCTER MUSCLE

manner. Finally, close the right nostril with the right thumb again, releasing the ring finger, and exhale through the left nostril. This completes one round. Begin with ten rounds and gradually increase to forty.

This exercise alone is extremely beneficial to the body. It is very quieting to the mind and strengthens the nervous system. It induces a wonderfully calm state, releases nervous tension, anxiety, agitation, anger and other disruptive emotions, and helps you sleep better. It also oxygenates the system, thus aiding in the circulation of energy and blood in the body. This in turn stimulates the proper functioning of all the internal organs. Continued practice of alternate nostril breathing will strengthen the lungs and breath control.

Skull Shining (*Kapala Bhati*)

Skull shining is a series of forced exhalations with the breath. Begin by inhaling quickly and lightly through both nostrils. Then quickly and fully exhale all the breath through both nostrils. Emphasize the exhale, letting the inhalation come as a natural reflex. Repeat this pattern for one round consisting of thirty exhalations. After each round, which should last no longer than one minute, rest and breath naturally. Then repeat the round. Begin with three rounds of thirty exhalations each and gradually increase to ten rounds of sixty exhalations each.

This method purifies the head area which calms the thoughts and the breath and aids the mind. As in alternate nostril breathing, skull shining helps release nervous tension, balance the emotions and circulate energy and blood in the body. It also strengthens the lungs and breath control.

Caution: Persons with high blood pressure or lung disease should not practice skull shining.

Fire Wash (*Agnisara Dhauti*)

This exercise is performed with all the air held out of the body. Begin by taking a normal inhalation and exhalation, letting all the air out from the body. Then while holding the breath out, pull the diaphragm up and toward the backbone and next release it suddenly. Repeat this in-and-out movement rapidly, as

long as the breath can be held out without strain, about thirty pulls. Then inhale gently. This makes one round. Start with three rounds, gradually increasing to ten. Begin with thirty pulls per breath and work up to sixty. It is helpful to lean the body forward resting the hands on your knees.

This method strengthens the "navel lock" frequently used in breathing exercises and creates heat at the navel center (manipura chakra), which purifies the nerve channels, stimulates the digestive system, increases gastric fire, strengthens the lungs and alleviates indigestion, abdominal diseases and menstrual disorders.

Horse Mudra (*Ashvini Mudra*)

This fourth exercise is an internal movement of the anal sphincter muscle. Begin by inhaling a complete and full breath and hold the breath in. Bend the head forward and press the chin tightly into the hollow of the neck while holding the breath (called *jalandhara bandha*—throat lock). Then contract and release the anal sphincter muscle rapidly and repeatedly. Hold the breath only so long as the following exhalation can be slow and controlled. Do not force your breath or length of holding. Begin with three rounds of thirty pulls each and increase gradually to ten rounds of sixty each. The horse mudra strengthens mula bandha, the anal lock, which increases concentration, strengthens the reproductive glands and stimulates the gastric fire.

Intermediate Method

After performing the Four Purifications regularly for two to three months and when feeling comfortable with them, one may undertake the intermediate method. In the intermediate method, the Four Purifications are done in such a way that there are no "resting breaths" in between; that is, they are done consecutively without a breath or rest in between.

To do this, do ten to thirty rounds of alternate nostril breathing. After the last exhalation through the left nostril, inhale partially and immediately begin skull shining. At the end of one series of skull shining exhalations, inhale slowly and completely, then exhale all air, hold the breath out and do the fire wash. After a round of the fire wash, inhale completely, hold the breath and do the horse mudra. This entire series now completes one round.

After the horse mudra, exhale completely and immediately begin again with alternate nostril breathing, thus starting the next round. Do five rounds, gradually increasing the numbers of alternate nostril breathing and the duration of retention in each of the other three techniques.

Cupping

Cupping is a technique which was (and may still be) widely used by folk people in Europe as well as China. Cupping can be seen in the movie, *Zorba the Greek*, and can be read about in *Every Month Was May*, by Evelyn Eaton when she experienced it in France in the '40s.

Cupping is the treatment of disease by suction of the skin surface. A vacuum is created in small jars which are then attached to the body surface. The vacuum causes a drawing up of the underlying tissues into the cups, pulling inner congestion in the body up and out. When effective in its job, the skin will appear reddened and bruised after the cup is removed. This marking can take several days to disappear, but it will go away. The person should notice an immediate difference in condition, be it congestion or pain.

To do cupping, you will need several jars or cups with even and smooth rims. Good cups to use are the small votive candle holders easily found where candles are purchased. However, wine glasses or other light weight and thin glasses may be used. Bamboo cups are effective, too. Cups may also be purchased at the supply stores written at the end of this lesson. You will also need some cotton balls, forceps or other metal holder or stick for the cotton, or alternately a candle and some rubbing alcohol and matches.

Have the person and all your tools in place before starting. Then attach the cotton ball to the stick, tweezers or forceps and dip in alcohol. Hold the cup so its mouth opening is down or the flame can burn

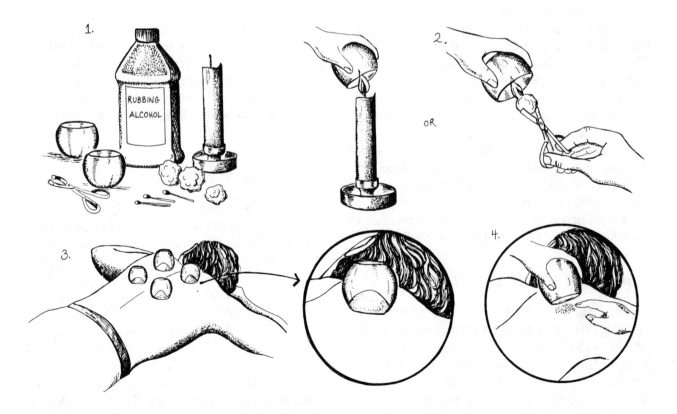

your hand. Ignite the cotton and, while burning, insert it into the mouth of the cup. If you are using a candle, hold the cup over the flame for a short time, then quickly place on the skin as above. This will evacuate some of the air, causing a partial vacuum within the cup. Withdraw the cotton stick and quickly place the mouth of the cup firmly against the skin at the desired location. Suction should hold it in place. Check by lightly tugging at the cup.

Be careful not to leave the lit cotton stick in the cup too long as this will cause a hot cup and could burn the person. Conversely, if the lit cotton is not left in long enough, suction will not occur and the cup will fall off when tugged gently. Practice will yield desired results, and it is easier to do than it may sound.

To remove, let air into the cup by holding it in the left hand and pressing the skin at the rim of the jar with the right. You may need to gently slide your pressing finger down and under the rim in order to break the seal. The cup should then pop off.

Cups should be retained in place from 5 to 15 minutes, depending on the strength of suction. Especially in hot weather, or when cupping over shallow flesh, the duration of treatment should not be too long. Often I have seen the cups pop off for no apparent reason. If the suction was good in the first place, then generally this is an indication that suction is not needed in that place, or there was too much body hair for the cup to hold. It is also possible for the cup to remain in place and still be unnecessary, and, if so, no redness or bruising will occur. Bruises occurring under the cups indicate where the congestion has been. I have also seen blisters appear which should be dressed and treated to prevent infection.

Cupping is done over areas where there is swelling, pain or congestion, either of energy, blood or mucus. Thus, it is good for edema, swellings, asthma, bronchitis, dull aches and pains, arthritis, abdominal pain, stomachache, indigestion, headache, low back pain, painful menstruation, coughs from excessive mucus, and places where bodily movement is limited and painful.

Cautions: Cupping should not be done during high fever, convulsions or cramps, or over allergic skin conditions, ulcerated sores, or on the abdomen or lower back of pregnant women. It will also be ineffective over areas with irregular body angles, where the muscles are thin, the skin is not level or where there is a lot of body hair.

For Supplies: Cups may be purchased from Chinese medical suppliers, some of which are listed in the Appendix, *Herbal Resource Guide.*

Dermal Hammer

A dermal hammer is an acupuncture tool which has a long handle supporting a head which holds a cluster of small individual needles. The needles are not sharp, but dull, and they can puncture the skin or not depending on the use. Several needles striking the skin simultaneously cause less pain and stimulate a wider surface area than does a single needle. They are more suitable for use on small children, those sensitive to pain and those who desire to treat themselves.

Other names for dermal hammers are seven star needle and plum-blossom needle, both having a different number and arrangement of needles. They may be purchased at acupuncture supply stores listed in the Appendix, *Herbal Resource Guide.* As an alternative, you can make a similar device by bundling together about 25-50 toothpicks and binding them with a rubber band.

The dermal hammer is rarely used over a single point, but rather is applied over a broad area, tapping across the skin more in the manner of pecking than puncturing. Where an area has been stimulated, the skin becomes reddened and moist. In general, it should not be painful or cause bleeding.

Dermal hammers are tapped over local areas of pain and congestion, over numbness, areas of hair loss, around sites of wounds and localized diseases, blocked areas where energy and blood do not flow, aches, spasms and local skin diseases. If acupuncture meridians are known, tapping can occur on the meridian following its flow to cause an effect to its corresponding internal organ. With this approach many internal and chronic diseases can be treated, such as headache, dizziness, vertigo, insomnia, menstrual disorders, hypertension and gastrointestinal disorders. Any acupressure or shiastu book should give diagrams and instructions on acupuncture meridians.

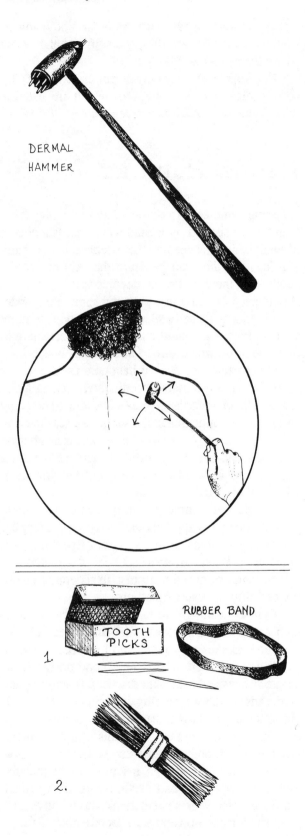

DERMAL
HAMMER

RUBBER BAND

TOOTH
PICKS

1.

2.

To use, hold the dermal hammer by its handle 1-2 inches from the skin, then lightly and repeatedly tap over the desired area with a flexible movement of the wrist. If you know acupuncture points or meridians it may be done over them, but just the general area to be treated will do. The tapping should be done continuously for 5-10 minutes, until the skin becomes red and moist. **Do not break the skin and cause bleeding.** (If you do, the dermal hammer must be sterilized before using on someone else.) Treatment may be repeated several times a day for many days or until the problem is alleviated.

If many areas of the body are to be treated or acupuncture meridians used, then generally the tapping follows a traditional sequence, which is: first do the center of the body, then the sides; first do the top of the body, then move down to the feet; first do the back, then the front. This sequence is traditional, whether using needles, moxa or dermal hammer.

Sterilization: Dermal hammers should be sterilized by cooking in a pressure cooker at 15 lbs pressure for 20 minutes before and after each use.

Cautions: Do not use on anyone who has a blood-carrying disease, such as AIDS. Do not break the skin and cause bleeding. If you are experimenting with the dermal hammer and cause the skin to bleed, be sure to sterilize it before using it on someone else. Do not use in areas where there are ulcerations or traumatic injuries, or during acute infectious disease or acute abdominal disorders.

For Supplies: Dermal hammers may be purchased from Chinese medical suppliers, some of which are listed in the Appendix, *Herbal Resource Guide*.

Enema Therapy

Enemas are important because of their ability to help eliminate many varieties of disease. The herbalist often sees the colon as the organ which must ultimately take the brunt of all our dietary excesses and deficiencies. Toxic wastes, when improperly eliminated from the colon, will accumulate along the inner lining and possibly harden to form gas pockets, becoming a natural breeding ground for the cultivation of undesirable parasites and bacteria.

With improper elimination, some of the wastes are reabsorbed back into the tissues of the body and are the primary cause of many chronic diseases. This can occur even if the person is having a daily bowel movement since this may still not be a complete elimination. Instead, the wastes gradually collect over a period of time and cause imbalance in the body's chemistry and electro-biological energy.

The function of the colon happens as a result of a neurological wave-like peristaltic motion. Because its action is movement, it involves the essence of vital nerve energy, and the peristaltic motion of the colon is then a general reflection of the tone of the entire body's nervous system. This peristaltic motion partially happens as a reaction to a naturally occurring irritation of bile which was previously secreted from the liver through the gallbladder into the small intestine.

The colon is known to harbor certain beneficial forms of micro-organisms which help in the breakdown of waste products. If undesirable strains of these microorganisms, or an unfavorable balance of beneficial bacteria, are allowed to develop, then the root of a disease process can be established.

Often it is not the bacteria directly which harm the body, but the bacterial wastes circulating or lodging themselves in surrounding tissues which are responsible for the development of other undesirable and harmful bacteria and viruses that then take hold at the place of least resistance in the body. Therefore, at the base of many acute and chronic illnesses is a toxic and imbalanced intestinal environment.

Enemas can have the effects of eliminating, calming, sedating, nourishing, cleansing and toning the entire digestive system. They are useful for alleviating and curing bodily pains, indigestion, gas, toxicity, colds, constipation, parasites, prolapsed colon and hemorrhoids, arthritis, rheumatism, fevers, hypertension, poor digestion and assimilation, nervousness and irritability to mention a few conditions, while the direct effect of enemas is to eliminate fecal waste and gas from the lower bowel.

Enemas can be given daily for 7 days in the Spring or Fall, with or without fasting or a special diet. Otherwise, they should be given no more than two to three times a week for therapeutic purposes, and/or once a month for preventive health mainte-

nance. Excessive and habitual reliance on enemas can cause weakness and should be avoided when it isn't necessary, especially by those who are already thin, weak or feel cold.

Individuals who have a strong constitution and/ or disease can be given eliminating enema therapy. Individuals with weak constitutions or disease can be given nutritive enema therapy. If an individual is unable to digest or eat, s/he can be sustained by regular injections of nutritive enemas consisting of meat, chicken, vegetable or grain soups which have been strained.

Administering Enemas

First, make the chosen enema formula, either a tea, soup or other liquid. Have all materials ready and at hand when you begin. Be sure the enema liquid is lukewarm right before using. If too cool or too warm it can actually cause gas and discomfort.

Fill the enema bottle first with one quart of tepid salt water and suspend it about 3 feet above you. Grease the tip with a little Vaseline or oil for smooth insertion. Now, lie on your back on the bathroom floor with the knees bent slightly and insert the tube into the rectum.

After inserting, allow the fluid to slowly enter the colon. If it stalls, it can be lightly squeezed, but it is better to avoid forcing the fluid into the colon too rapidly. After the entire amount is in, the tube is removed and you try to retain the fluid for 10-20 minutes. For some people it may be difficult to retain at first. With practice is becomes easier.

To encourage the solution to penetrate all areas of the colon, change position by first laying on the left side and then on the right side. Lightly massage the abdomen if desired, moving in a clockwise circular motion from the navel outward. This first solution is voided after about 10 to 20 minutes.

Then inject one cup of sesame oil, unless oil is already included with the prescribed enema solution. The oil will help dislodge the stuck fecal matter clinging to the sides of the colon and help the penetration of the remaining solution into all parts. Lastly, administer the prescribed enema, unless this has already been done in place of the straight oil.

Oils for Enemas

Many kinds of enemas are given using herbs, oils, soups and nutritional liquid substances, such as wheat grass juice or meat or chicken soup. These offset the possible depleting aspects of an enema while helping in the elimination process. Oils, such as sesame or castor, are specifically useful in enemas since they are calming to the nervous system. In general, oils are useful for the lining of the bowels and entire digestive tract as they help to improve suppleness, motility and digestive power.

Herbs for Enemas

The following list of useful herbs has been categorized into bitter, astringent, spicy and calming herbs. Bitter herbs aid in the release of bile, help parasites, hypertension, fevers and heat. The astringent herbs tone the intestinal tissue and aid in prolapse and hemorrhoids. Spicy herbs stimulate the circulation, aid digestion and eliminate gas. Calming herbs alleviate gas and calm the nervous system. Herbs from the four categories may be combined according to one's individual needs.

Bitter herbs: *wormwood, gentian, yarrow, turmeric, golden seal, oregon grape root, aloe, willow bark*

Astringent herbs: *comfrey root, slippery elm, bayberry bark, myrrh, cranesbill*

Spicy herbs: *black* and *red peppers, ginger, mustard seeds, cardamom, basil, oregano, marjoram, thyme, prickly ash, garlic, onion*

Calming herbs: *lavender, catnip, comfrey, valerian root*

A Balanced Enema Formula

Following is a most useful enema for diseases such as weak digestion, constipation, arthritis, rheumatism, cancer, leucorrhea, spermatorrhea and bladder and kidney diseases. It is best to give this enema for 7 consecutive days, which is all right to do as a special treatment once or twice a year. This is a traditional Ayurvedic (East Indian) recipe.

> 2 ounces anise seeds
> 1 ounce rock salt or
>   roasted sea salt (turned yellow)
> 1-1/2 quarts water
> 4 ounces sesame oil
> 4 ounces honey
> 1 ounce castor oil

Boil anise seed and salt from 3 to 5 minutes in water. Then strain and add remaining ingredients, stirring all together. Allow to cool to lukewarm temperature before inserting.

Specific Enemas—Eliminative

Parasites: Equal parts *garlic, wormwood* and *bayberry bark* in a tea.

Prolapsed colon and hemorrhoids: Equal parts *comfrey root, oak bark* and *prickly ash*.

Fevers, hypertension, excessive feelings of heat and burning: use herbs which are bitter, cooling, demulcent, calming, antispasmodic, nervine and sweet, such as *licorice root, slippery elm, catnip, valerian, basil, yarrow, marshmallow root, lobelia* and *chamomile*.

Specific Enemas—Nutritive

Weak digestion and assimilation, deficiency of favorable bacteria to aid in breakdown of food: use *fermented barley* or *whole grain water, tamari soy sauce* mixed with warm water, and *citrus rind* tea. The tea of any of these should be combined with a tea of *marrow, meat, chicken, sesame* or *olive oil, ghee* (clarified butter) and *salt*.

Nervousness and irritability: *catnip, comfrey leaf, valerian root, basil* combined with *sesame* or *olive oil, salt, honey* and a small amount of *castor oil*.

Wasting and general debility: soups of *bone marrow, chicken, meat, ginseng, dong quai* and *ghee* (clarified butter).

Harimake

A harimake is a type of "cummerbund" or wide band worn around the waist by the traditional Japanese. It is worn under the clothes, although the outer sash (called "obi") on kimonos serves the same purpose. The harimake protects the vital aspects of the body, the places where the root energies and fire reside. This includes the "hara," a place just below the navel, and the Kidneys and Adrenals, at waist level on either side of the spine on the back.

Protecting these areas is very important to the health and well-being of the entire body. This is where the energy, heat and immunity powers of the body come from. When constantly kept warm, they are supported in their functions and abilities to protect the body from stress, exhaustion and illnesses. A harimake does this and, as such, is considered an important aspect in preventing disease. I once met a black man who had been raised by a Japanese couple. He claimed he had worn a harimake all his life and had never had a cold.

While wearing a harimake all the time is preferable, it may also just be used for certain conditions as the need arises. Low back pain, frequent and/or copious urination, night time urination, poor circulation, coldness, low energy and vitality, poor appetite and digestion, gas and bloatedness with coldness, frequent colds and flus, frequent hair loss, bone and disc problems, lowered immunity and a general state of debility and hypofunctioning are all conditions in which wearing a harimake will help. It is also valuable to wear a harimake while pregnant to maintain strength and health. A Japanese woman I know of was horrified to learn that American women didn't wear harimakes while pregnant!

Harimakes are very difficult to obtain in America unless you know a traditional Japanese who can get them for you or if you go to Japan yourself. They are easily made, however, and may even be substituted by a vest that covers the waist and lower abdomen, or a scarf wrapped around these areas. I think the corsets of the past may have served this purpose. As all of

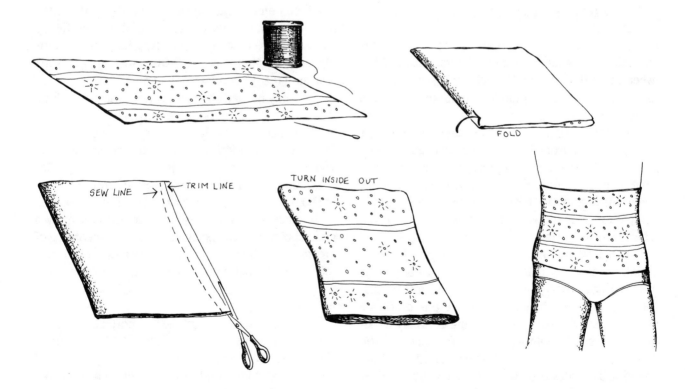

these can be bulky, however, it is well worth the small effort to make your own.

To make your own harimake, purchase enough stretch cotton (for summer) or stretch wool (for winter) material to fit snugly around your waist and hips without slipping. Keep in mind that it is to be worn under your clothes next to the skin. The material should be wide enough that it covers your hips, navel and waist, about 12" for most people. It is possible to use double this amount and then fold it in half for extra warmth and protection. Now sew the two ends together to form a tube, perhaps sewing it a little tighter at the waistline to conform to your figure better. This is then slipped on your body and pulled over your hips and waist for wearing.

Use your harimake daily, or wear when you experience any of the conditions mentioned above. I often wear mine to bed on a cold night and stay toasty warm this way. Of if I or my patients feel a susceptibility to colds or flus or any lowered resistance at all, the harimake goes on until the symptoms pass.

Journal Writing

It is being more and more acknowledged these days that there exists an inseparable interconnection between the body, mind and emotions. Disease is often caused by blocked and hidden emotions which are allowed to fester and then move into the body as disease. Many people do not have an outlet for their feelings, either from lack of a listener, appropriate environment or ability within themselves to express what they are feeling. By writing in a journal, one is given this safe outlet for expressing exactly what is going on inside, allowing the release to occur before it builds up and affects the body.

Journal writing is a wonderful therapy which has definite indirect effects on the physical body. It is different than diary writing where one records the events of the day. In journal writing one describes any feelings, ideas or thoughts being currently experienced. Since the journal is for your eyes only, you may express any feeling, thoughts or ideas about anything desired, knowing that no one will ever see it unless you so choose.

Writing in a journal is different than just thinking or feeling; it becomes a vehicle for expressing these thoughts and feelings. Expressing creates a flow from what is inside you to the outside. Doing this then starts an entirely different process going. For one, you are no longer keeping your thoughts and feelings inside, bottled up, unacknowledged or unknown. For another, you are providing an outlet, a doorway, a thoroughfare, if you will, for the thoughts and feelings to travel. This creates a bridge between your subconscious, superconscious and conscious minds which allows a release to occur, inner connections to reveal themselves, new ideas to flow, hidden emotions to arise or past experiences to emerge, all of which can form new meanings and awareness in yourself.

It is amazing what comes when starting to write in this fashion. I am always surprised by the outcome at the end of a journal writing session. It is constantly revealing and nourishing. Using journal writing in this fashion allows an incredible healing to occur for when emotions are given vent and thoughts are provided a channeled pathway, a release occurs on the emotional and mental levels which then affects the body. The journal may also be used to specifically write about your healing process, asking and answering such questions as: Do I truly want to get well? And am I ready? Am I willing to do what is necessary to make any needed changes? If not, what is blocking this? What do I feel about it and why?

There are a few helpful tips on keeping a journal. First, purchase a journal book which is attractive to you, one which you will enjoy looking at and holding. Doing so will draw you more often to opening the book and writing in it. Next, keep it in a secure yet easily accessibly place. Near your bed is usually a good choice so it can be available for the recording of dreams upon awakening. Since dreams are a direct reflection of what you are feeling and thinking at the time, they are further input and revelations of your waking writings.

When to write is another important consideration. As in all things, it is best to establish a routine if possible. This will ensure frequent regular use of your journal. Many find that right before bed is especially beneficial. It is a good time to process what has occurred during the day and plan ahead for the next day. This unloads the mind and heart, leading to a more restful and sound sleep. At this time problems can be offered to the subconscious and superconscious for solutions during sleep.

Regardless of what routine is set, journal writing is an essential tool during times of stress, mental or emotional upset, creative blocks and so forth. For this reason, I would suggest carrying your journal with you wherever you go, so it will always be available when you need it.

When writing in your journal, remember that no one else will read it. This will provide you with an inner security that allows you to write whatever it is you really want to say. To help you write more openly, imagine you are talking to a friend, a person involved in the thoughts and feelings you are having or an imaginary person who can really listen and understand you, such as your guardian angel. Sometimes it helps to "talk" to a part of your body, or to a tree or another object of your choice. None of these are necessary, but they may help you to draw out more of your thoughts.

Lastly, trust the process of journal writing. Even if you think you are fully aware of all that you are feeling and thinking and so have no need to write anything down, go ahead and write it down anyway. You will almost always be surprised and amazed at what else comes up and seeks expression in spite of your original thought that there was nothing else there. Writing in a journal daily is an intensely personal and powerful process which can bring many emotional, mental, physical and spiritual benefits.

Moxibustion

Moxibustion is a method of burning herbs on or above the skin, usually at specific acupuncture points. The heat warms the energy (chi) and blood in the body and is useful in the treatment of disease and maintenance of health. Quite often pain and disease result from a blockage or improper flow of energy and blood, and moxibustion stimulates with heat to alleviate the original blockage and correct the flow. Moxibustion is wonderful for sprains, traumas and injuries. In addition, it stimulates and supports the immunity of the body and eliminates cold and damp, thus promoting normal functioning of the organs.

Although it can be made from a variety of herbs, moxa (short for moxibustion) is generally made from the mugwort plant (*Artemesia vulgaris*). This herb, while its heat is mild, burns easily and penetrates deeply beneath the skin into the body. It comes in a variety of forms, as the loose wool, in cones or as sticks, often called moxa cigars. It can be burned either directly on the body or over the surface.

For home use we will only learn how to use moxa sticks over the surface of the body. This is a safe and universally useful method. The sticks may be purchased at the addresses given in the Appendix, *Herbal Resource Guide*, and are not expensive. Moxa sticks may be made at home by picking and drying mugwort, then grinding it into a fine powder, sifting and filtering it to remove coarse materials and then repeating this entire process until a fine, soft, wooly powder results. It is then tightly rolled up in tissue paper to form a 6" long thick "cigar."

To use, remove the commercial paper wrapper (not the white inner paper) from the stick and light one end. Hold it about 1 inch from the surface of the skin over the chosen area, the distance varying with the tolerance of the person and the amount of heat stimulation desired. With this method the stick is held still and only moved when the heat level becomes intolerant. It is not necessary to withstand the heat beyond tolerance levels or to become burned. Heating to the threshold level and then moving the stick away for a moment is sufficient.

If several points or areas are to be warmed, then the stick may be moved to the next place, coming back to the original point later. Normally, the moxa stick is burned from 5 to 10 minutes on each area or until the skin becomes red in the vicinity of the point.

Another method is to use a circular motion with the stick moving around and over the desired area. This spreads the focus of the heat over large surface areas and is especially good for soft tissue injuries, skin disorders and larger areas of pain. A third method is called "sparrow pecking"—the moxa stick is rapidly "pecked" at the point without touching the skin. This enables the heat to penetrate deeply and so is

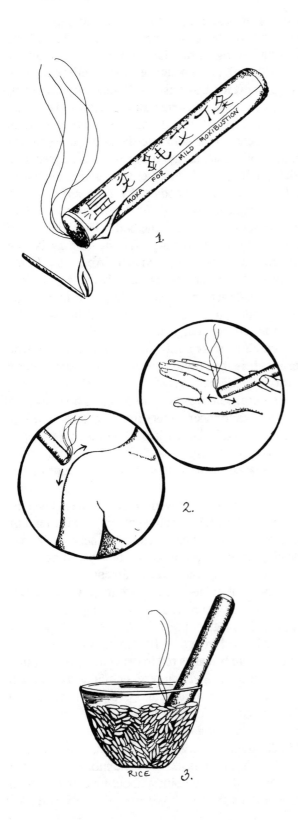

1.

2.

RICE 3.

good when strong stimulation is desired. Be sure to periodically tap the ashes off the stick into a container, as otherwise they will fall on the person's skin and burn.

Putting out the moxa stick is just as important as learning to use it. If not safely extinguished, it can easily continue to smolder and potentially cause a fire. Make sure the stick is no longer smoking before you leave it and turn your attention elsewhere.

To extinguish moxa sticks, either twist them down into a container of rice, place them in a jar and screw the lid on tight or wrap a piece of tin foil tightly around the lit end. With any of these methods you will not lose any of the stick. It is possible to cut off the burning end, or douse the cut end in water; however, much of the stick is then lost. Often one can find a small-holed candle holder which just fits the stick, and placing the lit end of the moxa down inside will effectively put it out. A major caution here is not to put the moxa stick out in dirt. Though this seems as if it will work, it doesn't. The moxa stick continues to quietly burn, potentially causing a fire.

The usefulness of moxa is endless. Be sure to save the moxa ashes to use in stopping bleeding, and the smoke can be used therapeutically, too (see the chapter on *Home Remedies* under *Ashes* and *Moxa Smoke* respectively). When used over the following areas, it can help the conditions indicated:

Chest: lung congestion, cough, cold, flu, allergies, asthma, bronchitis, mucus, difficulty in breathing and other lung complaints.

Upper abdomen: poor digestion, gas, poor appetite, nausea, vomiting, local spasms and cramps and food congestion. Caution—do not use over the right upper abdomen near the rib cage, as this is the residence of the liver, an organ already too prone to heat.

Middle abdomen: poor digestion, gas, diarrhea, local cramps and spasms, weakness, low energy.

Lower abdomen: gas, diarrhea, local cramps and spasms, bladder infections (without the appearance of blood), low energy, body coldness, lowered immunity, menstrual cramps and difficulty, frequent urination, nighttime urination, weakness, leukorrhea and other discharges, poor circulation and prostate difficulty.

Upper back: This will treat the same conditions as listed under "Chest," only this area is perhaps not as sensitive or vulnerable to treat on most people.

Middle back (waist level): kidney and bladder disorders, frequent and nighttime urination, low back pain, bone and disc problems, hair loss, knee and other joint pains, lowered immunity and resistance, poor circulation, coldness, weakness, low energy. Heating this area will raise the resistance and energy level of the entire body, thus aiding all other bodily organs and systems and any diseases being experienced. It is especially good for vegetarians who tend to have more internal coldness than others.

Lower back: low back pain, menstrual difficulties, leukorrhea, bladder infections and diarrhea.

Joints: local pain and swelling, arthritis, aches, soreness, local injuries, coldness and congestion.

Other body parts: Moxa is useful over other body parts where there is tension, soreness, ache, arthritis, cramps or spasms or any type of blockage, and where healing is not occurring.

Cautions: A few cautions do exist in using moxa, including not over the liver as indicated above under "Upper abdomen"; do not burn the person; do not use when a fever exists; do not use over areas of inflammation or infection; do not use over the lower back or abdomen of pregnant women; avoid use in the vicinity of sensory organs or mucous membranes; if an area is numb or there is little feeling or poor circulation, take special care not to over-use on those areas because the person cannot feel as well in those places and burning could easily occur.

If for some reason the person does get burned, then a blister will form. Take care not to let small blisters break. The fluid will be absorbed without infection. Large blisters may break and so should be dressed to prevent infection.

Note: An interesting note here is the use of moxibustion for injuries. Western medicine usually defines any injury as inflammation and thus promotes the use of ice over the affected area. Seemingly heat would be contraindicated in these situations.

Yet, from the viewpoint of Chinese medicine, the opposite is true. While ice numbs and stops the heavy influx of inflammation and infection-fighting cells, thus decreasing the pain, the long-term results are blocked energy and blood (which coldness causes), a slower healing process and a longer-term pain. and coldness slow down circulation and congeal the blood, just as ice on a river stops the flow of water on the top. The flow of energy is then blocked, also.

With the application of heat (the sooner the better), fresh energy and blood are immediately brought to the location for healing with continued circulation. The heat also alleviates the pain and actually quickens the healing process, especially over the long run. This is true of wounds, too. The only time moxa should not be used in these cases is where a true inflammation occurs, and this will be indicated by extreme redness of the skin and possible pus formation. For injuries such as broken bones, ice can be used first, alternating with moxibustion.

I will give you an example. My family and I were playing volleyball with some friends. One person got her hand smashed by the ball, and the pain was excruciating. We immediately obtained some heat (no moxa was on hand, but we found a person with a cigarette) and applied it over her swollen and painful fingers. Within five minutes the pain had lessened substantially, and after 15 minutes she could play volleyball again! With ice she would have remained out of the game with dull aching fingers for quite a few days.

As another example, I have treated numerous people with injuries where with the use of ice the problem and pain were slowly subsiding over several weeks time. Yet, with the use of moxa, the condition and pain were lessened substantially within days to a week. Experiment with using heat on injuries rather than ice, and see how effective it is for yourself.

Other: If moxibustion is not available and heat is needed, a hot water bottle, or stones or bags of sand or salt heated in an oven or on a woodstove are good alternatives.

For Supplies: Moxibustion supplies may be purchased from Chinese medical suppliers, some of which are listed in the Appendix, *Herbal Resource Guide.*

Nasal Wash

Nasal wash is a procedure of washing the nostrils out with a water or herbal solution. This can be done to wash just the nostrils, or to additionally wash the throat. Doing this aids sinus congestion and infections, stuffy nose, difficulty of breathing through the nose, sore throats and especially recurring sinus and throat infections. It may be done on a preventative basis once a day first thing in the morning, or several times a day in the case of an infection. This is traditionally done by yogis in India, when it is called *neti*, to help clear the air passages for their breathing practices.[2]

To do a nasal wash you will need a water container that has a small spout, such as some watering pots have. Alternatively, a bulb syringe, squeeze bottle, eyedropper or turkey baster work fine. Fill this with about 2 cups water or herbal solution. Place the end of the spout in the right nostril while you tilt your head to the left. Now slowly pour the solution into the nostril, making sure it comes out the left nostril, rather than the one it is going in. You may have to adjust your head or tilt it more to make sure this happens. Continue doing this for half the solution. Be sure to locate yourself over a sink or pan for this therapy!

Now reverse sides, inserting the spout into the left nostril while tilting your head to the right and making sure the solution comes out the right nostril. Use up the rest of the solution on this side. At first it may seem difficult, if not impossible, for the solution to come out the opposite nostril. This is because of the mucus blockage in the airways at the root of the nose. With repeated attempts, however, it will come out the opposite side and create a wonderful clearing of your nasal passages. You will be amazed at how well you can breathe afterwards.

Another method involves pouring the solution alternatively through the right and left nostrils and having it run down the throat and out the mouth. For this, the head needs to be tilted backwards so the solution doesn't go out either nostril but down the throat instead. This method treats the throat directly. Often recurring and chronic sore throats, tonsillitis and other throat infections occur because the bacteria that cause them stay in the passages between the nose and the throat. These bacteria cannot be reached with the traditional gargle or throat medication. Using a

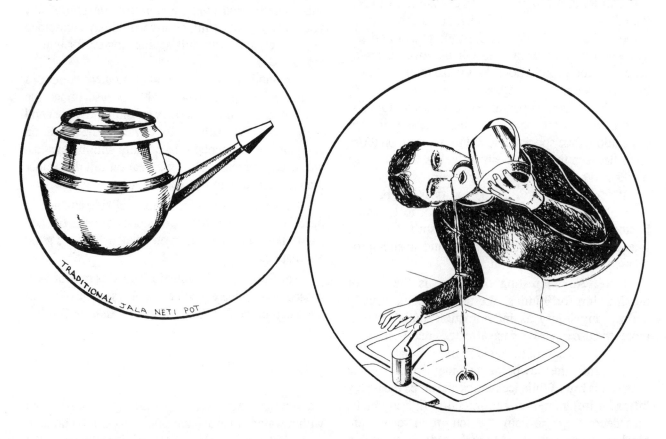

TRADITIONAL JALA NETI POT

nasal wash so it runs down the throat is about the only (comfortable) way to reach it.

Using a warm salt water solution with a nasal wash is effective in preventing and clearing up infections and inflammations. It kills the bacteria causing these, as many people who have experienced a warm salt water gargle heal their sore throats can attest to. Alternatively, an herbal tea may be made and used as the wash instead. Good herbs to use include antibiotic, alterative and anti-inflammatory herbs, such as *echinacea, chapparal, red clover, dandelion* and *goldenseal* (which is especially valuable since it tones the mucus membranes) and astringents, such as *raspberry, calendula* and *squawvine*. A small amount of demulcent may be added, like *marshmallow* or *licorice*, to soothe inflamed and irritated tissues. Make up your own customized solution and experiment to find your favorite ones.

Singing

Singing may sound like a strange therapy to include here but it truly has many wonderful benefits, even for those who claim they can't carry a tune. Through singing you may strengthen your digestion, heal bodily ailments and rejuvenate your being. It can benefit tremendously on all levels of being—physical, emotional, mental and spiritual.

Singing helps uplift our vibrations, stabilizes emotions, gives joy and generally lifts the spirits. Whenever depressed or feeling off-balanced, sing, for it will center, ground and dissipate depression. Singing spiritually oriented songs or chants will intensify these effects even more. It is known now that laughter is a great healing agent in serious diseases. Singing has similar affects upon the body-mind complex.

Singing directly affects the physical body. In Oriental medicine every organ complex is associated with an emotion, color, sound, taste, function and so on. Singing is the sound of the Earth element, encompassing the Spleen, Pancreas and Stomach organs. This is not surprising considering that singing makes use of the diaphragm, which is located in the middle of the torso right next to these organs. Through the act of singing, therefore, one is actually strengthening these organs and helping their individual functions.

According to Oriental medicine, the Spleen, Pancreas and Stomach function together in the process of digestion, which includes the breakdown, assimilation and transportation of food and drink. In Ayurvedic (East Indian) medicine, digestion is considered the key to health. A poor ability to digest and/or assimilate food is known to be at the bottom of all disease. The first signs include gas, tiredness, lethargy, diarrhea or constipation, weakness and heaviness. But the root problem can move deeper causing anemia, allergies and lowered immunity to diseases on the one hand, or hypertension, asthma, allergies and arthritis on the other, to mention just a few affected conditions. Focusing on singing to strengthen the digestive process can have far-reaching benefits.

Singing also stimulates the circulation of energy throughout the body. It does this by activating the Earth element, which is one seat of energy in the body, and by a renewed circulation of air that occurs through the breathing process involved in singing. Both refresh and rejuvenate by bringing in fresh blood, air and energy to every cell in the body.

Singing before and after you eat will especially help the digestion, but one may sing at any time of day to affect the emotions, spirit, diseases and cells. It does not matter if you don't know any specific songs, just sound any tune that comes into your mind. Make up your own words if you want, or use the traditional "la-la" to whatever melody you like. Although singing spiritual songs and chants does help uplift the body's vibrations, singing any tune or simple words will be of benefit. Therefore, make it a practice to include singing in your daily routine and see for yourself how it heals and increases your sense of well being.

Smoking

Smoking therapy is a method of filling a pipe with herbs and smoking them to relieve internal conditions. It is effective for coughs, asthma, sore throats, insomnia, restlessness, bronchial congestion and in helping to quit the smoking of tobacco. Smoking provides immediate, but temporary, relief for these conditions. Herbs are smoked for therapeutic purposes and contain no nicotine or other addicting substances.

To smoke herbs, place a small amount of the chosen herbs in a corncob pipe. Fill the lungs with smoke and then fully exhale it. Inhale the smoke about 6 to 10 times for a single treatment.

The most commonly used herbs for smoking are *coltsfoot, rosemary, mullein, yerba santa, sarsaparilla, uva ursi, licorice, hops, passion flower, chamomile, rose petals* and *comfrey*. Here are some other herbs smoked for specific purposes:

Quitting tobacco smoking: *Lobelia*, also known as Indian tobacco, is smoked. It contains lobeline, which is similar to nicotine but does not have the same set of effects. Thus it reduces the sensation of need for nicotine but does not provide the effects that lead to addictive smoking. A good combination to help in quitting smoking is equal parts *coltsfoot, lobelia* and *mullein*.

Insomnia and restlessness: *Mugwort* and *catnip* have been smoked for their calming effects.

Sore throats and hoarseness: *Licorice* is a good herb for this. Also adding licorice to any smoking formula will give it a sweet flavor.

Asthma, lung congestion, bronchitis and cough: A formula of *coltsfoot, mullein, wild cherry bark, comfrey* and a bit of *lobelia* is very effective.

Cooling menthol: *Peppermint* may be smoked or added to any other formula.

Caution: The smoking of herbs should only be an occasional practice, done with proper concern for the ability of the lungs to remove smoke particles and tars that are an inevitable result of burning plant materials. For more chronic ailments, smoking should be combined with internal therapies and herbs to treat the root cause of the condition.

Smudging

Smudging is a Native American term for cleansing the body and aura with the smoke of burning herbs. This is actually a similar usage to incense, for both uplift vibrations and alter the atmosphere. Rather than using stick incense, however, the Native Americans burn loose dried herbs in a bowl or shell. They then take the smoke with their hands and direct it around their bodies, sacred objects and homes.

I highly recommend the use of this therapy ritual on a regular basis as it is beneficial in so many ways. First, it is a way of centering the body, mind and spirit and of focusing on the moment and what is about to be undertaken. It clears the mind of all previous activities and wholly (holy!) prepares one for the next. It creates a one-pointed attention to the matter at hand or object being smudged, and this in turn funnels the mental, emotional and spiritual energies in a focused and attentive manner, a sure way to create success or a positive outcome to whatever is being attended to.

Next, the smudging smoke itself affects all levels of being. It attunes the spirit to higher rates of vibration, calms the mind and nervous system, harmonizes the emotions and purifies the outer physical body. When done in a group, it aligns each individual's energy with the whole. Smudging serves as a ritual, providing a group focus and preparatory rite.

With all this in mind, smudging is effective for any number of things. Smudging oneself is foremost and can be done in the morning to prepare for the day ahead, at night to clear the day's activities from one's being and prepare for a sound nights sleep, whenever feeling upset, angry, depressed or emotional in general, before an important meeting, in preparation for a trip or other undertaking, or before a discussion with another person to mention a few examples.

Smudging in group meetings before dialogue starts, in businesses, during gatherings or any other type of group focus is beneficial not only for the individuals being smudged, but also for the group as a whole. Each person becomes centered, thus aiding communication and listening skills. The shared ritual also helps unite the individual participants and enables them to let go of all previous thoughts and experiences, preparing to fully be present for the group focus.

Smudging is also effective for objects. Cars (especially before trips), important letters, houses, offices, stores and work tools such as computers or typewriters all benefit from smudging. This occurs through the one-pointed focus and intention during this ritual as well as the protective and purifying smoke of smudge.

To smudge you will need smudging herbs, a bowl or abalone shell, which was traditionally used by many tribes, and matches. The herbs used by the Native Americans vary according to what is sacred in their region. *Sage, mugwort, cedar, juniper* and *sweet grass* are most commonly used. The herbs may be used alone or mixed together. If you can find any of these locally, then harvest and dry some for your own use. Otherwise, you may purchase *white sage* at an herb store and this will work well. Some teachers state that each of these herbs will affect the body and aura differently. This may be so, but for our general use any of these mentioned herbs will be fine.

Place a small handful of the dried herb or herbs in a bowl or abalone shell. Then light with a match, and, when the herbs are burning well, blow out the flame. The herbs will continue to smolder, producing the smoke. Now to begin smudging, always smudge your-self first so that you are clean and prepared to smudge others. With your hands, take the smoke and pull it over your body four times, in representation of the four directions. Take it over your head, your torso, your back and lower body. Be sure to coat your entire body with the four passages of smoke. If you want, you may silently say a prayer at this time, which will reinforce and intensify what you are doing.

If smudging other people, do them next. Hold the bowl or shell in front of each person and wait while the person takes the smudge four times. Then proceed to the next person in a clockwise direction until the entire group is done. If anyone enters later, be sure to smudge him or her also. If you have a feather, it can be used to help fan the smoke toward the person and keep the smudge burning.

If smudging objects, do so after any people involved are smudged. Then using your hand or a feather, brush the smoke over, around and under the object. Be as thorough as you can in coating the object or objects with the smudge. If smudging a room, house, car or similar object, start in the east

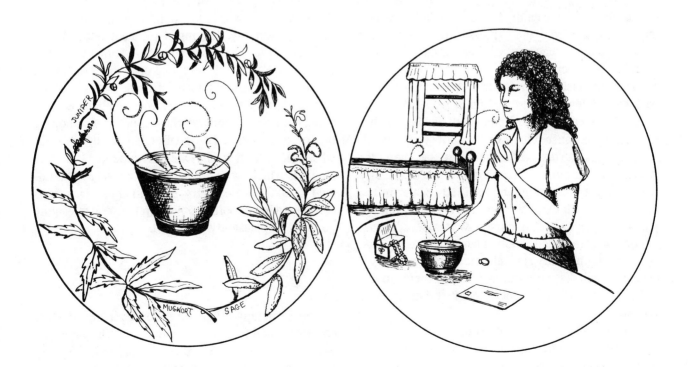

and move clockwise, permeating the areas with the smoke.

When smudging indoors, be it people or objects, be sure to open a window or door slightly to allow for adequate ventilation and a place for the "impurities" to go. This is especially important to do where there are a lot of negative vibrations. This is a good practice in any case to help circulate the smoke and air the area. You might smudge closets and/or cupboards, windows, doors, attics, fireplaces and basements along with rooms and objects. Mentally or verbally asking any negativity to move on and inviting goodness in can enhance the effects of smudging.

At times the herbs stop burning, and you may have to relight them. This can be avoided if you make sure they are thoroughly burning at the start before extinguishing the flame and if you periodically fan the burning herbs with your hand or feather.

When finished smudging, you may leave the bowl or shell in a safe place and allow the herbs to burn out. Or it may be placed outside and left burning until out if the smoke gets too strong. When cooled, it is a good practice to scatter the ashes on the ground around a plant or tree as a symbolic gesture of returning the smudge plants to the earth. This acknowledges where the herbs came from and expresses thankfulness for the earth's gifts, a way of giving back to the earth what has just been received.

I continuously hear wonderful stories from people who have integrated the smudging ritual into their lives. One woman had a tremendous dislike for her job, mainly because it involved a lot of typing which she didn't like to do. So she smudged her typewriter several days in a row and gradually came to actually enjoy her job. Something had shifted for her in the process of smudging which enabled her to accept her job as it was. Another person was a receptionist whose duties included handling customer complaints. After smudging daily several times this person's job became much less stressful as the customers "magically" became more patient, tolerant and pleasant to deal with.

I know of another woman whose friends owned a drug store in a small town. For some reason their business kept falling off until they were in serious trouble of losing the store. When my friend was asked by them to help in any way she could, she thoroughly smudged the store. No customers were in at the time and the store gradually filled with the light smoke of the smudge. Within ten minutes, customers began coming in the store, many of whom commented on it feeling different and liking it better. Some people asked what was different, even suggesting that the store had been rearranged. From that time on, with repeated smudging, the store's business picked up.

By now many of you may wonder if you can really use smudge in your meetings, places of business or other common areas of mixed peoples. Many are concerned that others may think them weird or improper, or that their co-workers, for instance, may dislike the smell or be allergic to smoke. However, this is usually not the case for many reasons. For one, the Catholic Church has used incense for a long time, and so most people are either familiar with burning of incense or can understand its use. If you are smudging some thing or place and are questioned about it, just state that you are burning incense because you like the smell of it. Most people will even appreciate this and accept what you are doing.

Secondly, smudge has a light clean smell which dissipates quickly, leaving a pleasant odor. While smudging, the smoke can be seen, but that dissolves quickly, too. A window can be opened a crack until the smoke clears and this satisfies the needs of many people. I have never met nor heard about anyone being bothered by either of these aspects of smudging or, for that matter, being offended by the process when told what it is for. One or two people have had allergies which, with a window open, were not bothered at all. Give it a try even in those situations considered inappropriate or vulnerable. You may quite possibly be pleasantly surprised.

Sweating

Sweating therapy is used in the early stages of acute colds, flus and fevers to stimulate the elimination of toxins through the pores of the skin. It helps to cleanse the lymph system and eliminate mucus conditions, chills, colds and stubborn fevers. It relaxes the pores of the skin, stimulates a sluggish appetite and is beneficial for certain conditions like arthritis and rheumatism. For acute ailments it is used to stimulate and help the body's own natural defense system by raising the body temperature, which dilates the pores of the skin. This then helps the body eliminate a toxic condition before it penetrates the internal vital organs.

If we catch a cold, it means that our natural immune system is weakened and the energy of cold and dampness penetrates through the pores of the skin. This invading energy may stimulate the body to close up its pores and lock it into the system. The body's next recourse is to raise the surface temperature, dilate the pores and sweat out the invading negative energy.

Likewise, through poor eating and life style habits, one may create toxicity within the body, which lowers immunity to the invading energy of cold and damp. In these cases, sweating not only opens the pores to release the invading energy, it also eliminates toxins through the skin, rebalancing the system.

Sweating therapy is well known and highly used throughout the world. The sweat lodge of the Native Americans encompasses sweating therapy along with spiritual renewal. Hot rocks are placed in a depression in the lodge, and water is thrown over them, creating an intensely heating steam. Usually the lodge is placed near a stream or pool where the participants can periodically dip, further stimulating their circulation. This is accompanied with various healing chants and rituals to facilitate the healing.

The East Indians, through traditional Ayurvedic medicine, perform *swedan* treatments, a method of sweating therapy which consists of laying the person in a box that closes over all but the head of the body. In the bottom of the box an herbal steam is created which eventually causes a complete sweating of the body. Keeping the person's head out of the box is an important part as prolonged heat to the head (and genitals of men) can cause harmful debilitation. So long as an individual can breathe cool air, s/he can sustain heat for a longer period of time.

The traditional Swedish sweat includes sitting in a wet or dry sauna room with the individual periodically rolling in the snow for relief and further stimulation. There are also several home versions of sweat-

ing therapeutically used by the European, American folk and naturopathic traditions. It is these which we are going to explore for our use. They include the cool sponge method, the cold sheet method and the stool method.

There are two basic kinds of sweating therapy:

1) Sweating with fire, which includes saunas, tub baths, applications of dry heat with sand, applications of poultice and fomentations (raising the temperature only in a local part of the body) and the taking of hot stimulating liquids.

2) Sweating without fire, including being closed in an unventilated room, exercise and sun bathing.

Of these two, we are going to learn the sweating with fire method.

It is a good idea to give hot sweating teas during all three methods, consisting of warming stimulating herbs for those who also have a lot of chills and want to remain covered, or cooling stimulating herbs for those who have little to no chills and want to throw the bedclothes off. Examples of warming stimulating herbs are: *fresh ginger, cinnamon branches, cayenne, garlic, mustard, horseradish, angelica, lovage, scallion bulbs, ephedra, osha, sage* and *hyssop*. Cooling stimulants include: *the mints, lemon balm, catnip, elder, feverfew, chrysanthemum, bupleurum, yarrow* and *kuzu root*.

It is important to note here that high fevers can be dangerous and so should be reduced as quickly as possible. For all fevers it is essential to keep the head and male genitals cool, as too high a fever can destroy nerve cells in the brain and cause sterility in men. Be sure the person is drinking plenty of liquids so dehydration does not set in.

In undergoing sweating therapy, no heavy or solid foods should be in the stomach. Food would only take up the body's energy for digestion, and this then detracts from the body's ability and energy to fight off an infection.

The patient should also keep the feet warm. A good method for doing so is to dip a towel in a diluted solution of hot apple cider vinegar with grated ginger and/or garlic and wrap around the feet. Then apply either a heating pad, hot water bottle or hot brick

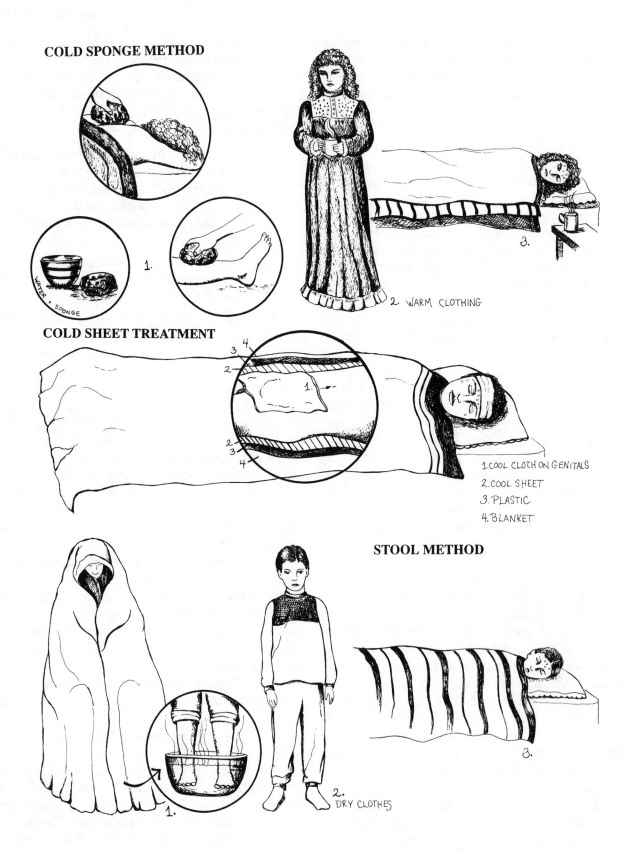

COLD SPONGE METHOD

WATER + SPONGE

1.

2. WARM CLOTHING

3.

COLD SHEET TREATMENT

1. COOL CLOTH ON GENITALS
2. COOL SHEET
3. PLASTIC
4. BLANKET

STOOL METHOD

1.

2. DRY CLOTHES

3.

against them to help keep warm. This is tremendously effective in helping normalize the circulation during acute fevers. After sweating therapy, one should rest quietly, avoid exertion and exercise and, if desired, take only light warm food and drink.

Contraindications for sweating therapy include:

1) Individuals who are too weak, obese, thin, severely debilitated or alcoholic.
2) Individuals suffering from hepatitis, jaundice and anemia.
3) Pregnant women.
4) Individuals who are in a state of shock, fright, grief, anger or other extreme emotional state.

Extreme sweating and sweating to the point of exhaustion can be counterproductive in its overall effects, especially for individuals who have weakened bodily conditions. The loss of salt can be severely depleting, as it tends to diminish the volume of plasma, causing hypotension, weakness, fainting and lowered immunity.

Cool Sponge Method

This method of sweating is a sure-fire treatment for breaking stubborn fevers, occurring either alone or with colds and flus. I have seen it break a two to three day old high fever in a child where nothing else would work. It is equally effective for adults—it saved me once in Mexico from spoiling too much of my vacation.

The cold sponge method simply uses a cloth or sponge and lots of blankets. The method is to completely sponge the sick person's skin off using room to cool temperature water, head to toe, as quickly as possible. Then just as quickly dress and put the person to bed covered by as many blankets as can be tolerated. This will cause the person to get even hotter, ultimately causing a sweat and breaking the fever.

The sponging off needs to be repeated every half to one hour until the fever breaks. It is important to do this process quickly. Otherwise a chill could set in, making the condition even more complicated. This is

not always a comfortable process for the patient, as the coolness of the sponge can feel rather shocking, but it is extremely effective. Be sure to keep the head and genitals (for males) cool by regularly applying a cool damp cloth to those areas. Administer appropriate sweating teas throughout the day.

Cold Sheet Treatment

In the cold sheet method the patient, with all clothes removed, is completely wrapped up in a large sheet wet with cool water. S/he is then wrapped in plastic (large garbage bags cut up will do) and immediately placed in bed under a large pile of blankets. The head (and genitals, if appropriate) are covered with a cool cloth and the person left to sweat. The cool sheet wrapped by plastic will draw heat out of the person's body, reducing the fever and releasing toxins causing the cold or flu. If necessary, repeat every several hours. Give stimulating herbal teas throughout the day.

When sweating has occurred for 10-15 minutes, then unwrap the person and dress in clean, dry clothes. Have the person go back to a clean, dry bed, covered adequately, to rest. Be sure to give plenty of fluids and simple nourishing food when appropriate.

Foot Soak Method

In this process, the person only removes shoes and socks, sits on a stool or chair and soaks the feet in a pot of hot water or herbal tea, such as ginger. The person is then draped with blankets from head to toe and encompassing the pot of hot water, leaving only an air hole for breathing. These are left in place until sweating is induced; then allow sweating to continue for 5-10 minutes. The person should then disrobe, be sponged off, dressed in clean dry clothes and put to bed.

As with all sweating methods, administer sweating herb teas while sitting on the stool. After sweating occurs give plenty of fluids, simple nourishing food and rest to build up the strength.

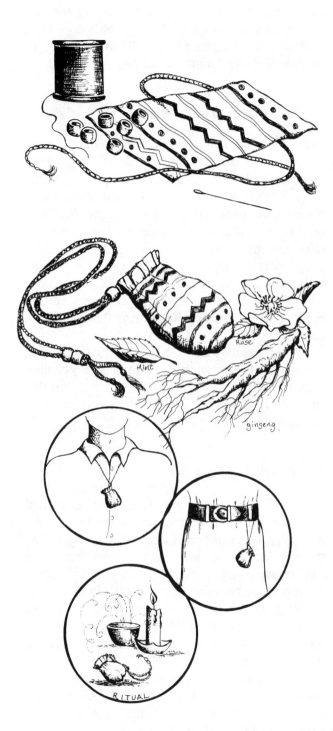

Talismans

Along with physical medicinal action, plants contain a subtle energy which is also healing. This subtle energy may be enhanced through the use of ritual or from strong intentions projected into the herbs. By combining both the gross and subtle energies, they may be worn on the body to transmit their physical effects and subtle energy intentions and to act as magnets for whatever energies are desired. Herbs worn on the body in this way are called talismans.

Talismans may contain plants along with substances from the animal and mineral kingdoms. Their use in this way is a known part of folk traditions worldwide. Very respected systems of traditional East Indian Ayurvedic medicine, Middle Eastern Unani medicine and traditional Chinese and Tibetan medicines make use of talismans. The Native Americans also use charms, rituals, talismans, amulets and sacred songs sung for special kinds of healing.

More often than not there is a solid scientific basis to so called old wives' tales. Many folk traditions uphold the wearing of certain plants such as garlic, ginseng and others to ward off evil spirits and contagion. My grandmother used to pin a small bag of asafoetida on my mother when she was a little girl to prevent her from catching colds. My mother says although it smelled horrible, it worked. I have since met many other people whose mothers did this or pinned a bag of camphor on them when they were children for the same purposes.

The odor of plants is usually based upon the presence of volatile oils whose purpose is either to attract beneficial insects or repulse harmful pathogens. Certainly the odor of many of these plants, though either unpleasant or pleasant to our senses, seem to be repugnant to various bacteria. It seems that in their effort to protect themselves from disease, the bruised plant inadvertently protects the wearer. Therefore for substances used in this way there is an empowerment that extends from the known to the unknown, making them very useful in transpersonal healing.

In making an herbal talisman you need to choose the herb(s) desired, make or purchase a little pouch for carrying the herbs and create a ritual for the "empowerment" of the talisman, or the transmission of intentions into the herbs. The kinds of plants selected can be based upon the known properties of the herbs. *Valerian root*, an herbal sedative, may be used for restoring peace between two people. The *dried pansy* or *periwinkle flowers* may be carried as a talisman of love. *Angelica root*, whose sweet scent was said to resemble the scent of angels, may be carried to prolong life. *Mugwort* is slept with at night in a dream pillow to reveal dreams and worn during the day to open intuitive knowledge of the future.

European mandrake has been used to promote fertility and wealth. *Vervaine* and *St. John's wort* may be worn to keep away evil influences of all kinds. The familiar *rose* is said to increase feelings of love and devotion for both the wearer and those with whom s/he comes into association. *Asafoetida, camphor* or *garlic* protects the body from colds or other "bugs," called invading pathogens in Western medicine, or "evils" by the Chinese.

The uses for talismans are many, and the pouches chosen will reflect the desired outcome. The plant may be directly carried or strung and worn around the neck. Or the herb(s) may be wrapped in a special leaf, cloth or leather pouch, which can then be held in a pocket, pinned on the shirt or worn around the neck. The way you choose will depend on whether you want a constant visual or tactile reminder of your intentions or a less obvious and more intimate connection with your talisman. What ever is done, I suggest making the carrier personally meaningful, such as using a silk string or an embroidered bag or utilizing something which has been given to you. This will make the talisman that much more special to you, thus increasing its effectiveness.

Ritual, the final step for making the talisman, is one of the most important ingredients, as an actual empowerment of the herbs can then occur through the will or strong intentions of the person transmitting them. The ritual is done to induce a deep meditative or intuitive state where we contact our Source, which is also the Source of the plant. The ritual creates a deep focus of intention, which is then transferred from ourselves to the plant, resulting in a powerful magnet and transmitter of healing properties.

Example rituals include lighting a candle, fasting with the plants, meditating, drumming and chanting, reciting prayers, smudging, blowing the breath on the herbs, sprinkling them with some special water from a sacred stream or river, adding a special stone or any other single or combination of ceremonies. Choose whichever rituals will create the alpha consciousness that generates the necessary energy to connect with the Source of Life.

Empowerment is the basis of the arts of shamanism and of herbal healing. The alpha state awareness, focused on the object of our intention, is integral to all spiritual healing. Therefore, after performing the ritual, hold the herb(s) or pouch of herbs in your hands and project your healing intentions into them, either verbally or silently. This will transfer your thoughts to the herbs, empowering them as talismans.

Then place the talisman on your body in whatever way you have chosen and carry it with you throughout the next several days and nights or until your healing intentions have been realized. You may desire to periodically reinforce your intentions in the talisman by creating more ritual with it, or refresh the herbs by adding fresh herbs to the talisman. If the latter is done, however, be sure to perform ritual again so that the new herbs become empowered with your intentions.

---

[1] The Four Purifications are thoroughly described and illustrated, along with many other valuable breathing and yogic techniques, in the *Ashtanga Yoga Primer* by Baba Hari Dass, Sri Rama Publishing, 1981 (Box 2550, Santa Cruz, California 95063).

[2] The yogic methods of *neti* are described in the *Ashtanga Yoga Primer* by Baba Hari Dass, Sri Rama Publishing, 1981 (Box 2550, Santa Cruz, California 95063).

III.
How to Obtain & Make
Your Own Healing Tools

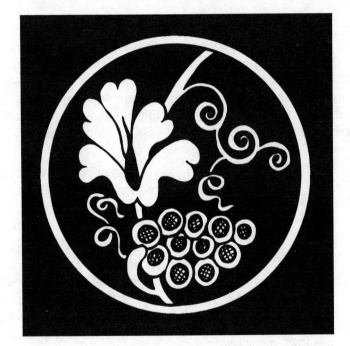

Harvesting, Preparing and Storing Herbs

The process of harvesting, preparing and storing herbs provides a very enriching and satisfying experience. Working with herbs directly teaches invaluable information about them which cannot be substituted by books. With some simple guidelines and understandings, it is also a great deal of fun.

Herbs are always more potent when handled with care and reverence. As with all healing tools, intention and concentration of purpose are of primary importance. Ideally, this should involve all aspects of the use of herbs, from the growing and harvesting of herbs in the wild, to the actual process of drying and rendering them into various traditional preparations.

Harvesting Herbs

Harvesting and preparing your own herbs is a wonderful experience and gives direct contact with the herbs in their growing environment. You may pick herbs you grow in your own garden or go into the fields, woods or mountains to obtain them. Harvesting a plant which grows wild in nature without any cultivation is called wildcrafting. This provides the purest and best source for making herbal medicines while giving the wildcrafter an enriching experience with nature. The essence of wildcrafting is harvesting plants in a manner that increases their number and health.

When wildcrafting herbs, it is important to follow certain procedures to ensure that the plant populations are not destroyed in the process. Because of indiscriminate harvesting practices in the past, sev-eral native herbs in America are already endangered, such as goldenseal, wild American ginseng and lady's slipper. Thus, it is important to develop sound, ethical harvesting practices where the gatherers have the environment's and plants' best interest in mind. Following are several guidelines for picking and processing your own herbs, whether they are wildcrafted or grown yourself:[1]

1. Bring along gloves, cutting knives, shears, string and large bags to carry your harvest home. Avoid wearing hard-soled shoes, as they may cause delicate hillside ecosystems irreparable damage.

2. Try to discover "secret" favorite areas for picking certain herbs away from common highways subject to pollution by car exhaust and traffic. Also try to harvest in areas not used by other herbalists. Do not pick herbs growing near high tension electric wires (this may cause mutation), on lawns or in public parks that have been fertilized, downstream from mining or agribusiness, or around parking lots and any possible areas sprayed with chemicals, herbicides or pesticides. Be especially wary about picking herbs in fragile locations. One irresponsible wildcrafter can easily destroy a rocky hillside or streamside environment.

3. Generally, pick the various herb parts at their prime therapeutic state:

    Roots and rhizomes: in the early spring before the sap rises and after seeding and in the early morning before the sun hits, or in the late autumn when the sap returns to the ground and the aerial parts have died back.

Barks and root-barks: in the Spring or Fall when they easily peel from the wood.

Seeds, fruits and berries: when fully ripened and mature.

Leaves and stems: when fully matured, usually before full development of the plant's flower.

Flowers: just as they are fully developed, that is, when aromatic principles are easily smelled, or oil content is evident, and before the fruiting and seeding stages.

Saps and Pitches: in the late Winter or early Spring.

Buds: when sticky.

It is usually best to pick herbs in the early morning after the dew has dried and by 12:00 noon as this is when the life force is at its strongest. Later in the day the plants may wither and wilt under the stress of the sun and so have weaker energy.

4. Before picking, develop a ritual of making an offering to the mother plant, generally the biggest and healthiest herb of the group. Perhaps quietly state your use for the plants' lives and ask that they surrender their healing properties for your reverent use in healing. Do not ever pick the mother plant, as this is the guardian of all the rest.

The offering should be something important to you—corn, rice, tobacco, even money, or a special prayer or song. This is a personal gift from you in exchange for the plants' sacrifice of life. Such rituals help to foster a non-greedy attitude in ourselves as well as encourage the plant to offer up their full subtle healing potential.

A simple prayer which may be used is: "O Sacred Herb, I honor your healing powers, asking your permission and guidance in picking your children today for the healing of _____ and any other who may be in need of your healing energy."

5. Harvest herbs in such a way as to not deplete or inhibit their future growth and development; take only what you immediately need for yourself or those to whom you are going to give them. Try to pick where there is an abundance of a particular herb, and only take about one-third by thinning so the plants are assured of repropagating themselves. Do not harvest the same stand year after year. You may need to

tend the area by thinning, cleaning the area and preserving a selection of grandparent plants to seed and guard young plants.

Never gather an endangered or threatened species, such as goldenseal, American ginseng and lady's slipper. Check your local herbarium or botanical garden for a list of these plants. Harvest no more than 10% of the native and 30% of the naturalized plant species from that area. Gather only from abundant stands. Taste, but don't swallow a plant you don't know. Have positive identification of the plant before harvesting. Use identification keys or a specimen when necessary.

Spread any seed that you don't need to help propagation, especially when taking roots. When digging roots be sure to fill the hole you made in the ground. Replace foliage and dirt around the harvested area. It may be necessary to gather foliage from nearby unharvested plants and spread it around. If harvesting leaves, don't pull the roots. Flower pruning of certain plants will increase root yields as well as foliage. Keep your picking places secret so they will not be crudely plundered by others.

6. When getting barks from trees, only take longitudinal strips and never strip a complete circumference around the tree as this will kill the tree. Only pick from the smaller branches.

7. As we gather herbs it is good to understand the effects they have in healing the earth where they grow. There is a scientific basis in all this: farmers traditionally have known how to tell the condition and quality of the soil by the kind of weeds that appear there. For instance, the common garden purslane is a very abundant plant in our garden. This is because it has the ability to retain moisture which tends to sink too rapidly below the surface of the soil in our garden.

As another example, the herb horsetail *(Equisetum species)* grows in boggy soil with a high acid content from decaying organic matter. Horsetail is a diuretic and alterative. It helps to control excessive moisture as well as neutralize acidity. Interestingly, other herbs with known detoxifying or alterative properties, such as plantain, malva and chickweed, help to control soil acidity to some extent.

Leguminaceous herbs such as lupine, peas, clover and alfalfa volunteer themselves on nitrogen depleted soil because of their ability to fix nitrogen into the soil through a peculiar biological activity of their roots. Such herbs are highly nutritive and protein-rich foods for animals and humans.

Harvesting According to the Moon

Many herbalists attach further astrological importance to the actual month and day that is optimum for harvesting individual herbs. The great Nicholas Culpepper stated in his 16th century *Complete Herbal*:

"Such as are astrologers (and indeed none else are fit to make physicians) such I advise; let the planet that governs the herb be annular and the stronger the better; if they can, in herbs of Saturn, let Saturn be in the ascendant; in the herbs of Mars, let Mars be in the mid-heaven, for in those houses they delight; let the moon apply to them by good aspect, and let her not be in the houses of her enemies; if a plant of the same triplicity, if you cannot wait that time neither, let her be with a fixed star of their nature."

An easier rule of thumb is to pick herbs following the moon phases. The moon passes through every one of the 12 signs of the zodiac once every month. Some of these signs are good for planting, while others are better for harvesting. If you want to follow the moon in harvesting your herbs, then you will need a current moon guide which will tell you what sign the moon is in every day of the current year.

To harvest herbs according to the moon phases pick as follows:

Above-ground parts (flowers, twigs, fruits, leaves and stems): Pick in the Spring or Summer and between the new and full moons (the first and second quarters). At these times it is best to pick these plant parts when the moon is in the signs of Aries, Gemini, Leo, Sagittarius or Aquarius.

Barks: Harvest in the Spring or Fall, at the third quarter during the waning moon. Pick when the moon is in the signs of Aries, Gemini, Leo, Sagittarius or Aquarius.

Root and Rhizomes: Pick in the Spring or Fall between the full and new moons (third and fourth quarters) and especially on the new moon. At these times it is best to pick them when the moon is in the signs of Aries, Gemini, Leo, Sagittarius or Aquarius.

Of course all of this implies a knowledge of astrology. However, it demonstrates the cosmological interrelationship of plants with the celestial bodies. Each plant exists as a channel of sun and moon energies as well as that of perhaps every star in the universe. These cosmic energies influence the diversity of colors and forms of all plant life on this planet.

Preparing Herbs

1. Gently wash the herbs first if needed, scrubbing roots well and rinsing barks. Usually flowers, leaves and seeds don't need to be washed. Instead, shake them to get bugs and dust off. Then slice any roots into small pieces.

2. Dry your herbs in a shaded and well-ventilated area, either spreading them out on screens or sheets. Avoid wire screens and newspaper print. It is important to keep most herbs out of the sun or else they will scorch and lose their medicinal properties. Some barks, except wild cherry, may be dried in the sun, as the sunshine activates their medicinal properties. If they are too close to each other, they will take too long to dry and mold or turn brown, losing much of their healing value. Also, do not dry them too quickly, especially if the plants contain natural oils.

Herbs may also be gathered together and tied in a bundle (with a diameter no bigger than 1-1/2") near the end of the stem. Suspend upside down from a ceiling beam or wall. This lets the plant's sap run from the stems to the leaves and flowers while drying. Hang in a well-aired, dry and shady place for several weeks, or until completely dry. The flowers can then be crushed off separately, or leaves easily stripped off and dried. All plant parts are dry when brittle. You can pinch the lowest part of hanging plants to check this, or cut a large sample root in half to see if the center is dry.

3. Crush and "garble" (clean) your harvested herbs so that you can easily store them. Leaves are best removed from their stems by running your hand along

the stem from its top towards its bottom. This strips them off easily without ripping them or the stem.

4. Usually fresh herbs are best to use for teas, alcoholic extracts and so forth. Exceptions are some barks, such as Cascara, which must be aged for a year to bring out its best qualities, and in making salves, when it might be best to use dried herbs so that there is no water from the herbs which can later cause spoilage.

Storing Herbs

Herb potency is destroyed by heat, bright light, exposure to air and bacteria. Therefore, store herbs in well-sealed or tightly capped and dark-colored jars or containers. Place them in a cool, dry place away from windows, direct sunlight, the stove or other places of high heat. Be sure to label the herbs and any herbal preparations. Include the name of the herb(s), name of the preparation, if the herbs were wildcrafted, organically grown or store bought, the location, the date and any other relevant information you think necessary.

The shelf life of dried loose herbs is from one to two years, and some parts, like barks, last much longer and even improve with age, such as cascara bark. Broken or crushed herbs lose their value more rapidly than whole, uncut herbs. If herbs begin to lose smell, taste and/or color, they are best used in an herbal bath rather than as medicine. Herbs bought at the store, especially if whole, should last about 1 year in a well-sealed jar. Herbs which you harvest and dry yourself can last from 1-2 years. Herbs with a lot of oils will lose potency first, while roots and barks will keep their medicinal power longer.

In the chapter, *Herbal Preparations,* the storage life of each type of preparation is given as part of its directions. In general, however, herbal teas keep about three days when tightly bottled and refrigerated. When reheating, do not boil the tea. Tinctures and wines last for 7-10 years. Vinegar extracts last 3 years or more if stored in a cool dark place.

Oils last up to seven years if a small amount of Vitamin E or benzoin tincture is added to the oil to preserve it. They also need to be stored in tightly covered jars and kept in a cool place. Likewise, salves last for 5 years or more when preserved and stored in this way.

Powders last from 3 months to a year or two at most depending on how well they are stored. Powders particularly need to be well-sealed to prevent exposure to the air and kept in a cool, dark place. Herbal poultices, fomentations, washes, plasters, milks, gargles, gruels and potherbs are made as needed and not stored at all.

---

[1] Many of the following harvesting guidelines have been thoroughly outlined by the Rocky Mountain Coalition. See the Appendix on *Educational Resources, Herbalists* for their address.

Herbal Preparations

Having a thorough knowledge of the properties and uses of herbs in treating disease is important. However, knowing how to use and apply the herbs is just as important in effectively treating those diseases. The choice of method used will depend on a number of factors, but through familiarity with the nature of the different preparations, one will be able to choose the method that best suits each particular ailment, individual and herb used.

It is very enriching to make your own healing tools. There is something special about making and using your own handmade preparations. Using Nature's plants and creating preparations with them is a healing process in itself. This then empowers us to care for ourselves and others.

When making any of these preparations, grasp this opportunity to become very familiar with each herb used by researching its properties in good herbal books. If picking them fresh, be sure of your identifications. Learn the herb's specific methods of use and any possible contraindications. Be aware of the form the herb should be in for each method of application, whether a powder, leaf, root and so forth.

In treating conditions, it is often more effective to combine several remedies for greater effect. For example, when treating a lung complaint, one could first use a liniment or healing salve as a chest rub, then place an herb pack or fomentation on the chest. Or in treating a wound, one could use an antiseptic to wash it, followed by the application of a soothing healing salve or a poultice.

In making herbal preparations be sure that all of your utensils, strainers, cheesecloth and such are very clean. Most metal containers will add metallic "salts" to herbal solutions, diluting and altering their properties. Even stainless steel does this, but to a much lesser extent than other containers such as iron, aluminum or copper. Iron pots are specifically recommended, however, when the "salts" of that metal are desired as part of the medicine. If glass or enamel containers are not available, stainless steel is the next choice.

For long-term storage, use enamel or glass containers, not metal. Bottles or jars are best if dark-colored to exclude sunlight. They can be sterilized by boiling them for 10 minutes or washing in a dishwasher. Use cheesecloth for straining; some grades can be washed and reused. For very fine straining, use coffee filters. If very small particles still get through, let the formula sit for a few days first, and the particles will settle to the bottom. Then decant the liquid into a new bottle and discard the sediment.

If you are purchasing the herbs you use, it is better to get whole herbs. When herbs are powdered, they become aerated and immediately begin to loose effectiveness. Because of this, it is better to buy the herbs whole and then powder them yourself in a nut and seed or coffee grinder, or a blender/mixer when a recipe calls for powdered herbs.

Fresh herbs you pick yourself contain more water than dried herbs. In making salves and liniments, this water will need to be cooked out. Otherwise, the fresh herb is usually the most effective form of use. Fresh herbs should be used as soon as possible after picking. Collect as far from roads and freeways as possible, and free of rain or dew. Refer to the chapter *Harvesting, Preparing and Storing Herbs* for further information on collecting fresh herbs.

Bath

An herbal bath can be made just for a specific part of the body, such as the hands, hips or feet, or can be a full-body bath. Because the skin is the largest digestive organ in the body, it will readily absorb the herbal properties in the bath and affect the parts being submerged, but in a gentle way. Of course, the stronger the bath made, the greater and more rapid the effect will be. In the treating of infants, baths are especially useful and effective as the baby will assimilate what it needs through the skin without needing to take the herbs internally. Likewise, this is a safe method for treating the elderly.

Baths can help stimulate blood circulation, warm the body, heal infections and inflammations, help headaches, lower fevers, calm the nerves and relax, relieve chills and eliminate aches, pains, cramps and spasms, to mention just a few of their uses. In general, the less severe the condition, the less strong and frequent the bath needs to be, and vice versa. The effect the bath will have on the body depends on the herbs included, and they can be used singly, or several in combination. The only limits are your imagination.

Bitters

Bitters is a type of tincture or wine in which the herbs it contains are bitter in taste. This bitter principle stimulates the secretion of digestive juices and bile, thus activating digestion, bowel elimination and increasing appetite. Bitters are traditionally taken before meals just for these reasons. They are also antifungal, antibiotic and antitumor in action.

Good herbs to include in bitters are *gentian, citrus peel, angelica, barberry, burdock, dandelion, elecampane, turmeric, yellow dock, atractylodes* and *ginseng.* They taste better if some sweet carminatives are added also such as *anise, fennel* and *coriander seeds,* and rice syrup also makes the taste more palatable. The alcohol used may be *vodka, brandy* and *burgundy wine,* or a combination of any of these. To make bitters, follow all the directions for Alcohol Tinctures (see page 191), including the steps, amounts, dose and storage.

Bath

Method 1—yields a stronger bath:
1. Chop up or grate desired herbs.
2. Make an infusion or decoction, as appropriate (refer to teas later in this chapter).
3. Add tea to hot bath water.
4. Soak and enjoy.

Method 2—yields a weaker bath:
1. Chop up or grate desired herbs.
2. Place in a thin cloth bag and tie closed.
3. Tie bag under bath faucet and let hot water pour through bag in filling up tub, or simply place bag in tub.
4. Soak and enjoy.

Amounts: If using Method 1, make 2 gallons of herb tea. If using Method 2, use 2-6 ounces of herbs, depending on strength desired and herbs used. Weaker herbs need larger quantities while stimulating herbs can be used more sparingly.
Dose: Take baths as needed.
Storage: Bath herbs are not stored after use. A bath may be made from any herbs left on hand and is an especially good use for herbs stored a long time when their medicinal actions have weakened, usually within a year or two (depending on the form in which they are stored).

Bolus

A bolus is a suppository inserted into the rectum to treat hemorrhoids or various cysts, or into the vagina to treat infections, cysts, irritations and tumors. The herbs used in the bolus may include astringents, such as *white oak bark* or *bayberry bark*; demulcents, such as *comfrey root* or *slippery elm*; and antibiotics such as *garlic, echinacea, chaparral* or *goldenseal.* A binder is also needed, such as *ghee* or *cocoa butter,* both of which are also healing substances.

The bolus is usually inserted at night when the cocoa butter will melt due to body heat, releasing the herbs. Take precautions to protect clothing and bedding, and rinse away the external residue the following morning.

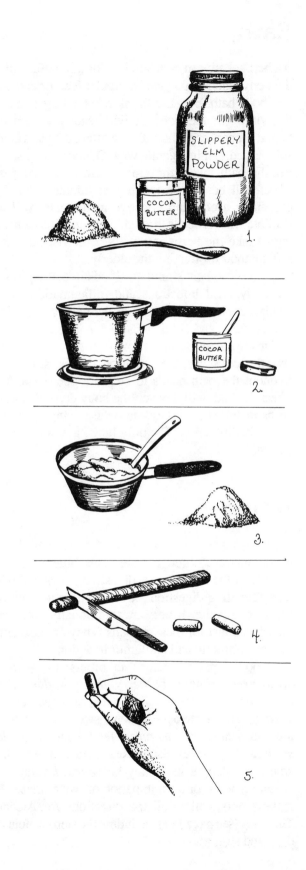

Bolus

Method 1
1. Powder desired herbs.
2. Mix herbs together in small bowl.
3. Add enough binder (ghee or cocoa butter) to form a thick, firm pie-dough consistency.
4. Roll mixture into a long strip about 3/4" thick.
5. Place in refrigerator to harden.
6. When ready to use, cut segment of mixture 1" long.
7. Allow to come to room temperature, then insert into rectum or vagina as needed.
8. Wear underwear or pad to protect clothing from possible leakage after bolus warms up in body. Do not rinse out.

Method 2
1-2. Same as Method 1.
3. Add binder to form a soft mass.
4. Roll a piece of aluminum foil around a pencil to form a tube. Remove pencil and crimp one end.
5. "Pour" the mixture into the tube, packing it down. Crimp open end.
6. Place in freezer. When it is to be used, cut off desired length and defrost.

Amounts: Mix 1 ounce of powdered herbs to approximately 1 tablespoon of binder. Add more herbs or binder as needed. Some herbs powder more coarsely than others and so will need more binder.

Dose: Insert a 1" segment 1-2 times a day. Before going to bed is a perfect time to use a bolus.

Storage: The bolus preparation should be made as needed and not stored beyond 5 days, unless kept in the freezer, in which case it will last 6 months.

Capsule

Capsules are useful when herbs are:
1. taken in small amounts, such as 1/2 to 3 grams (this is less than 1/9th of an ounce!);
2. bitter tasting or have a lot of mucilage;
3. taken regularly for a long period of time.

Capsules are a good method for taking herbs individually as well as in formula. Only the stronger-tasting herbs should be used in capsules. It would not be possible to take enough mild-tasting herbs to be effective. Also, do not mix mild-acting herbs, except those which are mucilaginous, with more potent herbs in a capsule, since the mild herbs will only dilute the potent ones and then not be present in sufficient quantity to provide the desired effect.

To use capsules, herbs may be either root, bark, leaf or flower. They need to be powdered first as they will constitute a more concentrated dose and are easier for the body to assimilate. You can purchase herbs already powdered, but it is best to buy them whole or cut and powder yourself. This way the effectiveness of the herbs won't be lost.

Capsules come in several sizes: most common are small "0" and large "00" caps. The smaller "0" size is best for children and "00" size is better for adults. Take with meals or herbal tea. Whenever a formula calls for using capsules, one may take pills instead, using twice as many pills as capsules to get about the same dose (see section on "Pills"). Another method is to wrap the powder in rice paper to the appropriate pill size.

Congee

Congee is a well-cooked, soupy grain or type of fortified porridge. It is a very therapeutic food which is perfect during convalescence from sickness, for treating acute diseases, strengthening the digestion and assimilation ability, general debility and low vitality. Congee gives strength and energy to the whole body and helps those who cannot digest carbohydrates or keep any food down. Traditional Chinese families serve it to the whole family on a weekly basis with herbs added to enhance the immune system and strengthen digestion.

Capsule

1. Powder herb(s) by placing small amount(s) in a nut & seed blender or coffee grinder.
2. Place powdered herb(s) in small bowl. If using more than one herb, combine and blend well with spoon.
3. Separate two parts of capsule and press each through powder to side of bowl so powder is forced into capsule. Continue until both ends are filled.
4. Carefully close capsule ends together and place in another bowl. Continue until all powder or capsules are gone.

Amounts: 1 ounce of herbs fills about 60 "0" caps or 30 "00" caps. One "00" capsule holds a little more than 1/2 teaspoon dried powdered herb, which is equivalent to 1 teaspoon dried whole herb.

Dose: Take 1 "0" capsule for children or 2 "00" capsules for adults 2-3 times daily. Take capsules with room temperature water or meals.

Very strong herbs, such as cayenne, are ingested in smaller doses or combined with other herbs. Herbs such as goldenseal, mandrake, poke and lobelia should be taken in smaller quantities, as larger doses of these can be either distressing or possibly harmful when taken over a long period of time (weeks or months). They are preferably taken by adding them in smaller quantities to a larger formula.

Storage: Store in tightly sealed jar in cool dark place. As stated before, herbs begin to deteriorate shortly after they've been powdered. Yet, when put into capsules they will keep approximately 1 year.

A congee is made with a grain, usually rice, water and your personally chosen herbs. It has a long cooking time over low heat which slowly and thoroughly breaks down the grain so that it is extremely easy to digest and assimilate. Thus, the body gets the most nutrients out of it possible, which is perfect for weak digestive power that can't break down or assimilate food well.

Ideally enamel, clay, glass or good quality stainless steel is used. Do not use aluminum, iron or water-soluble metal pots. The herbs chosen can vary from week to week to satisfy your current needs. Sometimes herbal tablets are broken down and used instead of fresh herbs, although the fresh ones are best. Examples include *lycii berries*, *codonopsis, dong quai, red dates, astragalus, cornus, licorice* and *ginger*.

Congee

1. Fill large pot with water, grain and herbs. Cover pot.
2. Bring to a boil, then turn down heat to lowest possible setting.
3. Cook slowly and gently, about 6-8 hours.
4. Congee is done when soupy, but thick, porridge consistency.

Amounts: Use 1 cup grain to 9 cups water and 1 ounce (28 grams) herbs. The herbs should be whole and not powdered. Rice is the best grain to use.

Dose: Eat as needed, a bowl at a time.

Storage: Congee keeps refrigerated for a day, but is better not kept longer than that. Gently reheat before eating.

Fomentation

A fomentation, sometimes called a compress, is an herbal fluid wrapped on the body and kept warm. It benefits swellings, pains, colds, flus, stimulates fresh blood circulation and warms the area where placed. Herbs that are too strong to be taken inside the body can be put on the outside, and the body will then slowly absorb the herbs in small amounts. A *ginger* fomentation is an excellent remedy for sore throats or back, as it is warm and relaxing.

In helping restore vitality to a part of the body that has been immobilized or weakened by a disease, the hot fomentation can be alternated with a shorter application of cold water. Heat serves to relax the body and open the pores, while cold stimulates the body and causes contraction. The alternation of hot and cold will revitalize the area.

Fomentation

1. Make tea out of herbs, either infusion or decoction.
2. Dip small cloth (such as washcloth) into tea and let soak 5-10 minutes to absorb tea.
3. Using pair of tongs, lift cloth out of tea. Quickly wring out and put over part of body where fomentation is desired.
4. Immediately cover cloth with towel. Place hot water bottle or heating pad over towel and cover everything with another towel so all is kept warm.
5. Leave on at least 20 minutes. If using castor oil and you plan to leave on overnight, then protect bed with several towels or plastic covering before lying down.

Amount: Make about 2-4 cups of tea for the fomentation, using 2-4 ounces of herbs respectively, depending on body area covered and number of fomentations to be done.

Dose: You may want to put a fomentation on more than once. Fomentations can be left on for 20 or more minutes; then another cloth soaking in tea can be placed over the same area. Leave second compress on for another 20 or more minutes. Fomentations can be applied as needed. Be sure to keep them warm.

Storage: Fomentations are not stored, but made when needed.

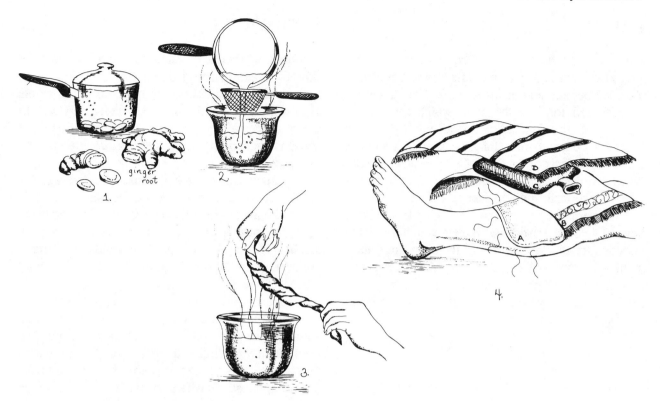

Gargle

A gargle is a tea which is used to stimulate circulation in the throat area and heal inflamed tissue. The tea is made of demulcent, anti-inflammatory, antibiotic, analgesic and antiseptic herbs. Examples are: *goldenseal, myrrh, cayenne, licorice, prickly ash, ginger, echinacea, cloves, calendula* and *marshmallow*.

Gargle

1. Choose desired combination of herbs.
2. Follow steps for tea, using infusion, decoction or combination of both as appropriate for chosen herbs.
3. Gargle as needed.

Amounts: Use 1 ounce herbs to 1 pint water.
Dose: Gargle once an hour in acute cases or as needed.
Storage: It will keep two days in the refrigerator.

Gruel

A gruel is a thick, soupy mass of herbs. It is made this way for easier ingestion and is a good way to take herbs when any other form of taking herbs is inappropriate, such as tinctures, capsules or teas. *Slippery elm* is most often taken this way for people who cannot keep any food or herbs down at all.

Gruel

1. Powder herbs in nut & seed or coffee grinder or blender.
2. Pour a little water at a time into herbs while mixing.
3. Stir until a thick, soupy consistency.

Amounts: The amount of water needed will vary according to the herbs used. In general, use 1/8 cup water to 1 ounce powdered herb.
Dose: Take in teaspoonful doses as able (if slippery elm), or take 1 teaspoon three times per day.
Storage: Keeps two days when refrigerated.

Juice

When a fresh herb is triturated (that is, crushed, ground up thoroughly or pulverized) the liquid in a plant is liberated and this is its juice. This juice is a concentrated form of the plant which can be extremely valuable for healing application. *Chickweed* juice is wonderful for itching, scaling skin such as eczema, psoriasis or dandruff. *Comfrey* and *plantain juices* are used as a wash for cuts, scrapes, burns, eczema, psoriasis and other skin conditions.

The herbs are best triturated in a blender or juicer. Several juicers are on the market which are quite effective for this. With some of them the juice automatically pours out of the juicer; with others you have to strain and press it out yourself. Alternatively, the fresh herb may be crushed and pounded and then hand strained.

Juice

1. Place herbs in blender or juicer with enough water to mix smoothly.
2. Blend thoroughly to a pulp.
3. Strain juice into container.
4. Place herb pulp in cheesecloth and squeeze hard to extract remaining juice into container.
5. Add glycerine to preserve.

Amounts: The amount of herb used varies according to the herb, the form it is in and how much you want to make. In general, be sure to use enough herb so that the blades in the blender are covered. Use fresh herbs. Use 1/3 of the amount of vegetable glycerine.
Dose: Use enough to cover the desired area.
Storage: Because juices give the most vitality of any preparation, they are quite perishable and so should be used immediately. However, they keep refrigerated a day or two in a tightly capped container. If vegetable glycerine is added, it will preserve for several years.

Liniment

Liniments are herbal extracts that are rubbed into the skin for treating strained muscles and ligaments, bruises, arthritis and some inflammations. Liniments usually include stimulating herbs, such as *cayenne*, to warm the area and increase the circulation, and antispasmodic herbs, such as *chamomile*, to relax the muscles.

Liniments may be made from *alcohol*, *vinegar* or *oil*. The application of alcohol can be somewhat cooling, while the liquid will evaporate quickly and leave the herbal principles in the skin. One can use a grain alcohol, such as *vodka* or *gin* (this yields a tincture—see section on "Tinctures"), or a *food grade (ethyl) alcohol* for external use. *Rubbing alcohol* may be used for externally applied liniments but is poisonous if accidentally taken internally. Vinegar acts as a natural astringent and as a preservative. It may be used directly or diluted to 50% strength with water. Oils are useful for extracting herbs with aromatic oils and for applications where one wishes to massage the area being treated (see section on "Oils").

Liniments

1-2. Same as steps 1 and 2 in making tinctures (see page 190.)
3. Pour alcohol, vinegar or oil over herbs into glass jar.
4-6. Same as steps 4-6 in making tinctures.

Amounts: Use the same amounts as in tinctures.
Dose: Because liniments are applied directly onto the body, there is no specific dosage for their use. However, do not overuse as they can be messy in excess.
Storage: If made with alcohol, liniments will keep as long as tinctures. Store them and vinegar liniments in the same way. If made with oil they will keep about one year. Store in glass jars (dark are best) in a cool dark place.

Essential oils may be added to liniments to act as stimulants, aromatics and carminatives. Use caution in working with them, however, since some of them are vesicants (cause blisters), and others cannot be taken internally. Avoid rubbing them near the eyes.

Possible Formulas

The following are some of the possible essential oils which can be added to either plain or herb-extracted oil for liniment use:

bay	*juniper*
birch	*mustard*
cajeput	*nutmeg*
camphor	*peppermint*
cayenne	*rosemary*
clove	*sage*
cinnamon	*thyme*
eucalyptus	*turpentine*
ginger	*wintergreen*

Herbs good for liniments include:

bay	*marjoram*
bayberry	*myrrh*
cayenne	*oregano*
cumin	*sage*
chaparral	*thyme*
ginger	*wormwood*
lobelia	

tion: *cardamom, comfrey, fenugreek, licorice, marshmallow, slippery elm, turmeric, astragalus, citrus, jujube dates, lycii berries* and even *ginseng.*

Milk

Method 1—simple and quick form:
1. Powder desired herbs in nut & seed or coffee grinder or blender, or use whole.
2. Add herbs to milk in a pan, stirring well.
3. Slowly heat milk and simmer for 5-10 minutes over low heat.
4. Strain large herb parts if desired. Cool and drink as is.

Method 2—traditionally done in Ayurvedic medicine in India:
1. Combine 1 ounce whole herbs, 1 cup milk and 4 cups water in pan.
2. Bring to boil and cook slowly over low flame until all water is evaporated.
3. Strain and cool.

Amounts: Use 1 teaspoon herbs to 1 cup milk in Method 1.
Dose: Drink 1 cup, 2-3 times a day.
Storage: Milk will last 1-2 days refrigerated.

Milk Decoction

Decoctions may be made with milk as well as water. Milk is a nourishing and building food and augments the tonic and nutritive effects of herbs. It is cooling, sedating, helps stop bleeding, reduces inflammation and antidotes hot, pungent herbs. With demulcent herbs it soothes the mucous membranes. Milk decoctions are frequently prescribed in Ayurvedic medicine.

It is best to use raw milk for this preparation. The addition of a little ginger or cinnamon helps counteract any mucus-forming tendencies it may cause. It may also be followed by a teaspoon of honey for this purpose. Several herbs are wonderful as milk decoc-

Oil

Herbal oils are a method of extracting the active principles of herbs into an oil. Used on the outside of the body like liniments, they are good for sore and aching muscles, cuts and stings and are wonderful for massage. My whole family loves to be massaged regularly with herbal oils. Spices, mints and other strong-smelling herbs are especially good to use in oils. The best herbs to use are those whose major properties are associated with their essential oils. Powdered herbs make oils gritty, so whole or cut herbs are used instead.

Generally there are two kinds of herbal oils used: one is soothing, emollient and healing, and the other is warming and stimulating. Oils which are soothing

Oil

Method 1:

1. Rub fresh or dried herbs between palms of hands to break down herbs (called "bruising" herbs).
2. Place herbs in glass jar.
3. Pour chosen oil(s) over herbs. Cover jar with a tight lid.
4-6. Same as Steps 4-6 for making alcohol tinctures. (See page 191.)
7. Add tincture of benzoin or Vitamin E as preservative.

Method 2—quicker:

1. Same as Step 1 above.
2. Place bruised herbs in oil in a pan. Slowly heat and cook herbs gently until crispy, about 1/2 to 1 hour. Cook roots first, then add leaves and flowers last. Keep pot covered.
3-5. Same as steps 4-6 for making alcohol tinctures. (See page 191.)
6. Same as Step 7 above.

Method 3—lengthier, but yields a superior oil. The proportions of herbs to oil is different, and water is added to extract additional medicinal properties into the oil. This is an Ayurvedic (East Indian Healing) method of making herbal oils:

1. Same as Step 1 above.
2. Place 1 part herbs, 4 parts oil and 16 parts water in a pan. Gently heat all ingredients together until water is evaporated.
3-5. Same as steps 4-6 for making alcohol tinctures.
6. Same as Step 7 above.

Amounts: Use 4 ounces dried herbs or 8 ounces fresh herbs to 1 pint of oil. Add tincture of benzoin (1/4 tsp. per cup oil) or Vitamin E (400 IU per cup oil) as preservative.

Dose: Oils do not have a dosage limit since they are used on the body. Overuse, however, can be messy and stain clothes or furniture.

Storage: Oils will last about 1 year. Store in glass jars in a cool, dark place.

and healing are usually made with such herbs as *comfrey, calendula, sage, lemon balm, lavender* and other similar herbs. These herbal oils can be used over the entire body or specific areas needing treatment. Oils which are warming and stimulating are made by adding pure essential oils such as *cinnamon, thyme, cajeput, camphor, eucalyptus, peppermint, ginger* or *wintergreen* to name a few. These herbal oils are generally used over specific areas where treatment is needed.

The best oils to use are olive or sesame because these warm the skin and keep longer. A few other oils are nice to add in smaller amounts such as apricot, almond and avocado. Experiment with these oils until you find your favorite combination. Besides their therapeutic effects, pure essential oils of lemon, mint, orange, rose and so forth can be added to the vegetable base to make an excellent massage oil. When the oil is made, a bit of tincture of benzoin or Vitamin E oil needs to be added as a preservative.

Paste

An herbal paste is also called an electuary or herbal candy because it is mixed with sweeteners and tastes good. Children especially like to take herbs this way. In fact, in East Indian Ayurvedic medicine, herbs are often administered powdered and mixed with a little honey as a carrier. Various sweeteners may be used such as *honey, glycerine, raw sugar* or *rice syrup,* and often *ghee* (clarified butter) is added for aiding digestion and assimilation.

Cinnamon, ginger, licorice, cardamom, black pepper, lemon balm, echinacea, chamomile, calendula, mullein, comfrey and *plantain* are sample herbs which may be made into pastes, although all herbs may be used in this manner. A traditional Ayurvedic paste, called *Trikatu,* contains *black pepper, long pepper* (pippli) and *ginger* and is fabulous for cold, flus, mucus congestion, lung ailments, sore throat and cough, all from coldness.

Paste

1. Powder desired herbs in nut & seed or coffee grinder or blender. If using fresh herbs in a blender, add a little water.
2. Place in bowl and add enough sweetener to form a paste.
3. Store in covered glass container.

Amounts: Use 1 part herbs to 2 parts sweetener, although this varies if the herbs are fresh or dry. For fresh herbs, dry sweeteners can be used, and for dry herbs, use liquid sweeteners. If the mixture is crumbly, add more sweetener; if too sticky, add more herbs. The mixture will harden with age, so make it just thick enough that it won't easily drop from a spoon.

Dose: Children—take 1/2 teaspoon 3 times a day; Adults—take 1 teaspoon 3 times a day.

Storage: Herbal pastes store well in tightly covered glass jars from 3-5 years if honey or glycerine and dried herbs are used. It may be a shorter time for other sweeteners. Fresh herbs, because they contain some water, will start spoiling in about 3 months.

Pill

Herbal pills are used for more chronic illnesses and during periods of convalescence. They are used in the same way as gelatin capsules but have the advantage of being prepared entirely with herbs. For strict vegetarians they are advantageous since most capsules are made from animal gelatin. Powdered herbs are used in pills but do not need to be as finely ground as those for capsules.

Any formula which can be taken in tea or powder form may also be taken as pills. Fun to make, they are also a tasty treat if *licorice* or *slippery elm* powders are added, since both are sweet. Both of these are also good binders, helping to hold the pill together. About 10% of the mixture needs to be a binder, and whole wheat flour is also commonly used.

Pills

1. Mix and powder herbs in a nut & seed blender or coffee grinder. Place powders in mixing bowl.
2. Add binder to mixture.
3. Slowly add water and mix to form a dough. Note: wet dough will take longer to dry.
4. Roll dough into little balls about size of pea and place on cookie sheet spaced apart.
5. Pills may be eaten now, but it is best to dry them so they will keep much longer. Place cookie sheet in warm air away from open windows (so they won't get dirty); leave to dry overnight or about 10 hours, depending on how wet balls are. You can also put cookie sheet in oven on low heat for about an hour or two until dry, but do not burn.

Method 2—a sweeter pill, good for sucking and coating the throat with honey, having antibiotic and anti-phlegm properties:

1-2. Same as above
3. Instead of water, add enough honey to form pills.
4-5. Same as above

Method 3—takes longer and requires more care in cooking, yet it yields a superior and more effective pill:

1. Make strong herbal tea from chosen herbs.
2. Strain, then cook down the strained liquid to thick, paste-like consistency. Do not burn or overcook (this will alter or destroy its properties).
3. Cool. Scrape mass from bottom of pan.
4-5. Same as above.

Amounts: 1 ounce of powdered herbs makes about 30 pea-sized pills.

Dose: Pea-sized pills equal about half the dose of a "00" gelatin capsule. Therefore, for children, use 1 pea-sized pill per "0" capsule, usually taking 1 pill 2-3 times per day; and for adults, use 2 pea-sized pills per "00" capsule, usually taking 4 pills, 2-3 times a day.

Storage: Store in a tightly covered glass container for up to a year in a cool, dark (but not wet) place.

Plaster

A plaster is an herbal mash that is wrapped up in a protective cloth or combined in a thick base material such as *slippery elm*, oil or Vaseline and then placed on the skin. It is first placed in the cloth or oil because the herbs used in a plaster are stronger and might burn or extremely irritate the skin if they were put directly on it. *Mustard* and *garlic* are two common examples.

Plasters are good for muscle spasms, swelling, arthritis, rheumatism, tumors, fevers, mucus congestion in the chest, bronchitis and pneumonia. They can be used in treating enlarged glands and organs (neck, breast, groin, kidney, liver, prostate) and various eruptions (boils, abscesses).

A plaster should be kept warm, either by replacing it often with a fresh hot one, or by placing a hot water bottle or heating pad over it. Don't rewarm a used plaster and don't store.

Plaster

1. Choose herb(s) and powder in blender or nut & seed/coffee grinder.
2. Add a little bit of hot water, herbal tea, liniment or a tincture to powdered herbs and mix to form a thick paste. If all herbs are not powdered, make them into tea first and add some to rest of powdered herbs.
3. Spread paste on thin piece of cheesecloth. Wrap up until paste is well-enclosed in cloth. Place on skin where wanted. Keep warm with hot water bottle or heating pad. Change frequently if needed.

Amount: This depends on the area to be covered, and if fresh or powdered herbs are to be used. For an area 4" x 4" use approximately 1/2 ounce powdered herb(s) and 2 tbsp liquid.

Dose: Plasters may be applied continuously and overnight as needed. Some need to be reapplied and kept on for several days. Usually, however, they are applied from 20 minutes to several hours or longer.

Storage: Plasters are made as needed and not stored.

Poultice

A poultice is an herbal pack applied directly on the skin. It should be kept warm, either by replacing it often with a fresh, hot one, or by placing a hot water bottle or heating pad over it. Don't rewarm a used poultice and don't store. Some poultices do not need to be kept warm, such as for bites, stings or wounds.

A poultice may be made with fresh herbs. Bruise and crush the fresh plant to a pulp and heat. Then follow steps 2-3. A poultice can also be made when you are in the wild. Pick leaf of herb, wash off and chew up, but don't swallow. Spit out and put directly on skin where wanted. Cover up so it won't fall off.

Poultice

1. Choose herb(s) and powder in blender or nut & seed/coffee grinder.
2. Add a little bit of hot water, herbal tea, liniment or a tincture to powdered herbs and mix to form a thick paste. If all herbs are not powdered, make them into tea first and add some to rest of powdered herbs.
3. Put paste on skin. Cover right away with gauze bandage and tie or tape in place. Or spread paste on gauze first and then apply to skin area. Leave there several hours or overnight. If needed, replace with another poultice until problem is healed. Keep warm with hot water bottle or heating pad.

Amount: This depends largely on the area to be covered, and if fresh or powdered herbs are to be used. For an area 4" x 4" use approximately 1/2 ounce powdered herb(s) and 2 tbsp liquid.

Dose: Some poultices need to be reapplied and kept on for several days. Usually, however, they are applied from 20 minutes to several hours or overnight.

Storage: Poultices are made as needed and not stored.

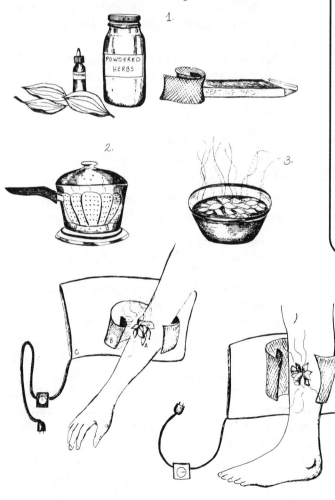

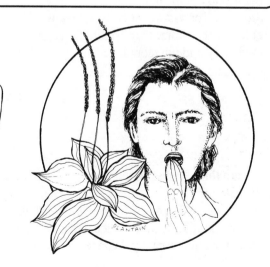

Potherb

Potherb is the term used when an herb is steamed and eaten as a vegetable. Many herbs have traditionally been eaten and enjoyed this way for hundreds of years, such as *nettles*, *dandelion leaves*, *comfrey*, *marshmallow* and *plantain*. Usually only the leaves of the plant are used. Because herbs contain many vitamins, minerals and other important nutrients, they are a valuable addition to the daily diet. Leafy greens in general aid the assimilation of grains, detoxify the blood, decongest the liver and provide the vitality of chlorophyll to the body.

Potherb

1. Place a steamer basket in pot with a little water in bottom.
2. Wash leaves well, place in steamer basket and cover.
3. Bring to boil, then simmer for 5 minutes.
4. Remove and eat.

Amounts: Stuff the pot full of the greens.
Dose: Since most people eat little, if any, greens in their diet at all, there is no end to the amount of greens you can eat. Once or twice daily is ideal.
Storage: The vitality of cooked greens is lost quickly; therefore, they should be eaten immediately and not stored.

Salve

A salve is a thick herbal oil that can be put on the skin and left there. Used for bites, stings, cuts, sores, scrapes, burns and other skin problems, salves heal the skin quickly. They also reduce pain and eliminate itching almost immediately. Whenever my child gets a cut or scrape, he asks me to put salve on it right away. Then after it has been on a few minutes, he usually forgets the hurt was ever there! Salve works especially well for me, too, on mosquito bites, cuts, sores and much more.

Salves can be made with fresh, dried, whole or powdered herbs. They are easy to use: place your finger in the salve and spread it on the sensitive area. Salves are a good first aid remedy to have on hand or to take on a trip.

The herbs included may be kept as simple as one to three, or made more complicated by combining many herbs, keeping them in the desired proportion of effectiveness. Salves can be made to address a single condition, such as itching, dryness, cuts, beauty and so on, but a general all-purpose salve may also be concocted.

The oils used should be readily absorbed by the skin. Sesame and olive oils are generally best although ghee (clarified butter) may also be used. Possible oils include:

Non-drying oils (saturated fats-oleic acid): *coconut, avocado, castor, apricot, cocoa butter, olive*

Semi-drying oils (unsaturated-linoleic acid): *wheat germ, sesame, safflower, sunflower*

Drying oils (unsaturated-linolenic and linoleic acids): *soybean, linseed (flax)*

Non-drying oils are best for dry skin and massage as they do not absorb as readily as the semi-drying oils. Try combining both types (for instance, sesame and olive). Castor oil is a nice addition to salves, as it is very thick and an excellent healing oil. However, add only in small amounts as it is very sticky.

In addition to these ingredients, any herbal tincture may be included to enhance the salve's healing power. For example, calendula tincture added to calendula flower salve makes its healing properties stronger. Lastly, some Vitamin E oil or tincture of benzoin (a tree resin) needs to be included to preserve the salve. Both are healing for the skin.

Salve

1. Make herbal oil with desired herbs. (See "Oil" section on page 182.)
2. Pour strained herbal oil into pot and gently heat to simmer.
3. Melt beeswax in old pot (because it is messy).
4. When beeswax is melted, pour into herbal oil. Mix well.
5. Add Vitamin E oil or tincture of benzoin.
6. Test salve for hardness: take teaspoon of salve oil and blow on it until hard. Or put teaspoon of salve oil in refrigerator for a minute. When it looks hard, test with finger to see how it feels. If too hard, you won't be able to spread salve; add a little more oil to salve. If too soft, it will feel mushy; add a little more melted beeswax to salve. In either case, test salve oil until you get desired hardness.
7. Right away pour oil into small jar or tin, for it will start to harden immediately. Wash out pots with hot water as soon as possible. Put tight lid on salve container.

Amounts: For about 4 ounces of salve, use 2 ounces of dried or powdered herbs, or 4 ounces of fresh herbs to 1 cup of oil, and 1-1/2 ounces beeswax. Add 1/2 teaspoon of Vitamin E oil or benzoin tincture as preservative.
Dose: Since salves are rubbed directly on the skin and are not taken internally, there is no dosage limit. However, too much salve could be messy.
Storage: Salves will keep for as many as 5 years. But I find my salve is used so much it doesn't have a chance to last that long!

Soup

Herbal soups are traditionally made in China on a weekly basis to keep the body and immunity strong and to prevent colds, flus and other seasonal "bugs."

Soups are similar to congee in that the herbs are cooked with food. However, they are made into a soup form and not cooked down for hours. Soups generally contain some form of meat, vegetables, grains and water along with the herbs. Typical herbs include *codonopsis, jujube dates, peony, fu ling, lycii berries, atractylodes, ginseng, astragalus, cornus, dioscorea* and *dong quai.*

Soup

1. Place herbs, meat (if desired) and water in large pot.
2. Bring to boil, then lower heat and cook slowly for 1 hour.
3. Add raw vegetables during last 10 minutes, or sautéed ones (they maintain their own flavor and so taste better this way) at the end.
4. Add cooked grain.
5. Cook all together another 5-10 minutes.
6. Serve and eat.

Amounts: Use 1 ounce herbs to 1 pot soup. Add more or less water accordingly for a thick or watery soup.
Dose: Eat once or twice a week.
Storage: As with all food, it is best to make and eat it fresh rather than refrigerate it.

Sun Tea

Sun teas are commonly made today, usually with black tea. A sun tea made from herbs can be delicious, however, and just as refreshing without the caffeine of black tea. They impart the medicinal properties of the herbs used, making your herbal medicines an enjoyable experience.

Because sun teas are a type of infusion, they are usually made from the leaves, seeds and flowers of plants. Roots and barks are generally not used this way as they need cooking to extract most of their properties. *Lemon balm, chamomile, mint, licorice, fennel, comfrey, plantain* and *calendula* all make nice sun teas.

Sun Tea

1. Wash leaves or flowers well and place in clear glass jar.
2. Fill jar to top with water, then screw on lid tightly.
3. Place jar in sun for 4 or more hours, as desired.
4. Strain and drink.

Amounts: Use 1 cup herb mixture or 12 tea bags for 1 gallon jar. For a medicinal tea, use 1 ounce herb to 1 pint water. For a strong tea, leave jar in sun the entire day; for a weak tea, just leave 4 hours.
Dose: Drink 3 cups a day or as desired for beverage.
Storage: Store refrigerated up to 3 days.

Syrup

1. Make tea of herbs wanted in syrup using 1 quart of water and 2 ounces of herbs.
2. Slowly simmer tea until only half remains, about a pint.
3. Strain through tea strainer. While still warm, add 2 ounces honey and/or glycerine. Stir well until dissolved.
4. After cooling, pour into glass bottle with tight lid. Keep in refrigerator.

Amounts: Use 1 quart of water and 2 ounces of herbs. For a simple syrup add 2 ounces of honey and/or glycerine. This syrup will last about 1 month if refrigerated. For a syrup that lasts unrefrigerated a year, use 2 pounds sugar to 1 pint of herbal tea. When finished, you will have about 1 pint of syrup.
Dose: Children—take one teaspoon of syrup as needed; adults—take 1 tablespoon of syrup as needed.
Storage: Always keep syrups in refrigerator. They will keep about 1 month, if simple, a year otherwise.

Syrup

A syrup is used to treat coughs and sore throats, relieve tickling and irritation of the throat, loosen phlegm, facilitate expectoration and heal and soothe the throat and lungs. Syrups work well for these situations because they coat the area and keep the herbs in direct contact with problem areas.

Syrups are fun and easy to make. Either fresh or dried whole herbs can be used. You don't want to use powdered herbs because they will taste gritty. The sweetener added can affect the properties of the syrup somewhat. White sugar is depleting to the body's immunity and can rob it of calcium and other important nutrients. *Honey*, on the other hand, adds medicinal properties of cutting mucus and soothing sore and inflamed conditions, whereas a little bit of *whole sugar*, *fructose* or *glycerine* adds energy to the body without depleting it.

Tea

Herbs that have a mild flavor and are taken internally are usually made into tea. Herbal tea can be taken medicinally and also as a beverage. Herbal teas taken medicinally can have the strongest effects and are, therefore, appropriate for the most serious illnesses. To be this effective, however, the proportion of herbs to water is much greater than generally realized. Rather than the typical 1/4 oz of herbs to 1 cup of water as in a beverage tea, the medicinal dosage is 1 oz of dried herbs to 1 pint of water (or 1/2 oz herbs to 1 cup of water). Anywhere from 2 to 3 oz of herbs should be used if they are fresh.

Teas are made from fresh or dried herbs, either cut or whole. If you are using a fresh herb, it should first be rubbed between the palms of your hands, or broken up in a mortar and pestle (called "bruising" the herb), to help release its active ingredients. Powdered herbs can be used in a pinch, but they do not taste as good and are gritty in tea form.

Teas should be made in such non-metallic containers as glass, earthenware or enamel pots. Stainless steel is all right to use if the others are not available. Whenever possible, spring or purified water, rather than tap water, should be used.

There are two basic methods of preparing teas: infusion and decoction. An infusion is used with delicate plant parts: flowers and soft leaves. It is also used with herbs that have strong smells and contain volatile oils, such as mint. Decoctions are used with herb parts that are sturdy and need to be broken down: course leaves, stems, roots and barks. Herbs that do not have much smell or volatile oils are also used in this way. Decocting herbs dissipates any volatile oils.

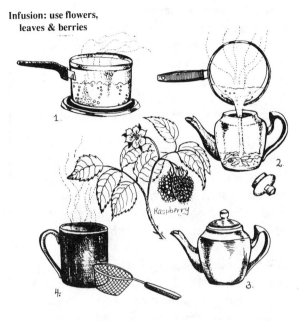

Infusion: use flowers, leaves & berries

Tea

Infusions:
1. Bring water to boil and turn heat off.
2. In the meantime, put herbs in tea pot or container.
3. Pour boiled water over herbs in container.
4. Put tight lid on to keep the volatile oils from escaping and put in warm place.
5. Let sit (steep) for 15 minutes.
6. Strain tea by pouring herb water through strainer into cup and drink.

Decoctions:
1. Place herbs directly in water and stir well.
2. Bring water to boil, then turn heat down to simmer.
3. Simmer herbs for 30-60 minutes (30 minutes for course leaves, up to 60 minutes for stems, roots and barks). Usually water will decrease by half through evaporation.
4. Strain tea by pouring herb water through strainer into cup and drink.

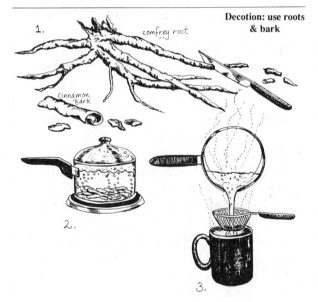

Decotion: use roots & bark

Tea

Infusions and Decoctions:
Occasionally an infusion and a decoction should be combined, since a formula may include soft leaves and flowers along with roots and barks.
1. Prepare the decoction first.
2. Strain and use this liquid for infusion.

Amounts: Use 1 ounce of dried herb to 1 pint of water for both types of preparations. This is similar to 1-2 tablespoons of herb to 1 cup of water. If fresh herbs are used, use 2-3 times amount of herb due to high water content, or stuff the pot with the herbs and then add water to cover.

Dose: Drink teas warm; or, to cause sweating, hot. Normally 1 to 2 cups (children) or 2 to 4 cups (adults) of tea are taken per day. In acute cases (illness comes on strong and suddenly), drink 4-6 cups of tea per day. Often frequent small doses of 2-3 tablespoons every 1/2 hour are more effective than a few large doses, especially for children. In chronic conditions (illness is mild and ongoing for a while), use 2-3 cups per day, taking 1 day per week off from the herbs. For long-term usage or fluid restrictions, herbs may best be taken in tincture form. (See *Herbal Extracts* section.)

Herb teas can be made in larger amounts and stored in the refrigerator for up to 3 days. Very bitter or stimulating herbs are used in smaller amounts of herb to water, such as 1/4 to 1/2 ounce herb to 1 pint water. Tea can also be poured into a dropper bottle and carried throughout the day, taking a few dropperfuls every several hours. This is very effective for administering herbs to children.

Storage: Herbal teas may be made in large batches of 1 quart to 1 gallon and stored up to 3 days in tightly sealed container in refrigerator. Comfrey is an exception to this as the high protein content causes it to go bad more rapidly.

Tincture

In a tincture the medicinal parts of herbs are extracted by one of the solvents alcohol, vinegar or glycerine. This process is called *maceration*, the solvent is called the *menstruum* and the herbs are called the *marc*. The final result is called the *extract* or *extractive*. The purpose of the menstruum is to pull the medicinal constituents of the plant into the solution and be preserved by it.

Tinctures are concentrated medicines so only a small amount should be taken at one time. They are useful for bitter-tasting herbs, those too strong to drink in teas or for herbs taken over a long period of time. They are good for herbs which do not extract well in water but do better in alcohol. Having a long shelf life, they are also convenient when stored in small bottles and carried with you wherever you go. A tincture is my favorite method for taking echinacea, as I can carry it with me everywhere, and it's always ready to use when needed. It is safe for children to take tinctures in lower dosage with adult supervision.

Tinctures are often made on the new moon and strained on the full moon so that the drawing power of the waxing moon helps to extract further herbal properties. This is similar to the pull the moon has on the ocean, creating tides. You can follow the moon cycle in making tinctures, but it is fine to make them at other times, too.

Tinctures may be made with either alcohol, vinegar or glycerine. Alcohol is an excellent extracting agent, drawing out both the volatile oils and alkaloids of plants. It is also a preservative. One can use a grain alcohol such as vodka or gin; or, if only external use is intended, as in liniments, a rubbing alcohol.

Vinegar acts as an astringent and a natural preservative for use in liniments and is a useful tincture for those who cannot tolerate alcohol. However, it only extracts the alkaloids from plants. Glycerine is a preservative and extracts properties from plants as alcohol and water do, but not as strongly. It is also antiseptic, emollient, soothing and acts as a drawing agent. Because it is sweet, it is wonderful for children's medicines.

Alcohol Tincture

Vodka is the best alcohol to use in tinctures due to its lack of color and taste. Also, dried herbs use 50% alcohol and 50% water, which is fairly equivalent to 100 proof vodka. Because fresh herbs have water in them, normally 70-80%, this needs to be taken into account, and the alcohol-to-water ratio then varies per herb. In general, use the same amount of alcohol and decrease the amount of water by how much is in the plant.

Because this gets confusing and varies per plant, the instructions here are for using the vodka alcohol-to-water ratio for both dried and fresh herbs. This yields a perfectly adequate tincture for home use.[1] It is better to powder the herbs, as this allows for better extraction. However, as always, powder them right before use rather than purchasing them already powdered.

Possible Formulas

Many herbs are very effective in tincture form; these are only a sampling:

- *myrrh* is one of the finest natural antiseptics
- *bloodroot* applied externally helps fungus on the toes and peculiar skin diseases
- *echinacea* helps fight off colds, flus and infections
- *lobelia* is an anti-spasmodic
- *cramp bark* is for menstrual cramps
- *valerian* is a pain killer and nervine, good for teething or calming baby, to help calm and sleep for adults
- *scullcap* is excellent for sleep and calming the nervous system.

Vinegar Tincture

Vinegar extracts are tinctures made with vinegar instead of alcohol. Although vinegar does not draw as many medicinal properties out of herbs as alcohol, it is still an excellent method for herbs that contain alkaloids and for those people who cannot ingest alcohol in any form. It does not work well for herbs that contain acids, since vinegar is an acid. For this reason, vinegar extracts are called acidic tinctures. Any herbal which lists biochemical ingredients will tell you which herbs contain acids or alkaloids.

Alcohol Tincture

1. Powder dried herb(s) by placing in blender, nut & seed or coffee grinder.
2. Mix powders together and place 4 ounces of dried herbs (cut or powdered) in glass jar. If using fresh herbs, bruise 8 ounces herbs and place in glass jar.
3. Pour 1 pint vodka over herbs in jar. Cover with tight lid.
4. Every day shake jar so herbs and alcohol mix together. Do this for at least 2 weeks.
5. After 2 weeks, strain tincture by covering kitchen colander with piece of cheesecloth. Place colander in big bowl. Pour herbal alcohol into colander. Herbs will collect in cheesecloth while liquid will run through into bowl. If there are still herbs in liquid, strain again. Squeeze herbs in cheesecloth to wring out any extra liquid remaining.
6. Pour contents of bowl into clean glass jar and cover tightly. This is your tincture. You can also pour into eyedropper bottles, making it easier to carry and take.

Amounts: Use 4 ounces of dried whole, cut or powdered herbs to 1 pint of vodka. For fresh herbs, use 8 ounces herbs to 1 pint of vodka.

Dose: For children 5 drops of tincture twice a day is an average dose. If milder herbs are used, then up to 10 drops can be given, twice a day. For adults 10 to 40 drops of tincture are taken 2-3 times a day. The best way to take tinctures is to put drops into 1/2 cup of water and drink water. If you don't want the alcohol, put drops in 1/4 cup of boiled water and alcohol will evaporate, leaving the herbal essence.

Storage: Because of their antibacterial properties, tinctures will last up to 10 years. They should be kept in tightly sealed bottles (brown dropper bottles are best) in a cool, dark place.

Vinegar Tincture

1-2. Same as steps 1 and 2 in making tinctures.
3. Instead of alcohol, pour apple cider vinegar over powdered herbs in glass jar. Use alone or combine with equal amount of water. For example, if using 1 pint of liquid, use 8 ounces of vinegar and 8 ounces of water. This makes extract less strong, however.
4-6. Same as steps 4-6 in making alcohol tinctures.

Amounts: The same proportion of herbs to liquid applies as for alcohol tinctures.
Dose: The same dosage applies as for alcohol tinctures.
Storage: If well stored in dark bottles and a cool dark place, these will last for 1 to 3 years.

Glycerine Tincture

1-2. Same as steps 1 and 2 in making tinctures.
3. Instead of alcohol, pour vegetable glycerine over powdered herbs in glass jar. Use alone or combine with 3/4 amount of water. For example, if using 1 pint of liquid, use 9 ounces of glycerine and 7 ounces of water. This makes extract less strong, however.
4-6. Same as steps 4-6 in making alcohol tinctures.

Amounts: The same proportion of herbs to liquid applies as for alcohol tinctures.
Dose: The same dosage applies as for alcohol tinctures.
Storage: If well stored in dark bottles and a cool dark place, these will last for 1 to 3 years.

Glycerine Tincture

Glycerine tinctures, also known as glycerites, have a sweet taste and so are good for children's remedies. They are also beneficial for anyone not able to take alcohol, even in small doses. Vegetable glycerine is a preservative and draws properties out of herbs somewhere between water and alcohol. It is often added to alcoholic tinctures to ameliorate the harsh effects of tannins.

Toothbrush

A natural toothbrush from nature is easy to find and use. It is also quite fun, especially for children, and can be very effective in cleaning the teeth. Even today, this is the way many people throughout the world keep their teeth and gums healthy, such as the Native Americans and East Indians.

The twigs contain volatile oils which stimulate blood circulation, tannins that tighten and cleanse gum tissue and other nutrients, such as vitamin C, which maintain healthy gums. *Bay, eucalyptus, oak, pine, fir* and *juniper* all work well for this.

Toothbrush

1. Locate an appropriate tree and pick a smooth twig.
2. Peel bark off with fingers.
3. Chew one end until bristly as a toothbrush.
4. Clean teeth and gums with this toothbrush.

Amounts: Use about a 3" twig.
Dose: There is no limit. This is great to use while hiking, or otherwise away from your normal toothbrush.
Storage: These are picked and used immediately.

Wash

A wash is essentially a tea that is used externally on the body, such as an eyewash or mouthwash. Some washes are used on other parts of the body for skin irritations or ailments or to lower fevers, as in sweating therapy. Babies are often treated with washes, as this is a convenient and easy way to get the herbs into a young child. Antipyretic herbs used this way can lower a child's fever.

Echinacea, goldenseal, eyebright and a pinch of *cayenne* make a good eyewash. *Mint* and *myrrh* make an effective mouthwash. *Chickweed, comfrey* and *plantain* can be used as a body wash for skin conditions, or *boneset* and *chrysanthemum* to lower fevers.

Wash

1. Follow steps for tea, either infusion, decoction or both as appropriate for the herbs being used.
2. For body wash: soak washcloth in tea and wash the desired area (or whole body for infants) repeatedly. Let wash dry on body.
3. For mouthwash, take 1/3 cup tea and swish around in mouth, then spit out.
4. For eyewash, put tea in eye cup (found in most drugstores), cover over eye, then tilt head back. Roll eye around and blink frequently to let fluid get on all parts of eye.

Amounts: Use 1 ounce herb per 1 pint water.
Dose: Use eye and body washes every hour in acute conditions.
Storage: Like teas, washes last up to 3 days when refrigerated.

Wine

Herbs are often made into wines and taken like a tincture this way. In fact, some Taoists have been known to live on herbal wines and nothing else. Needless to say, the herbs used in these instances are rejuvenative, tonic and supportive of all the body's functions. This truly shows that herbs are simply special foods.

Wines are often put in attractive bottles and left on display (when not being used!). Because whole herbs are used, they can be seen floating in the wine, which can make for interesting conversation at times. As such, they make wonderfully unusual gifts. Generally, tonic herbs are used for their strengthening and fortifying effects on various organs in the body. These include *ginseng, codonopsis, dong quai, lycii berries, hawthorn, astragalus, jujube dates, peony, atractylodes, cornus, schisandra, dioscorea* and *ho shou wu.*

There are two ways to make an herbal wine. One, which is simple and easy, entails making a tincture of the herbs in *brandy, burgundy* or *rice wine.* The other involves making a wine from scratch with the herbs, water, yeast and sugar. Dandelion and fruit wines are well known in this form. As this is complicated and entails some detailed instructions and care, this method is not described here. However, you may investigate doing this on your own by asking at a beer or wine making store for instructions and equipment and by using herbs in the process.

Wine

1. Place whole herbs in bottle.
2. Pour alcohol over herbs to fill bottle.
3. Tightly cap and shake vigorously.
4. Place in cool dark location.
5. Shake well every day for 2 weeks.
6. Don't strain, but leave herbs in bottle and take as needed.

Amounts: Use 1 ounce herbs to 1 pint alcohol.
Dose: Take 1 teaspoon 3 times daily (the alcohol may be evaporated off by putting the dose in 1/4 cup water that has just been boiled).
Storage: Wines keep for a long time and can keep for a good 10 years or more.

---

[1] If you desire to produce professional tinctures or to get exact solvent information on the individual plants, you will need to study *King's American Dispensatory* by Harvey Wickes Felter and John Uri Lloyd, published 1983 by the Eclectic Medical Publications, Portland, OR.

How To Shop for Herbs

In the past an herbalist would obtain herbs by going into the fields, forests, meadows and mountains to identify and then harvest what was needed. These were then used fresh or dried and stored for later use. Today, many herbalists still do this, yet more often than not a few wildcrafters or growers harvest the herbs and send them to other herbalists, stores or manufacturing companies. While it is ideal to learn plant identification and the use of fresh herbs, most people beginning, or even well into the knowledge of using herbs, depend on stores for their herbal sources.

At this point some of you may think, "I live in a rural area. There's not an herb store here, there's not even a health food store around!" You don't need to let this stop you. When I lived in Jackson, Wyoming, local often meant driving five hours to Bozeman, Montana, for what I needed.

Herbs and health food products can be obtained in many ways. Often they are found in small sections of natural grocery stores, body product shops, nutrition centers, even some supermarkets. Driving five hours or however long it takes to go to your local shop is possible, too. It just means organizing and planning ahead and stocking up for a long time when there. There are also several mail order stores available where most bulk herbs, even Chinese, and some formulas can be obtained. Some of these are listed in the Appendix, the *Herbal Resource Guide*. It is also possible to set up a co-op with friends and neighbors to order herbs in quantity for better prices, and then share. Or open a small store yourself!

Perhaps in time your situation will give you inspiration to grow in your own garden what you most often use, or to learn to identify what grows locally. Do not overlook the possibility of someone in your area who already knows about and uses herbs. Quite often there's a crone, wildcrafter or intensive gardener you can hear about through word of mouth and seek out for information and possible training. Our split from using herbs in our lives is not that far gone yet. My mother still tells me of folk remedies my grandmother used on her, and my husband remembers several natural therapies his mother gave him!

Once you find your herbal source, knowing what form you want to use is the next step. Entering an herb or health food store for the first time can be rather bewildering. All your senses are immediately greeted with jars, bottles of all sizes, containers filled with different supplements, smells of strange herbs, pretty potpourris, rows and rows of vitamins and much more. Not knowing where to go first, or even where to begin looking for what you came in to get, you may head to the checkout counter and ask a sales person, "Where can I find mullein for my child's cold and cough?"

The response can be even more confusing: "Do you want mullein leaves or flowers? What form do you need, bulk herb or capsule? Or do you want a glycerine extract? Perhaps a cough syrup would be best? We also have mullein in several formulas to help colds and coughs, like these cough syrups, these tabulated formulas, these Chinese patented formulas, a child's glycerine syrup, these capsuled formulas...." On and on it can go! It is enough to make you give up and walk out of the store at that point. Yet, with some basic information, discrimination amongst these myriad forms is possible, if not even enjoyable. Following is a list of the various herbal forms with information on each to help you choose the right one for your needs. For the guidelines given below, refer to the chapter on *Herbal Preparations* which explains how each form is made and what it is used for.

Bulk Herbs

Bulk is the term used to indicate the dried herb itself, usually found in quantity in jars or bins. It can be whole, cut and sifted, sliced or powdered. Herbs in whole form, like seeds, flowers and some roots, are simply the dried parts as is. These herbs retain their potency the longest, yet they often need to be cooked longer or partially broken down for use. Cut and sifted means the dried herbal parts have been cut up and then sifted so any hard parts, such as twigs, are filtered out. Most herbs in bulk are in this form. They are already broken up for use and need less preparation time. On the average they maintain potency up to a year, although delicate and aromatic leaves and flowers break down faster than roots, barks and seeds.

Herbs which are sliced are usually roots, such as licorice or dong quai, as this helps partially break down the root and makes more of it available. As a general rule, whole roots need to be cooked much longer than sliced ones. When herbs are milled to a fine powder, their potency is made readily available. This creates a larger quantity of that herb and less needs to be taken of it. Yet, its resulting larger surface area exposed to the air oxidizes the herb faster, thus decreasing its potency rapidly. On the average, powdered herbs begin to loose some potency within three months, although they still maintain some effectiveness up to a year or two. They keep longer if well stored in tightly capped glass containers and placed in a dark location.

Whole, cut and sifted and sliced herbs can be made into any possible herbal preparation, although for capsules they are usually powdered. Powders are generally not made into teas, syrups or salves unless they are well strained, for otherwise they create a gritty texture. Bulk herbs are preferred by the Chinese and some Western herbalists who believe that cooking the herbs a long time and then taking them as teas is the most effective form over all others. The Western tradition uses tinctures more while Ayurveda prepares pills and pastes from the whole herbs.

When purchasing bulk herbs in any of these forms, you'll either need to place the desired amount in a bag provided near the herb jars, or take the jars themselves up to the counter to be weighed out by a sales person. Either way you will need to know how much of each herb you want, and this will depend on what you plan to do with it. Do be sure to check for good vibrancy of color, smell, taste and texture of the herb before buying it to make sure it is potent and hasn't set on the shelf too long and to make sure you are getting the herb you came in for.

Sometimes herbs are adulterated by substituting another cheaper and easier-to-find herb for the original one. This has happened to *Echinacea angustifolia*, commonly called Kansas snakeroot, which is sometimes substituted by Missouri snakeroot (*Parthenia integrifolia*), an entirely different plant. There are organizations now, however, whose job it is to promote and maintain herbal standards, including AHPA (American Herbal Products Association), AHG (American Herbalists Guild) and the Herb Research Foundation. For further guidelines, see the "Shopper's Guide to Quality Herbs" given at the end of this chapter.

Herbs will be available as the root, leaf, seeds, flowers, fruit, stems, bark, root bark or any combination of these. For some herbs only one form is used, such as ginger root or chamomile flowers. In others a combination can be found, such as the entire herb, including stem, leaf and flowers of yarrow, for instance. In still others, two different parts will be available individually, such as comfrey root and comfrey leaves. Whichever part you choose will depend on that part's particular effects and which effect you desire.

Capsules

When herbs are powdered, they are usually not taken as teas because of their inability to dissolve in the water and the resulting gritty texture. Instead, they are either used directly as the powder, or put into capsules. Herbs capsuled at the manufacturer lose their potency far less quickly than those found in bulk. Therefore, if using herbs in this form, obtain the capsules already made of the desired herb or formula, or get the bulk herbs and powder and capsule them yourself.

Capsuled herbs are an alternative to herb teas. For strong-tasting herbs, or when they are needed in larger quantities or more frequently than is practical for tea drinking, they are capsuled instead. Often they are taken as a supplement to other forms of herbal application such as teas, syrups and liniments.

The standard size capsule is "00," and the standard dosage is 2 "00" capsules, 3 times per day. They are made in other sizes, however, such as "0," small ones valuable for children and those who find it difficult to swallow pills, and the large "000" size, good for those who need larger amounts of the herbs and who can swallow them. Two tightly packed "00" capsules hold about one teaspoon (or 1300 mg) of powder (this equates to one teaspoon or 60 drops of tincture), two "0" capsules hold about 3/4 of a teaspoon (or 1000 mg) of powder, and two "000" caps hold about 1-1/3 teaspoons (1600 mg) of powder. Fluffier herbs, such as mullein or mugwort, don't compact as well, and so one capsule only holds about 200-400 mg of these herbs.

Most capsules are made from animal gelatin, although it is possible now to obtain some made from vegetable gelatin. As some people find it difficult to digest capsules, it is best for those who have any digestive difficulties to use this method sparingly. Capsules can be purchased loose in a jar, or by the package in 100-lot amounts.

Rice papers are also available and in the past have been the only available vegetarian method of taking powdered "capsules." They dissolve and digest better than capsules. If using them, simply sprinkle 1/4-1/2 teaspoon powdered herb in the center of the paper, then wrap, fold and roll the paper around it into as small a capsule form as possible.

In using powdered herbs it is important to be aware that, because in the powdered form you cannot see the original herbs, they are sometimes adulterated by adding a non-herb substance to make the powder go a longer way and to cut costs. Goldenseal has been known to have turmeric or oregon grape root powders added to it since they are similar in color, and cayenne has had sawdust added to it. Ginseng is probably another suspect here because it is so expensive. Therefore, when using powders, check the color, smell and texture for quality and ask the sales person about the source of their herbs and if they know they are unadulterated.

Tablets

Herbal tablets are made by powdering the herbs and mixing in a binder, or something that holds it together, and a hydrous substance (containing water) that allows the tablet to be broken down when combined with water. Finally, a vegetable oil is lightly sprayed on the surface for smoothness in swallowing the tablet. Binders include guar gum, from the guar plant, slippery elm, acacia bark or dicalcium phosphate, derived from the mineral calcium. Usually magnesium sterate, an inert neutral substance, is added in the process to keep the powders flowing through the tabulating machines, as otherwise they tend to cake up. Lastly, actisol (a wood pulp fiber) is added which soaks up water and causes the tablet to break apart.

In another process of tabulating, called wet-granulation, the herbs are soaked in water and spun dry to result in small granules which are pressed together into a tablet. Many Chinese pills are made this way. Because the tablet holds together better and breaks down more easily during digestion, only 1-3% additives are necessary in this process versus 5-15% in the standard tabulating method. However, the herbs used will also determine the amount of binders added, as fluffy herbs, such as mullein, need more to hold them together, whereas gummy or moist herbs, like rehmannia, need less. Overall, the wet granulation process is less commonly found and store employees can determine directly from the companies which way their tablets are made.

Tablets are very convenient to take, can travel anywhere with you, like tinctures, but don't have the alcohol problem, can be taken frequently and in large doses more easily than teas and contain more herb than in capsule form. They also have less surface area exposed and so preserve better than powders. People with weak digestion, however, can have a difficult time breaking down the tablets in their stomachs. Others don't want to ingest the binders added to create them. Some tablets can be too large to be easily swallowed, although they can always be cut in two or ground into a powder. The Chinese "tablets" or pills usually come so small, however, that 10 to 20 need be swallowed at one time for the proper dosage. Taking the tablets with warm water aids their absorption and assimilation.

Most manufacturers now consciously exclude yeast, dairy, corn, soy, wheat, sugar, starch, salt, preservatives, artificial colors or fragrances from the tablets and use vegetable rather than animal sources for the binders and coating. For those with sensitivity to any of these, be sure to read each company's label to see what it is made of.

Caplets

Caplets are small tablets the size of a capsule. They provide the advantages of a tablet while being easier to swallow. Because they are so small, however, more needs to be taken to equal a standard dosage, about double the amount, unless the contents are more potent than normal from the addition of concentrated extracts, for instance.

Tinctures

Tinctures are a popular way to take herbs because there is no concern over loss of potency, and the herb or formula itself is very convenient to take and readily available. In Europe and Australia where herbs are legally given in clinics, it is most often in tincture form (whereas the Chinese give teas and East Indians give pills). There the tinctures are mixed together to create the desired formula.

Tinctures are extracts, and two basic types are available: the liquid extract and the fluid extract. The liquid extract uses a 1:5 or 1:10 ratio of herb to liquid, meaning that 1 gram of herb is extracted with either 5 or 10 milliliters of liquid. Fluid extracts use a 1:1 ratio, or 1 gram of herb is extracted with 1 milliliter of liquid. (In a 1:1 ration the weight of the herb equals the volume of alcohol. For example, 8 pounds of fresh herb are used per 1 gallon of alcohol, which is 8 pounds.) Thus, fluid extracts are much more concentrated and are usually only found in clinics where they are diluted before given as medicine.[1] The bottle should state whether it is a tincture or extract, and if it doesn't, it is most likely a tincture.

While one form is more concentrated than another, it is really not as important as how the herbs are extracted and by what solvent (*menstruum* as it is technically called). The solvents normally used are alcohol, water, vinegar and/or glycerine. Whichever is chosen depends on which one most effectively extracts the most properties from the herb. The most common are water and alcohol since they extract both the volatile oils as well as the alkaloids in the herbs. Sometimes glycerine is included with the alcohol and water, and it extracts certain properties from some herbs that the other two don't. Vinegar extracts are far less common as they don't extract the volatile oils or acids, and they don't preserve as long. Yet, some people prefer them, as they don't contain any alcohol.[2]

A tincture would be chosen over a bulk or capsuled herb in several cases since they are: a concentrated form of the herb, so less needs to be taken; ready to take without further preparation; potent; can be easily and quickly combined into formula; store well up to 10 years; very quickly enter the blood stream; usually affect the body the fastest. Tinctures are especially effective for circulatory problems because they enter the blood stream very efficiently.

While this sounds as if tinctures should be the best way to take herbs, they do have their drawbacks. The Chinese believe that most healing properties are obtained when herbs are cooked a long time and taken in tea form. Further, alcohol is a problem for those who are sensitive to it or have any liver problems. In these cases it is best to emphasize other herbal forms or take the tinctures less frequently. It is possible, however, to put the dose of tincture in a cup of water that has just boiled, which evaporates off most of the alcohol and makes tinctures more accessible to those negatively affected by alcohol.

Dry Extracts

Dry extracts yield a concentrated herbal product in which the herbs are first cooked down into a strong decoction, then dried by blowing air over the top of the herb until all the liquid is evaporated off. The material left is then granulated. This concentrates the potency of the herbs and increases their biological availability. Yet, it can also cook off all the volatile oils which have many important medicinal properties. Some manufacturers have found a way around this by cooking the herbs in a closed container which catches the volatile oils and adds them back in.

Because this latter method maintains and concentrates all the plant's constituents, it is rather a potent method of taking herbs and formulas. Yet, it also concentrates any chemicals they possibly contain if they are not organic, such as pesticide and herbicide residues, sulfites and bacteria. Some herbalists believe the medicinal action of the plants themselves helps ameliorate this, but for those who have environmental sensitivities, it can be a problem unless organic herbs are used.

Like powders, more surface area of the herbs is exposed in dry extracts, and thus some people believe they lose their potency faster than other preparations. Others think that because the moisture is taken out of the herbs they preserve well. In either case, they can be a highly potent and effective way to take herbs. Because they are 2-5 times stronger than the powdered herbs, less needs be taken, about 2 teaspoons per day.

Freeze-Dried Extracts

Freeze-dried herbs are dry extracts in which the fresh plants are directly frozen themselves in a low moisture area, such as a freezing machine and/or dryer, which takes out all of their moisture content. This results in highly concentrated herbs with all of the constituents included. They are also instantly available and concentrated, so less is needed. They can be easily taken mixed in water and are absorbed quickly by the body. Yet they have the potential problem of dry extracts, where chemical residues are also concentrated unless the herbs used are organic.

Dry Concentrate Extract

This is a third type of dry concentrate in which a liquid extraction (usually alcohol and water) is performed first rather than the herbs being cooked. The herbs are then pressed out, and half of them are added back in to the liquid, all of which is then dried and powdered. This results in a very strong powder, nearly two times that of regularly powdered herbs. Yet, as in regular powders it can loose its potency quickly as it is exposed to the air.

Standardized Extracts

In these extracts a standard is set for the active principles of every herb included in the extract. That specified amount of active principle is then guaranteed to be found in every batch of extract produced. Yet, the amount of active principle in an herb can vary according to where and when it is grown and picked. Not every dandelion plant found contains the same amount of inulin, for instance. Thus, to standardize an extract containing dandelion, it is often necessary to add back an additional amount of the extracted active ingredient inulin to the batch to match that set standard.

Many herbalists object to this because what some set as the active ingredients perhaps leaves other important constituents out, such as dandelion's other components of lactupicrine and a bitter principle. The whole herb contains all these ingredients in their found proportions for a reason, perhaps to counterbalance the other active principles. Thus, a potentially chemically unbalanced herbal product can result when one component is added to increase its quantity in the extract. However, this does provide a guaranteed potency of that herb.[3]

Syrups

Syrups are taken internally for sore throats, colds, flus, coughs, mucus congestion and other lung and throat complaints. They are made from a water extract of usually stimulating, expectorating and soothing herbs to which is added some form of sugar that forms a thick liquid and sweetens. The sweetener added can affect the properties of the syrup somewhat. White sugar is depleting of the body's immunity and can rob it of calcium and other important nutrients. Honey, on the other hand, adds medicinal properties of cutting mucus and soothing sore and inflamed conditions, and a little bit of whole sugar, fructose or glycerine adds energy to the body without depleting it.

Syrups can be taken alone or with other herbs internally. They are especially helpful in treating children's lung and throat complaints since they taste good. In fact, children often "need" them regardless of their lack of cough or throat symptoms!

Syrups can go bad quickly and so should be checked for mold before ingesting.

Liniments

Liniments are herbal extracts, like tinctures, made from alcohol, vinegar or oil that are rubbed into the skin for treating strained muscles and ligaments, bruises, arthritis and some inflammations. They usually contain stimulating herbs which affect blood circulation, such as angelica, myrrh or calendula; antispasmodic herbs, like lobelia, to relax the muscles; anti-inflammatory herbs, such as goldenseal or myrrh, to counteract inflammations; or astringent herbs, like witch hazel, to contract the tissues.

Most liniments are made from rubbing alcohol and so should never be taken internally. A few are made with vodka and so can be taken internally like tinctures. Therefore, it is very important to read the label and determine which type of alcohol that particular liniment contains.

Salves

Salves are solidified herbal oils used externally on cuts, sores, bruises, wounds, injuries, bites, stings, itching areas and other skin conditions to heal the skin quickly. Whenever there's a skin condition, a salve is a good form to choose either alone in more

simple cases, or along with herbs internally for more serious situations.

Salves are usually made by extracting the herbs into an oil, adding a preservative such as Vitamin E or Benzoin tincture, both of which are naturally occurring, safe and healing for the skin. Keep mixing in melted beeswax to solidify the salve. The salve's application will depend on the herbs it contains and their properties and uses. Comfrey and calendula are two herbs frequently found in salves.

The oils used in a salve can also help determine its medicinal properties. These are described under salves in the chapter on *Herbal Preparations*.

Cremes

Cremes are like salves but without the addition of beeswax to solidify them. They also have more water and possibly rubbing alcohol in them. Cremes are used as a soothing and healing lotion which spreads easily and absorbs into the skin. Calendula is commonly found this way.

Oils

Herbal oils are used on the skin, like liniments, for sore and aching muscles, cuts and stings and for massage. They can be soothing and healing, or warming and stimulating. They are applied in small specific areas, or over the entire body. Like liniments, oils are only used externally.

Essential Oils

Essential oils are made by extracting the volatile and other oils out of the herb and bottling them separately. This can lead to a powerfully effective remedy. Yet when just the essential oil is used it represents only one part of the plant and that may not be the most relevant one for certain conditions.

Essential oils are very strong in their effects, tastes and smells and so should be used with care. Usually several drops of the essential oil are added to a neutral oil base, such as sesame oil, and this combination is taken internally or used externally instead of the essential oil directly itself, although it can be taken straight. Either way, only one or two drops are needed for each dose. They can be placed directly on the tongue, in water and swallowed, rubbed into the temples for headaches or massaged into other parts of the body for specific purposes. This should be done with care, however, as it can cause burning or irritation if too strong for sensitive skin.

Teas

Along with using bulk herbs in tea form, many packaged teas are available in either loose herb combinations or tea bags. Usually these are enjoyed as beverages, but some are intended for medicinal use. Since the ratio for medicinal teas is 1 ounce herb to 1 pint of water, one tea bag per cup of water is insubstantial to say the least. Therefore, medicinal teas are usually made from bulk herbs. However, if one wants to use any of the tea bag formulas as a healing tea, it is best to brew three to four bags of the tea per cup, and if the formula contains roots and barks, it should be simmered in the pot first for 15-20 minutes.

Tea companies are beginning to differentiate their teas from others by saying they do not contain dioxins in their tea bags. Dioxin is a toxic chemical which is produced through the chlorine bleaching process of the tea bags. This can be avoided by bleaching the tea bags through a 100% oxygen process. Likewise, if the teas do not have any artificial colorings, flavorings or preservatives in them, they will say so on the package.

Soups

Whole herbs are sometimes packaged in a formula intended to be cooked as a soup. Such herbs are usually effective for building the energy, blood and/ or resistance of the body. They are cooked for a long time in a soup with typically a meat, such as pork, ox bones, beef or chicken, and vegetables added.

Sprays

Herbal sprays are a liquid form of herbs which are sprayed on specific areas of the skin. They are used to treat skin conditions of various sorts, like salves and cremes, but the liquid evaporates quickly, leaving the herbal essence on the skin. Usually the herbs are extracted first and then added to a base of water and rubbing alcohol. The sprays are in liquid form and not under pressure and so do not release fluorocarbons into the atmosphere as most commercial sprays do.

Potpourris

Potpourris are a combination of pretty and pleasant-smelling herbs which are placed in a bowl on a table or other conspicuous location. They add visual charm and delightful smells to any room. Though not used medicinally, their aromas can have some effects. Aroma therapy is practiced by a few herbalists who believe that the smells of specific herbs affect a person's emotions and sense of well-being. Often essential oils are added to enhance the herbal aroma, and artificial coloring may be added, too. Sometimes they are put in pillows for sleeping, such as hops or mugwort, to induce sleep or enhance dreams.

Homeopathics

Homeopathics, another valuable form of herbal application, is a method in which an herb, when given in miniscule amounts, will cure the same symptoms it causes when given in excess. The remedy itself is prepared by diluting the herbs in alcohol repeatedly, each time shaking it for quite awhile. This is then repeated until the desired dilution is reached. Some herbs are diluted so greatly that no trace of the original herb is found in the resulting remedy. Yet, its essence remains and still affects the body. Most remedies are single herbs, although some are made up of herbal combinations. When given in tiny milk sugar pills, they are a wonderful way to take herbs, especially for children. They are also found in tincture form. However, while they are being taken, herbs with volatile oils, such as camphor and peppermint, should be avoided, as it is believed they cancel the effects of the remedy. Some believe garlic can do this, too.

It is interesting to note that while most herbal products cannot make claims on what they are good for, homeopathics can. This is because they were once the main medicines used in Western medicine before drugs were created, and so the remedies were already passed and accepted by the system at that time.

Herbal Body Products

While not used for healing, herbs are now made into shampoos, conditioners, lotions, deodorants, soaps, creams, hair sprays, massage oils and bath lotions, bubbles and oils. Usually the body products are grouped together separately from the bulk herbs, but may be in the same location as the formulas and pills.

Formulas

Many herbs can be seen in combinations specifically geared toward healing a particular ailment. Such formulas are found in all forms of herbal remedies: bulk herbs, capsules, tinctures, tablets, salves, syrups, liniments, oils, teas, cremes, sprays, homeopathic remedies and Chinese pills. Knowing which form and formula to take may be confusing. But with some guidelines, this process can be understood.

The form an herbal formula is in will give some immediate indication of its use. For instance a salve is for a skin condition, a syrup for the throat or lungs, cough or cold and a capsule for an internal effect. Next, look carefully at the formula's contents. Each herb will have some common effect or will target treatment for the same area of the body. A few of the herbs in the formula will have a supplementary effect, such as a stimulant to help move the herbs into and through the blood and thus the entire body more quickly, and an antispasmodic to help calm the nerves and/or muscles. For specific information on how to create and understand formulas, see the chapter *Herbal Properties, Constituents, Families and Formulas*.

Some herbs you will be more familiar with than others, and this may help you choose one formula over another. Particular manufacturing companies are noted for their sound formulations, organically produced herbs, experienced herbalists on the staff for product quality and support and/or other qualities that set them apart from other companies' formulas. Thus, you may prefer formulas created by one particular company.

In order to locate the formula you want, it may be difficult to discern amongst all the bottles available. Many formulas are often categorized by their manufacturing company, so you have to go through each company's products to look for one that will match your needs. Some can be found where vitamins or homeopathic remedies are located. Others can be mixed in with other products and categorized according to their use. For example, an herbal gum and tooth tincture might be found separately by the toothpastes and floss. Sometimes the Chinese formulas are separated from the Western in bulk, pill and formulated forms.

Although Chinese and Ayurvedic (East Indian) herbs are still new to most herbalists in this country, they are more frequently being found now in herbal stores. Some are in single bulk herb form, but most are found in formulas, either traditional ones or else new ones in combination with Western herbs. Purists believe that Chinese or Ayurvedic herbs should not be mixed with Western herbs. Other herbalists feel that certain particular Chinese or Ayurvedic herbs have unique abilities which no known Western herbs can provide yet, and so they are included in formula with Western herbs for their unique uses. Korean Ginseng is a well known example.

All formulas are specific for certain conditions and ailments and usually the package will say so. Because of the current legal restrictions in the United States on prescribing and diagnosing, most herbal formulas cannot usually state their exact uses and indications, as this may then be construed as prescribing and diagnosing. Those formulas that do make claims for specific uses can do so because they have a certain percentage of herbs included which have been laboratory studied, tested (usually on animals) and approved for having an effect on some part of the body. Thus they can say the formula is good for that specific effect while the rest of the herbs included are listed as inert (or inactive) ingredients.

Therefore, most formulas go by numbers, letters or some name suggestive of their use. For example, "River Of Life," a Planetary Formula distributed by Threshold, is a poetic name for a blood-cleansing formula, while "LBT," distributed by Nature's Way, stands for Lower Bowel Tonic and indicates this formula is beneficial for the bowels and constipation.

It can be frustrating to see many formulas coded this way and not know for what the formulator had intended them. Therefore, getting to know the herbs that make up the formula will tell you what it is good for. For herbs that you are unfamiliar with, the sales person or a store library is often available for help and explanation. Do not hesitate to consult either of these.

Selecting Herbal Preparations

Each method of preparing an herb has its advantages and disadvantages. There is no one best way to take an herb for each person. And, the vehicle in which they are delivered can have some influence on their effectiveness since each vehicle has a medicinal quality. Therefore, it is helpful to know the special effects of each preparation as well as its advantages and disadvantages in order to select among them.

In traditional Chinese medicine fire can be used to treat fire, water to treat water, and earth to treat earth. Thus, tinctures (alcohol is fiery) are especially effective for the blood and circulation, teas (water preparations) have a special effect on the urinary system and on perspiration (causes sweating), and powders, tablets, capsules and pills (the herb itself or "earth") are especially beneficial for the digestive system (earth element). Tablets and pills made with dicalcium sulfate as their major binding agent will have the additional quality of a sinking or descending energy which lowers fevers, is calming and brings the herbs to the lower part of the body.

Syrups, because they have demulcents in them, adhere to surfaces they come in contact with longer and therefore are more useful for the throat and mucus linings. Because dry extracts are like a food, they are effective for the digestive system and build and strengthen the entire body. Ayurvedic herbs are usually prepared in a base of honey, glycerine or ghee, and each of these will have a different effect: honey is warming and cuts mucus, reduces weight and immediately assimilates into the blood stream; ghee cools heat, balances and aids digestion; and glycerine is absorbed by the cells more fully. Herbs cooked in soup form also build the body and assimilate more fully because they are taken as food.

Although each preparation has its special effects, it also affects the rest of the body. In Chinese medicine teas are made to treat most every physical ailment. Therefore, any tea can be taken for any ailment although it will have a special effect on the urinary system and for sweating.

Every type of preparation can have its disadvantages, too. Alcoholic preparations (tinctures, internally used liniments) are made according to an alcohol-to-water ratio which varies according to each herb and which extracts most of its active principles. While standards have been set, not every manufacturer follows them, and, even when they do, all the active ingredients of the herb are not necessarily extracted. In contrast, taking the whole herb yields its full potential.

How strong the tincture is also matters. Concentrated fluid extracts, as used primarily in Europe and Australia, are highly concentrated, and therefore a good dosage of the herb is received from them. Fluid extracts (tinctures), on the other hand, are less concentrated, and so up to an ounce may be necessary to take as an equivalent dosage to taking the herbs themselves. That is a lot of alcohol, and most people don't know which herbs are safe to take in this amount anyway.

Tinctures have a definite advantage, however, in that they very quickly affect the body since the alcohol carries the herb immediately into the blood stream and is readily assimilated. Powders, tablets, pills and capsules are effective for taking bad-tasting herbs, for travel and for those who can't tolerate teas or alcohol.

Yet, they need to be digested well to be assimilated, and if digestion is poor very little of the herbs are then actually used by the body.

Teas, because they are liquid, assimilate faster and more easily than powders, pills, tablets and capsules. Yet for those who don't metabolize fluids well, who are puffy or have edema (swelling in the tissues), who have frequent urination or have poor digestion with gas, bloatedness and coldness, too many teas can aggravate any of these conditions. Eating the whole herb delivers a "food" to the body with all of its chemical principles intact, yet it may not be absorbed or assimilated well by those whose digestive power is weak. In these cases, alcoholic preparations and some teas may be the best choice. Therefore, each herbal preparation has it distinct advantages and disadvantages as well as its special effects. At the end of this chapter is a chart to help you distinguish between these factors for most herbal preparations.

When working with sales people, do remember that they cannot diagnose or prescribe for you. The best they can do is say what most people buy or find useful, their own personal experience, or what has traditionally been used in the past. Do not press them to make a choice or decision for you. They can help you choose which of the six companies to buy a tincture from or help you determine the differences between various formulas. But the ultimate decision and selection is up to you.

How you phrase the question will help determine the kind of answer you get. If you say you have colitis (inflammation of the bowel), for instance, you'll be given vague or useless information or told you can't be helped. Instead, it is more useful to ask, "Have you heard of any herbs useful for colitis or for symptoms of irritated bowels with blood in the stool or seen such information in a book?" Such an approach is much more likely to yield helpful information and direction and will not compromise the sales person.

Example

Now let's look at the example given at the beginning of this chapter of walking into an herb store and wanting to purchase mullein for your child's cold and cough. Whether you explore the shelves and their many herbal options or ask a sales person for help, you'll need to be able to discriminate among all the possibilities with the information just given.

Since you are dealing with a cold or cough, mullein leaves are the specific herb part you want. The flowers treat ear infections and will only be useful if the cold or cough is accompanied by this condition. If so, you'll want mullein flower oil along with any other mullein leaf remedies chosen.

Next, coughs respond well to syrups, as do children, so an herbal syrup with mullein is a good start, especially if the cough is more pronounced than the cold. Taking mullein internally in herb form is also good. A tea is possible as mullein is mild-tasting, and another cough/cold herb can be combined with it to enhance it's properties, like wild cherry bark. Honey can then be added to taste. All these herbs can be located in the bulk herb section.

Tinctures are usually not often given to children because of their strength and alcohol content, unless the alcohol is evaporated off. A glycerine tincture with mullein in it and other herbs geared toward a cough and cold is a good try and would be a possible substitute for a syrup, or a supplemental remedy for calming and quieting, if the child is very restless and upset. Small tablets, caplets or "0" capsules of mullein can also be beneficial.

A salve, creme, spray or herbal body product is not indicated here since they treat the skin, but an oil to calm and soothe may be rubbed over the chest and upper back to affect coughing spasms, and a liniment may be applied likewise to help clear stubborn white or clear runny mucus. Both of these types of mucus are from coldness and the warming and stimulating liniments will help warm the lungs and break up the mucus. The volatile oils from several strong-smelling herbs in the liniment will also help open the breathing passages and clear out the cold.

Essential oils are usually too strong for children to take unless diluted with a vegetable oil and given in one-drop doses. A homeopathic remedy may be available to help the cough and cold, although it will be difficult to determine if it has mullein in it. The label will say it is for coughs and colds and give the proper dosage for children. Potpourris may be a beneficial supplement to your healing program as it may lift the spirits of your child and provide a new interest.

Lastly, an herbal formula with mullein in it is beneficial to take internally along with the syrup and/or glycerine extract and oil and/or liniment. This will help correct the internal condition and imbalance in the body. Small pill formulas are good, as are "0" caps, caplets and tinctures given so they evaporate off in boiled water or tablets cut into smaller pieces. Extracts are easy for children to take and often come in formulas specifically for them. For very small children, the syrup, glycerine extract or tea form are best. In fact, herbal teas can be given by the eye dropperful for babies.

When choosing a formula make sure the other herbs it contains are also good for the lungs. Since mullein also has an astringent effect on the colon and hemorrhoids, it can be found in formulas with other herbs which treat the colon for that purpose. These would obviously not be appropriate for your child's cough or cold.

I have given an example for treating children as this requires taking more possibilities into consideration when choosing herbal remedies. Yet, when selecting something for yourself or for other illness conditions, the same approach and considerations apply. Lastly, when in doubt, do consult the sales person or store library. Take your time, and make this an adventure.

HERBAL PREPARATIONS

Form	Advantages	Disadvantages
Bulk Herbs	obtain the complete herb can be made into any preparation or herbal form desired making the preparation is healing in itself	can be adulterated cut & sifted lose potency over a year they need to be prepared to be used
Teas	whole herb is used no binders, additives, or capsules to digest flavorful herbs can be added to improve taste preparing teas is a time investment in the healing process no alcohol needs be ingested get most of the medicinal properties of the herbs obtain the strongest dosage from the herbs[4]	can be too much fluid can taste and smell bad can be inconvenient if using with tea bags one needs to use a lot of them for a medicinal effect if using tea bags, some contain harmful bleaching chemicals (dioxins) may not extract all the medicinal parts of the herbs
Tablets & Pills	contains more herb than in capsules preserves better than capsules and powders taste doesn't matter tablets can be cut into smaller pieces or ground into powder travels well; convenient easy to take and use the entire herb and all its medicinal parts is included no alcohol need be ingested	binders and other items added for tabulating process can be difficult to digest for those with weak digestion can be difficult for some people to swallow need to take a lot to equal the same dosage in tea form (see footnote 4)

HERBAL PREPARATIONS

Form	Advantages	Disadvantages
Capsules	the entire herb and all its medicinal parts are included taste doesn't matter herbs can be powdered right before ingesting travels well; convenient easy to take and use	adulteration very easy usually contains less herb than in tablets can be difficult to digest for those with poor digestion loses some potency within 3-12 months need to take a lot to equal the same dosage in tea form (see footnote 4)
Caplets	contains same amount of herb as capsule easy to swallow see other benefits of tablets	need to take twice as many caplets to get the same dosage as tablets see other disadvantages of tablets
Tinctures	travels well; convenient easy to take and use alcohol can be mostly evaporated off in boiling water doesn't lose potency stores a long time affects the body quickly	may not extract all the medicinal parts of herb alcohol content can be a problem for some people to take doesn't extract as many medicinal properties as teas do may not get enough for effective dosage if 1:5 or 1:10 liquid extract a 1:1 fluid extract can have undesirable side effects from taking too much
Dry Extracts	very concentrated, less needs to be taken travels well; convenient easy to take and use doesn't lose potency as fast as powdered herbs	not all the active principles of the herb may be maintained can have undesired concentrated chemicals loses potency faster than the whole herb or tablets
Freeze-Dried Extracts	highly concentrated, less needs to be taken maintains all active principles travels well; convenient easy to take and use	can have undesired concentrated chemicals loses potency faster than the whole herb or tablets
Dry Concentrate Extracts	*same as freeze-dried extracts*	*same as freeze-dried extracts*
Standardized Extract	a standard amount of active principles of an herb is guaranteed to be present in that preparation travels well; convenient easy to take and use highly concentrated need less dosage	possibly creates an imbalance of constituents in relation to each other as naturally found in the plant doesn't fully appreciate the role of other complex constituents and their dynamic physiological effects

HERBAL PREPARATIONS

Form	Advantages	Disadvantages
Syrups	usually tastes great travels well; convenient easy to use and take	sugar can be a problem for some to take limited application can go bad quickly
Salves	travels well; convenient easy to take and use	can be messy limited application
Cremes	*same as salves*	*same as salves*
Oils	*same as salves*	*same as salves*
Sprays	*same as salves*	*same as salves*
Liniments	travels well; convenient easy to take and use	odors may be bad to some people limited application
Essential Oils	*same as salves*	can be too strong-tasting, smelling or acting for some people only uses one part of a plant, and that may not be the most relevant for certain conditions
Soups	very effective for building and strengthening the body usually tastes good taking herbs in food form aids their assimilation cooking process can be healing to the patient	needs cooking over time
Potpourris	lifts the spirits potential healing effects from aroma therapy	limited application and very subtle healing potential
Homeo-pathics	travels well; convenient easy to take and use formulas state what they are good for if the wrong remedy, it has no ill effects and can offer some value as a placebo	knowledge and experience needed to use the individual remedies may be ineffective if it doesn't fully match the person's condition
Formulas	remedies for specific ailments available several formulas can be taken together to treat more individual conditions	you can't tailor your own individual formula

A Shopper's Guide to Quality Herbs

In purchasing bulk herbs quality and potency are two of the major elements desired. To recognize these and also guard against any possible adulteration of the herbs, there are certain principles to be aware of. Following are some simple guidelines that one may follow:

1. **Know your source.** By far the best assurance of herb quality is to know the origin of the herbs you use. This can mean their place of origin, growing conditions, the time they were harvested and by whom. For the average consumer, developing a relationship of trust with an herb store or retail distributor is a good first step.

2. **Observe the vibrancy of the herb's color.** Many root herbs, such as goldenseal powder, should have a bright golden appearance. If they are greenish, they may have been adulterated with their leaf, which contains chlorophyll but is lacking in the concentration of important alkaloids that are found in the root. Leaves should be relatively free of stems, have a bright green color, and not be crumbled from overhandling.

Flowers, such as chamomile, should also have a bright lively color. Seeds, such as anise, cumin, dill or fennel should have good size, weight and density and not appear shriveled or dried out. Fruity herbs, such as rose hips and hawthorn berries, should have a consistent reddish color and not be pale, faded, orange or yellowish which is a sign of their inferior quality. They should also not appear overly dried out or cracked.

3. **Test the scent and flavor.** Volatile oils in herbs are among the most sensitive, easily dissipated constituents. These oils are developed by the plant to ward off pests, and, in a sense, they perform a similar function in our bodies. Besides promoting sweating and circulation, herbs such as cinnamon, mint, anise and ginger have known antibiotic properties which are centered largely around their volatile oils. Before the advent of refrigeration, many of these spicy aromatic herbs were used on perishable foods to prevent spoiling. To be of maximum effectiveness, aromatic herbs should have a rich, characteristic odor that will be a sure indicator of freshness and therapeutic effectiveness.

4. **Whenever possible try to purchase whole herbs.** This is especially true of the more valuable herbs such as ginseng. Good quality ginseng is determined by its age (it should be at least 7 years old— this can often be found by counting the notches of the leaf stalk at the top), size, weight, density and scent. Powdered ginseng root, on the other hand, may be adulterated with roots of inferior quality or plain rice flour. Even a common herb like cayenne pepper has been adulterated with sawdust.

Be especially wary of the following commonly available herbs for adulteration: echinacea (*Echinacea angustifolia*), scullcap (*Scutellaria lateriflora*), prickly ash bark (*Xanthozylum spinosa*), sarsaparilla (*Smilax officinalis*), slippery elm powder (*Ulmus fulva*) and black cohosh (*Cimicifuga racemosa*). Finally, there are a number of herbs, such as lady's slipper (*Cypripedium pubescens*), which are forbidden to be picked in many states because they are endangered species. Be sure it is the true cultivated plant sold in the store.

5. **Don't hesitate to pay more for quality herbs.** Unless you grow or pick your own herbs it may be a mistake to assume that herbal medicine is "cheap" medicine. To be assured of the desired results, you must have enough of the genuine herb in a high-quality form. I have seen people go into herb shops and buy one ounce of an herb, for instance, to treat some acute ailment, while that one ounce may constitute only a single day's dosage. Even antibiotic treatments with strong drugs are not usually finished in one day.

Herbs such as echinacea are wonderful for inflammations and infections and will show results, with no significant side effects, during the first day. However, they must be taken properly (every two hours during an acute condition) for this to occur. For chronic conditions, herbs must be used three times daily for months.

6. **Buy only the necessary quantity.** It is, of course, cheaper to get a pound of good quality herb than to buy it in smaller amounts. Buying more than you intend to use, though, invites an accumulation of herbs that will loose their potency as they sit around. Most dried herbs are good for up to a year, provided they have not been previously stored for a long time

in the warehouse and are kept in tightly capped glass jars in a cool, dark place at home. (Avoid plastic bags and jars as they cause the herbs to go stale faster.)

---

[1] These terms can be confusing, and in England fluid extracts are not differentiated from liquid extracts; rather, every liquid extract is termed a fluid extract. Tinctures in North America usually mean they are liquid extracts. It should be noted, however, that tincture, fluid extract and liquid extract are still not fully agreed-upon terms and so can seem unclear and confusing.

[2] There are two main processes for making tinctures, maceration and percolation. In maceration the herbs soak for two weeks in the liquid menstruum and are then pressed to extract as much of the total liquid possible to form the tincture. In percolation, the herbs soak for three days in the menstruum, and then the liquid is allowed to drip out of the herbs at a determined and controlled rate until it has all passed through. While there are varying opinions about which is more potent,

the maceration method is generally recognized as preferred and stronger.

[3] All extracts will not necessarily state if they are dry, freeze-dried, dry concentrates or standardized. A sales person should be able to find out for you, however.

[4] Chinese teas often contain 40-250 grams or more of herbs. This cooks into four cups of tea, giving a dosage for 1-1/2 days (28.3 grams = 1 ounce). Two "00" capsules hold on the average about 1300 mg (or 1 teaspoon of powder) and two average sized tablets contain about 2000 mg of herb. Since approximately 8 ounces of powdered herbs equals 250 grams, it takes 40-50 capsules or 20-25 tablets to equal one ounce of herb. (Of course this varies according to the herb itself as some are very light and others heavy.)

This means 10-12 capsules or 4-5 tablets need be taken three times a day to be an equivalent amount of dosage in a Chinese herb tea. That can be a lot to swallow for some people. This is also not a true equivalency as the entire herb is being taken in capsule or tablet form, whereas only the medicinal constituents are taken in tea form.

Herbal Medicine Kits

An herbal medicine kit is a place to store herbal remedies for treating a range of common ailments. It can be a larger medicine chest for home use, or a smaller portable first aid kit. Having various remedies made up and stored together in one location can be invaluable for emergencies. It is also extremely helpful in preventing more serious ailments when you feel the first signs of a cold, flu, fever, stomachache, headache or constipation for example.

Making your own herbal remedies is one of the best ways to learn about herbs. The chapter on *Herbal Preparations* gives complete instructions for their preparation. Specific formulas are covered in the chapter on *Home Remedies*. If a remedy is not listed in either chapter, the formula is given. In some cases homeopathic remedies or Chinese prepared medicines are included because they are extremely effective for those conditions. Both may be found in larger health food stores and herbal shops; or, for Chinese prepared medicines, the Chinese sections of larger cities.

Several remedies are given for most of the conditions listed. This way you can choose which one best fits your situation. General instructions are also given on how to use each of these remedies. However, it is wise to read about the herbs in the chapter on *Knowing the Herbs* and perhaps keep their dosage information on a small file card in your kit.

How To Store

For home use, a large box or chest, or an allotted space on cabinet shelves, can be a good location for your herbal medicines. For travel, you can sew a small cloth bag or purchase a make-up bag found in most drug stores. Put tinctures, liniments, syrups and oils in small glass bottles. For travel, left-over shampoo sample bottles make great containers for these remedies. Put capsules and pills in small multi-compartment receptacles, such as pill boxes or fisherman containers. Salves, gels, powders and pastes store well in small tightly capped jars.

Keep track of the longevity of each remedy and replace when needed. The chapter on *Herbal Preparations* gives specific information on this. In general, tinctures, oils, liniments, salves, gels and pastes keep many years. Syrups, capsules, pills, bulk herbs and powders loose potency faster and so should be replaced every six months.

Other Things To Include

Along with the remedies listed, there are several other items of importance to incorporate in your medicine kits. These include alcohol wipes, an eye cup, file card guides on how to use the remedies (this comes in handy for those who might be able to help you!), a small first aid guide, gauze, adhesive tape, bandaids, butterfly bandages, needle and thread, stretch bandage for sprains, small scissors, tweezers and empty gelatin capsules. I always include a moxibustion stick with matches and foil (to put it out), a dermal hammer and a 2" piece of fresh ginger. Perhaps there are other items you personally use or feel important to include. Feel free to add what you want; customize your kit to fit your and the family's needs.

HERBAL MEDICINE KIT

Condition	Preparation	How To Use
athlete's foot & fungus	cinnamon, thyme, clove & tea tree oils	apply to affected area
antiseptic, antiviral	cinnamon, thyme, clove & tea tree oils	apply to affected area
bites—snake & insect	echinacea tincture	apply to bite; also take internally, 1 tsp every 2 hr
bladder infections	goldenseal capsules	take 2 every 2 hr
bleeding/ hemorrhage	tienchi, shephard's purse or yarrow; tincture; *Yunnan Baiyao* (Chinese)	apply directly to wound and internally as needed
bruises, sprains, muscle aches	liniment; calendula oil; moxibustion stick; *Tiger Balm* (Chinese)	apply to affected area as needed
burns/sunburn	aloe vera gel; calendula oil	apply directly to burned area
coldness	composition powder, capsules; angelica, cayenne & prickly ash capsules	take 2 caps as needed; not to exceed 8/day
colds/ flu	echinacea tincture; composition powder capsules; tree flower oil; garlic juice, oil or capsules	take dropperful echinacea and tsp garlic every 4 hr, or 2 caps composition powder every 2 hr, or 3 drops tree flower oil every 4 hr
colic	chamomile tea; Homeopathic *Calms*	1/2 tsp as needed; follow directions
constipation	bitters tincture; 1 part cascara & 1/4 part ginger capsules	take dropperful or 2 caps every 2 hr
coughs	syrup; licorice pills; mustard powder	1 tsp syrup every hr; pills as needed; make plaster with mustard for chest
cramps	antispasmodic tincture; caps of equal parts lobelia, scullcap, peony, valerian, black haw, 1/2 part cayenne	take 15-30 drops or 2 caps as needed; not to exceed 8/day

HERBAL MEDICINE KIT

Condition	Preparation	How To Use
cuts, scrapes infected wounds	salve of goldenseal, myrrh and calendula	apply as needed to affected area
depression	St. John's wort tincture; clary sage essential oil	take 15-30 drops tincture every 4 hr; take 1 drop oil in 1/4 cup water every 4 hr
diarrhea & dysentery	1 part each blackberry root mullein & goldenseal capsules	take 2 caps every 4 hr
earaches	echinacea tincture; mullein & garlic oil	1 dropperful echinacea every hr; 3 drops oil in ear every 2 hr
eye problems	eyebright and goldenseal tea preserved with tincture of benzoin; cineraria eye drops (available —Homeopathic distributors)	apply a few drops as needed
fatigue	equal parts ginseng, astragalus & siberian ginseng capsules; ginger fomentation	take two caps as needed; no more than 8/day; apply fomentation over waist on back
fever	equal parts boneset, chrysan-themum & scullcap capsules	take 2 caps every 4 hr
food poisoning	bitters tincture; Arsenicum homeopathic; Ipecac tincture (found in drug stores to induce vomiting)	mild—1 dropperful bitters every 2 hr or 5 homeopathic pills every 1/2 hr; severe— take Ipecac as directed
headache	antispasmodic tincture; tree flower oil;	15-30 drops tincture or extract as needed or rub oil into temples/forehead
indigestion, gas, bloatedness	bitters tincture; ginger capsules; *Curing Pills* (Chinese prepared medicine)	take 1 tsp bitters before meals; take 1-2 small bottles *Curing Pills* after meals
infections, inflammations	echinacea tincture; equal parts echinacea, goldenseal, chaparral & garlic capsules	take dropperful tincture every 15 minutes; take 2 caps every hr; no more than 8/day

HERBAL MEDICINE KIT

Condition	Preparation	How To Use
injuries/ accidents	Arnica oil or Arnica Homeopathic; *Rescue Remedy* (Bach Flower Remedy); *Yunnan Baiyao* (Chinese prepared powder)	follow directions given
insect repellant	oils of pennyroyal, wormwood, citronella, eucalyptus, rosemary	30 drops oil combination in 1 oz. vegetable oil; apply as needed
insomnia	antispasmodic tincture with scullcap & valerian	take 15-30 drops 1/2 hr before bed
malaria (prevention)	bitters tincture with *Artemesia anuum*	take 1 dropperful daily
nausea	ginger capsules; slippery elm powder; *Curing Pills* (Chinese)	take 2 caps as needed; make gruel of of slippery elm & take in teaspoon doses; follow directions
PMS	clary sage essential oil; chaste berry tincture	take 1 drop in 1/4 cup water or 15-30 drops tincture as needed
poison oak & ivy	green clay; tincture of equal parts witch hazel, mugwort, white oak bark, comfrey & plantain	poultice or tincture on affected area as needed
sore muscles	liniment	apply as needed
sore throat	licorice pills; composition powder; syrup; tree flower oil; ginger & cayenne powders; ginger fomentation	as many pills as needed; drink tea of composition powder; drink 3 drops tree flower oil in 1/2 cup water; ginger & cayenne gargle; fomentation over throat
teething	chamomile tea; Homeopathic *Calms*	drink 1/2 cup as needed; follow directions
urinary problems	equal parts uva ursi, dandelion, goldenseal, nettles & parsley	take 2 caps every 4 hr; no more than 8/day

IV.
Appendices

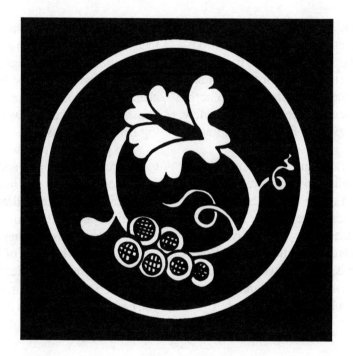

Symptoms and Their Herbal Remedies

The following symptoms are those mentioned in this book. They are not meant to be inclusive of all possible conditions, nor all possible herbs for that condition. Herbs are listed after each symptom which best help that problem. For the most part, only the herbs discussed in this book are included, although a few others which are very specific for certain ailments have been added.

I have divided the herbs up according to their warming, neutral and cooling energies. This will make it easier to decide which of the suggested herbs you should choose. After reading the chapter on *The Energy of Illness*, decide the energy of your condition. Then you can choose which herbs have the appropriate energy for your needs. In cases where an herb is becoming rare, such as goldenseal, research the other listed herbs as possible substitutes.

Once you have chosen your herbs, look each of them up in the chapter on *Knowing the Herbs* specific information on their usage, dosage, precautions and so forth. It would also be beneficial to reference the chapter on *Herbal Properties, Constituents, Families and Formulas* and review the instructions for creating herbal formulas.

It is important to discriminate which herbs with the correct energy are specifically appropriate for your needs. Do not just make up a formula with all the herbs listed. Instead, determine which of the herbs are most specifically suited for that condition. For example, to choose an herb listed under infections, look up to see what type of infection each given herb works for. Likewise, review what type of headache or indigestion those corresponding herbs treat. Then you can determine which herbs to use and how best to combine them together.

HOME REMEDIES			
Symptom	**Warm**	**Neutral**	**Cool**
Abdominal Pain	cinnamon, ginger, fennel	chamomile	————
Abdominal Distension	cardamom, cinnamon, citrus ginger, hawthorn	chamomile	————
Abscesses	————	————	dandelion, chaparral, echinacea, marshmallow
Acid Regurgitation	cardamom	slippery elm	pueraria, marshmallow

HOME REMEDIES

Symptom	Warm	Neutral	Cool
Acne	————	sarsaparilla, chaste berry	barberry, yellow dock, burdock seed and root
Addictions-drug and alcohol	————	————	scullcap, red clover
AIDS	————	reishi	American ginseng, St. John's wort
Allergies	astragalus	ginkgo leaf	————
Amnesia	————	zizyphus	————
Anal Itch	————	————	gentian, barberry, dandelion, gardenia, oregon grape, chickweed oil
Anemia	codonopsis, ginseng, dong quai, ho shou wu, cooked rehmannia	blackberries, raspberries, lycii, zizyphus	peony, yellow dock, nettles, dandelion
Anger	————	————	dandelion, burdock, scullcap, chrysanthemum, gardenia
Anxiety	fennel, ginseng, schisandra, jujube, dioscorea, cyperus, valerian	fu ling, zizyphus, sarsaparilla	black cohosh, scullcap, black haw, St. John's wort, peony
Appetite-loss of	cayenne, ginger, cinnamon, ginseng, jujube, fennel, angelica, elecampane, hawthorn, astragalus, citrus, atractylodes	Chinese wild yam	cascara sagrada, gentian
Appetite-too much	————	————	dandelion, comfrey
Arteriosclerosis	hawthorn	ginkgo leaf	
Arthritis	cinnamon, ginger, garlic, angelica, cayenne, aconite, prickly ash	calendula, black cohosh gingko leaf	barberry, burdock, nettle, red clover, oregon grape
Asthma	ginger, cardamom, garlic, ephedra, elecampane, schisandra, wild cherry	licorice, coltsfoot, reishi, ginkgo nut	mullein, comfrey, nettle, plantain, black cohosh

HOME REMEDIES			
Symptom	**Warm**	**Neutral**	**Cool**
Bed sores	_____	slippery elm	comfrey, marshmallow, echinacea
Bedwetting	parsley	ginkgo nut	burdock root
Bee stings	_____	_____	plantain, comfrey, echinacea, aloe
Belching	cardamom, ginger	_____	_____
Bites (see Insect Bites)			
Bladder Infections	ginger, parsley, garlic, astragalus	shepherd's purse	plantain, goldenseal, marshmallow, gentian, dandelion, nettle, uva ursi, gardenia, motherwort, burdock, chaparral
Bleeding (external)	cayenne, tienchi	calendula, yarrow, shepherd's purse	marshmallow, yellow dock
Bleeding (internal)	cayenne, tienchi , mugwort	yarrow, blackberry, raspberry, slippery elm, shepherd's purse, squawvine	gardenia, peony, nettle, comfrey, dandelion, marshmallow, uva ursi, mullein, American ginseng
Bleeding (uterine)	cinnamon, tienchi, mugwort, cooked rehmannia	shepherd's purse	peony
Bepharitis	_____	_____	eyebright
Bloatedness	black pepper, ginger, cardamom	_____	gentian, oregon grape
Blood Building and Strengthening	dong quai, ho shou wu, cooked rehmannia	blackberries, raspberries, lycii	dandelion, burdock, nettle, yellow dock
Blood Circulation (moves blood)	ginger, mugwort, tienchi, garlic, dong quai, cayenne, angelica, cinnamon, prickly ash, hawthorn, bayberry	calendula, ginkgo leaf	_____
Blood clots	angelica, tienchi	_____	red clover
Blood Poisoning	licorice	_____	dandelion, echinacea, goldenseal

HOME REMEDIES

Symptom	Warm	Neutral	Cool
Blood Sugar Level *(see also diabetes and hypoglycemia)*	fenugreek, schisandra	——————	comfrey, burdock
Blurred Vision	dong quai, ho sohu wu	lycii	chrysanthemum
Boils	fenugreek	yarrow, lobelia slippery elm	dandelion, echinacea, barberry, burdock, chickweed, comfrey, plantain, marshmallow, honeysuckle, chrysanthemum
Breast Sores, Cysts	——————	——————	dandelion
Broken and Fractured Bones	tienchi	chamomile	comfrey
Bronchitis	ginger, cardamom, garlic, elecampane, mugwort, wild cherry, ephedra	calendula, licorice, reishi, coltsfoot, slippery elm	comfrey, plantain, borage, eyebright, mullein
Bruises	turmeric, tienchi	yarrow, calendula	mullein
Burns	——————	calendula, chamomile, yarrow, slippery elm	plantain, comfrey, St. John's wort, aloe, echinacea, marshmallow aloe
Calming	valerian, jujube, schisandra	licorice, chamomile, fu ling, zizyphus	lemon balm, scullcap, peony
Cancer	——————	reishi	chapparal, echinacea, oregon grape, dandelion, red clover, burdock, goldenseal
Canker Sores	——————	——————	burdock
Carbuncles	——————	——————	burdock
Chicken Pox	——————	calendula, yarrow	dandelion, echinacea
Childbirth (after)	turmeric, hawthorn, ginger, dong quai, ginseng, cooked rehmannia	shepherd's purse	black haw, comfrey, uva ursi, black cohosh, motherwort
Childbirth (facilitates)	ginger	lobelia, raspberry	black cohosh, squawvine

HOME REMEDIES

Symptom	Warm	Neutral	Cool
Cholesterol	garlic, hawthorn	reishi	———————
Circulation (enhances)	angelica, ginger, bayberry, cinnamon, prickly ash, dong quai, Siberian ginseng	ginkgo leaf	peony
Cirrhosis	———————	———————	cascara sagrada, barberry, dandelion, milk thistle
Coldness	ginger, cinnamon, aconite, a little cayenne, Siberian ginseng, angelica, prickly ash	ginkgo leaf	———————
Colds	cinnamon, ginger, garlic, cayenne, angelica, bayberry, black pepper, cardamom, mugwort, ephedra	licorice, yarrow, coltsfoot, chamomile, sarsaparilla	lemon balm, peppermint, mullein, echinacea, pueraria, chrysanthemum, honeysuckle, feverfew
Colic	ginger, fennel, cinnamon, prickly ash, cardamom	chamomile	lemon balm, peppermint
Complexion	———————	blackberries	———————
Conjunctivitis			honeysuckle, yellow dock, goldenseal, marshmallow
Constipation	fennel, dong quai, ho shou wu	chamomile, licorice	dandelion, barberry, aloe, oregon grape, chaparral, gentian, cascara, sagrada, goldenseal, yellow dock, raw rehmannia
Convulsions	ginger	chamomile, lobelia	black haw, scullcap
Cough	ginger, cinnamon, citrus, ephedra, schisandra, bayberry, black pepper, wild cherry, codonopsis, garlic, cardamom, elecampane	yarrow, licorice, coltsfoot, lobelia, slippery elm, Chinese wild yam, ginkgo nut	comfrey, lemon balm, black cohosh, mullein, marshmallow, American ginseng
Cramps	ginger, cinnamon, cayenne, fennel, garlic, valerian	chamomile, licorice, calendula, yarrow	lemon balm, peony, black cohosh
Crying and Whining	———————	licorice, chamomile	lemon balm

HOME REMEDIES			
Symptom	**Warm**	**Neutral**	**Cool**
Cuts	tienchi	calendula, yarrow, chamomile	echinacea, plantain, comfrey
Cysts	——————	——————	dandelion
Dandruff	ginger	——————	chaparral, chickweed
Debility	aconite, astragalus, ginseng, codonopis	——————	American ginseng
Dental Carries	——————	——————	dandelion, chaparral
Depression	cinnamon, cayenne, cyperus	licorice, chamomile, fu ling, Chinese wild yam, zizyphus, chaste berry	lemon balm, bupleurum, St. John's wort, peony
Diabetes	elecampane, fenugreek, astragalus, codonopsis	licorice, Chinese wild yam	pueraria, dandelion, comfrey, marshmallow
Diarrhea	cayenne, cinnamon, aconite, bayberry, cardamom, prickly ash, hawthorn, schisandra, wild cherry, astragalus, atractylodes, citrus, ginseng, codonopsis, jujube	blackberry, raspberry, yarrow, Chinese wild yam	mullein, plantain, barberry, gentian, marshmallow, pueraria
Digestion (helps)	cayenne, cinnamon, garlic, ginger, elecampane, fennel, fenugreek, angelica, black pepper, fu ling, wild cherry, citrus, astragalus, mugwort, jujube, cyperus, codonopsis, hawthorn, parsley, prickly ash, turmeric, atractylodes, cardamom	yarrow, chamomile, slippery elm, Chinese wild yam	comfrey, dandelion, cascara sagrada, barberry, gentian, goldenseal, peppermint, feverfew
Dizziness	ho shou wu, valerian, cornus, cooked rehmannia	lycii, ginkgo leaf	peony
Dry Mouth	——————	——————	raw rehmannia
Dyes (use as)	——————	calendula, yarrow, chamomile	——————
Dysentery	cinnamon, cayenne, garlic, hawthorn, wild cherry	yarrow, mullein, blackberry, raspberry	plantain, barberry, goldenseal, marshmallow, honeysuckle

HOME REMEDIES

Symptom	Warm	Neutral	Cool
Dysmenorrhea	turmeric, bayberry, angelica, dong quai, mugwort, cyperus, ginger	calendula, chamomile, raspberry, yarrow	motherwort, squawvine, peony
Earache & Ear Infections	garlic, ginger	calendula, chamomile, lobelia	mullein, echinacea
Eczema	calendula, yarrow	——	dandelion, yellow dock, burdock, chaparral, chick weed, goldenseal, mullein, nettle, comfrey, red clover
Emphysema	wild cherry	coltsfoot	mullein, comfrey
Energy (gives youthful)	astragalus, ho shou wu, Siberian ginseng	reishi	——
Energy (low)	ginger, cayenne, jujube, ginseng, atractylodes, cinnamon, astragalus, codonopsis, Siberian ginseng	licorice, zizyphus, reishi, Chinese wild yam	nettle, American ginseng
Energy (moves it)	bayberry, ginger, cayenne, tienchi, citrus, cardamom, cinnamon	——	——
Epilepsy	——	sarsaparilla	black cohosh, peony, scullcap, turmeric tuber
Exhaustion	astragalus, ginseng, jujube, Siberian ginseng, dong quai	zizyphus, licorice, reishi	——
Eye Weakness or Problems	——	——	eyebright, chrysanthemum
Eyes (red and sore)	——	yarrow, calendula	honeysuckle, gardenia, dandelion, eyebright, goldenseal, scullcap, chrysanthemum
Fainting	valerian	——	——
Fat (excess)	——	seaweed (kelp)	chickweed
Fertility (see Infertility)			

\-			
	HOME REMEDIES		
Symptom	**Warm**	**Neutral**	**Cool**
Fever	ginger, fenugreek, garlic, mugwort, atractylodes, ephedra	calendula, yarrow, lobelia, sarsaparilla, chamomile	lemon balm, echinacea, gardenia, honeysuckle, barberry, borage, comfrey, chickweed, pueraria, dandelion, goldenseal, peppermint, red clover, bupleurum, American ginseng, chrysanthemum, raw rehmannia, feverfew
Flu	cinnamon, cayenne, garlic, ginger, angelica, mugwort, ephedra	licorice, chamomile, yarrow, coltsfoot, sarsaparilla	lemon balm, echinacea, mullein, goldenseal, peppermint, pueraria, honeysuckle, feverfew, chrysanthemum
Fluid Retention	parsley, aconite, astragalus, ephedra	fu ling	burdock, plantain
Food Stagnation	hawthorn, citrus, cyperus, ginger	————	peppermint
Forgetfulness	ginseng, schisandra, jujube, cinnamon, angelica, dong quai	ginkgo leaf, zizyphus, reishi	————
Frostbite	cayenne	————	mullein
Fungus	mugwort, angelica, garlic	calendula	————
Gallstones	————	————	dandelion
Gangrene	————	slippery elm	comfrey, echinacea, marshmallow
Gas	ginger, cinnamon, citrus, codonopsis, black pepper, fennel, cardamom, cayenne, parsley, cyperus, angelica	chamomile, sarsaparilla	gentian, motherwort, peppermint
Gastritis	wild cherry	————	gentian, marshmallow
Glandular Problems	————	licorice, sarsaparilla	kelp (seaweed)
Gonorrhea	————	sarsaparilla	————

HOME REMEDIES

Symptom	Warm	Neutral	Cool
Gout	————	sarsaparilla	burdock, red clover
Gums	bayberry, cayenne, prickly ash, cinnamon	————	————
Hair (graying)	ho shou wu, dong quai	————	————
Hair (growth)	————	blackberries	————
Headache	cayenne, cinnamon, ginger, cardamom, valerian	ginkgo leaf	peppermint, scullcap, pueraria, chrysanthemum, feverfew
Hearing Acuity (enhance)	cornus	ginkgo leaf	————
Heartburn	————	————	gentian, goldenseal
Heart Tonic	cayenne, hawthorn, aconite, ginseng	reishi	motherwort
Hemorrhage	cayenne, tienchi	raspberry, yarrow	nettle, turmeric tuber
Hemorrhoids	ginger, calendula	yarrow, shepherd's purse	mullein, plantain, comfrey, chickweed, goldenseal, bupleurum, yellow dock, cascara sagrada
Hepatitis	schisandra	reishi	dandelion, echinacea, plantain, oregon grape, gardenia, barberry, gentian, milk thistle
Hernia	fenugreek	————	————
Herpes	————	sarsaparilla	aloe, dandelion, yellow dock, gentian, lemon balm salve
Hiccoughs	elecampane	————	————
High Blood Pressure	hawthorn berries	ginkgo leaf, reishi	dandelion, echinacea, chamomile, plantain
Hives	————	————	chickweed tea and oil

HOME REMEDIES			
Symptom	**Warm**	**Neutral**	**Cool**
Hoarse Voice	cardamom	coltsfoot, licorice	mullein
Hyperacidity	codonopsis	slippery elm	pueraria
Hypertension	cayenne, hawthorn berries	ginkgo leaf, reishi	scullcap, gardenia, chrysanthemum
Hypoglycemia	———————	licorice	dandelion, burdock, pueraria
Hysteria	valerian	———————	black cohosh, black haw, lemon balm, motherwort, scullcap, peony
Immunity (increases)	astragalus, codonopsis, cinnamon, ginger, ginseng, bayberry, schisandra	reishi	echinacea, American ginseng
Impotence	ho shou wu, aconite, cornus, cinnamon, ginseng	raspberries, lycii, blackberries	———————
Indigestion	angelica, black pepper, cardamom, parsley, fennel, jujube dates, hawthorn, garlic, ginger, turmeric, atractylodes, citrus, cyperus	chamomile	peppermint, gentian, dandelion
Infantile Convulsion	———————	licorice, chamomile	lemon balm
Infections	garlic	yarrow, calendula, lobelia, slippery elm	echinacea, plantain, dandelion, goldenseal, honeysuckle, comfrey, burdock marshmallow, chaparral
Infections (bladder and kidney)	garlic, ginger, parsley aconite, astragalus	shepherd's purse	plantain, burdock, marshmallow, gardenia, motherwort, nettle, uva ursi, chaparral, dandelion, goldenseal, gentian
Infections (ear)	garlic, ginger	calendula, chamomile, lobelia	mullein, echinacea
Infertility	mugwort, aconite, ho shou wu, dong quai, ginseng, cooked rehmannia	blackberries, lycii, chaste berry	motherwort

HOME REMEDIES

Symptom	Warm	Neutral	Cool
Inflammations	cayenne, garlic, turmeric	yarrow, slippery elm	echinacea, plantain, honeysuckle, borage, comfrey, dandelion, goldenseal, burdock, chickweed, chapparal, marshmallow
Inflammation (bowel)	bayberry	slippery elm	mullein, honeysuckle, marshmallow
Inflammation (nose)	——————	——————	eyebright
Influenza (see Flu)			
Injuries	dong quai, tienchi, prickly ash, turmeric	calendula	aloe, gardenia
Insect Bites or Stings	——————	——————	aloe, comfrey, plantain, chickweed, echinacea
Insomnia	hawthorn, mugwort, ginseng, valerian, ho shu wu, jujube, schisandra, cooked rehmannia	licorice, chamomile, reishi, zizyphus	lemon balm, scullcap, raw rehmannia, gardenia
Irritability	jujube	chamomile, zizyphus	chrysanthemum, gardenia, burdock, dandelion, bupleurum, scullcap, turmeric tuber, barberry, American ginseng, raw rehmannia
Itching	mugwort	——————	chickweed oil, chapparal, gentian, yellow dock
Joint Pains	garlic, ginger, cayenne, prickly ash	calendula, chamomile	marshmallow
Knee Pain	cinnamon, cornus, ho shou wu, prickly ash	lycii	——————
Kidney Infection	garlic, ginger, aconite, parsley, astragalus	shepherd's purse	motherwort, gardenia, plantain, burdock, marshmallow, uva ursi, goldenseal, gentian, chapparal, nettle, dandelion

HOME REMEDIES			
Symptom	**Warm**	**Neutral**	**Cool**
Laryngitis	cayenne	coltsfoot, licorice, slippery elm	_____
Leukorrhea	garlic, ho shou wu, schisandra, mugwort	sarsaparilla, lycii, yarrow, Chinese wild yam, ginkgo nut, raspberry leaf	gentian, goldenseal, peony, squawvine
Liver Enlargement	_____	reishi	aloe, barberry, dandelion, burdock, bupleurum, milk thistle
Lockjaw	_____	lobelia	_____
Longevity	hawthorn, garlic, astragalus, ginseng	licorice, reishi	marshmallow, American ginseng, chrysanthemum
Low Back Pain (see Pain)			
Low Blood Pressure	garlic, ginseng	_____	_____
Malnutrition	astragalus, jujube, ginseng, cooked rehmannia	Chinese wild yam, lycii, slippery elm, reishi, raspberries, blackberries	American ginseng, comfrey, marshmallow
Measles	_____	calendula, yarrow	dandelion, pueraria, peppermint
Memory (see Forgetfulness)			
Menopause	valerian, dong quai	chaste berry	_____
Menstruation (delayed)	ginger, mugwort, parsley, angelica	calendula, chaste berry	motherwort
Menstruation (excessive)	bayberry, mugwort, cornus	yarrow, blackberry, raspberry, shepherd's purse, chaste berry	plantain, squawvine
Menstruation (lack of)	angelica, ginger, mugwort, parsley, cayenne, turmeric	chamomile, chaste berry	black cohosh, peony, motherwort, squawvine
Menstruation (regulate)	ginger, mugwort, turmeric, cyperus, dong quai, cooked rehmannia	blackberries, calendula, raspberries, chaste berry	black haw, peony, motherwort,

HOME REMEDIES			
Symptom	**Warm**	**Neutral**	**Cool**
Migraine	——————	——————	feverfew
Minerals (high in)	——————	——————	dandelion, comfrey, nettle, yellow dock, scullcap
Miscarriage (habitual)	mugwort	——————	black haw
Morning Sickness	fenugreek, cardamom, atractylodes	raspberry	black haw
Mother's Milk (decreases)	——————	yarrow	mullein, plantain
Mother's Milk	fennel, fenugreek	chaste berry	dandelion, marshmallow
Motion Sickness	ginger	——————	——————
Mouth Sores	——————	——————	raw rehmannia, echinacea, goldenseal, gardenia, chrysanthemum
Mucus (excessive)	ginger, cinnamon, black pepper, wild cherry, fennel, elecampane, fenugreek, cayenne, bayberry, citrus, cardamom	coltsfoot	comfrey, borage, chickweed, nettle, mullein
Mucus (irritated membranes)	——————	licorice	borage, mullein, comfrey
Mumps	——————	——————	echinacea, mullein
Muscles, sore	prickly ash, ginger, tienchi	chamomile, lobelia	St. John's wort
Nausea	ginger, cinnamon	chamomile	——————
Nerve Pain , Neuralgia (see Pain)			
Nervousness	jujube, fennel, garlic, fenugreek, hawthorn, mugwort, valerian, wild cherry, aconite	licorice, chamomile, lobelia, sarsaparilla, slippery elm, zizyphus	lemon balm, peony, black cohosh, scullcap, motherwort, black haw, St. John's wort

HOME REMEDIES			
Symptom	**Warm**	**Neutral**	**Cool**
Night Blindness	——————	lycii	——————
Night Sweats	cornus, schisandra, cooked rehmannia	zizyphus	American ginseng, peony
Nocturnal Emission	cooked rehmannia, cornus, schisandra, ho shou wu	lycii, ginkgo nut	——————
Nosebleeds	tienchi	yarrow	——————
Numbness	aconite, tienchi, bayberry, cayenne, cinnamon, prickly ash	——————	——————
Pain (abdominal)	ginger, cinnamon, cayenne, dong quai, aconite, cyperus, turmeric, prickly ash, fenugreek	chamomile, lobelia	motherwort, black haw, bupleurum, peony
Pain (chest)	aconite, cyperus	——————	bupleurum, peony
Pain (cramps)	cinnamon, cayenne, ginger, prickly ash, valerian, aconite, turmeric	licorice, lobelia, chamomile	motherwort, lemon balm, black haw, black cohosh
Pain (knee)	ho shou wu, cornus, cinnamon	lycii, calendula	——————
Pain (low back)	cinnamon, ginger, garlic, fenugreek, ho shou wu, cornus, aconite	lycii, lobelia	burdock, dandelion
Pain (nerve)	——————	licorice, chamomile	St. John's wort, scullcap, black cohosh
Palpitations	dong quai, ginseng, cayenne, cooked rehmannia, hawthorn, valerian,	licorice, fu ling, zizyphus	motherwort
Parasites	garlic, mugwort	sarsaparilla	chapparal
Pharyngitis	——————	——————	comfrey
Pleurisy	angelica	licorice	comfrey, marshmallow
PMS	parsley, turmeric, cyperus	chaste berry	motherwort, peony, skull-cap, aloe, bupleurum, black cohosh, dandelion

HOME REMEDIES

Symptom	Warm	Neutral	Cool
Pneumonia	ginger, cayenne, cinnamon,	licorice, yarrow	lemon balm, borage, comfrey, mullein, marshmallow, chrysanthemum
Poison Oak and Ivy	————————	yarrow	echinacea, dandelion
Poor Memory (see Forgetfulness)			
Post Partum	hawthorn, rehmannia, ginseng, dong quai	lycii	black cohosh, motherwort, black haw, uva ursi
Pregnancy	fenugreek, atractylodes	raspberry, lobelia	black cohosh, sqwawvine, black haw
Premature Ejaculation	cornus, lycii, ho shou wu	raspberries, blackberries	————————
Prolapsed Organs	astragalus, ginseng		black cohosh, bupleurum
Psoriasis	————————	sarsaparilla	comfrey, red clover, yellow dock
Quench Thirst	ginseng	licorice	————————
Rashes	————————	chamomile, calendula, slippery elm	echinacea, dandelion, burdock, red clover
Rejuvenative	astragalus, ginseng, garlic, fenugreek	licorice	marshmallow, chrysanthemum, American ginseng
Relaxing, Calming (see Nervousness)			
Restless	ginseng, jujube, valerian, schisandra	licorice, chamomile, fu ling, zizyphus	lemon balm, gardenia, scullcap, St. John's wort, peony, burdock
Rheumatism	ginger, calendula, cinnamon, prickly ash, angelica, garlic Siberian ginseng, cayenne	sarsaparilla, reishi, ginkgo leaf	bayberry, burdock, St. John's wort, black cohosh
Scabies	————————	————————	chapparal
Sciatica	aconite	————————	St. John's wort
Seboria	————————	————————	chickweed, burdock

HOME REMEDIES

Symptom	Warm	Neutral	Cool
Seminal Emission	cornus, rehmannia	————————	————————
Senility	————————	ginkgo leaf	————————
Shortness of Breath	astragalus, codonopsis, ginseng	————————	————————
Shock	ginseng, tienchi		
Sinus Problems	ginger, bayberry, cardamom, black pepper	————————	————————
Skin Eruptions and Problems	angelica, fenugreek, mugwort, prickly ash	calendula, slippery elm, sarsaparilla, yarrow	echinacea, plantain, chickweed, dandelion, borage, aloe, burdock, nettle, red clover, yellow dock, comfrey, oregon grape
Skin Tears	————————	calendula, yarrow, chamomile	comfrey, plantain, echinacea
Smoking (Stopping)	————————	lobelia	mullein
Snake Bites	————————	————————	echinacea, dandelion
Sores	astragalus	calendula, yarrow, chamomile, slippery elm, sarsaparilla	comfrey, plantain, echinacea, marshmallow, chickweed, gardenia
Sore Throat	ginger, bayberry, cayenne, garlic	licorice, slippery elm	echinacea, comfrey, honeysuckle, raw rehmannia
Spasms	angelica, valerian, garlic, ginger, fennel, cinnamon	chamomile, lobelia	black haw, motherwort, scullcap, peony
Spermatorrhea	cornus, ho shou wu, cinnamon	raspberries, ginkgo nut, Chinese wild yam	————————
Spider Bites (see Insect Bites)			
Spleen Enlargement	————————	————————	barberry, dandelion
Splinters and Slivers (draw out)	————————	————————	plantain, comfrey

HOME REMEDIES

Symptom	Warm	Neutral	Cool
Spontaneous Sweating	atractylodes, cornus, astragalus, schisandra, ginseng	Chinese wild yam, zizyphus	peony
Sprains	cayenne, ginger, tienchi	calendula	comfrey
Staph	garlic	————	honeysuckle, comfrey, plantain
Stiff Neck and Shoulders	cinnamon	————	pueraria
Stomach ache	ginger, cinnamon	yarrow, licorice, chamomile	dandelion
Stomach Ulcer (see Ulcers)			
Stones (gall)	parsley, turmeric	————	oregon grape, dandelion
Stones (kidney)	parsley	————	dandelion, plantain, nettle, marshmallow, uva ursi
Strep Throat	————	licorice	honeysuckle, gardenia, echinacea, marshmallow
Stress	fennel, schisandra, Siberian ginseng, cinnamon	licorice, chamomile, reishi	black cohosh, dandelion, black haw, lemon balm, borage
Styes	cayenne	————	burdock, honeysuckle, gentian, goldenseal, eyebright, scullcap, yellow dock, chrysanthemum
Sunburn	————	————	aloe, mullein, plantain
Swellings	prickly ash, tienchi, parsley, astragalus	————	borage, honeysuckle
Swollen Glands	————	————	mullein, echinacea, red clover
Syphilis	————	sarsaparilla	mullein, red clover, echinacea

HOME REMEDIES			
Symptom	**Warm**	**Neutral**	**Cool**
Teeth and Gums	bayberry, cinnamon, prickly ash	——————	——————
Teething		licorice, chamomile	lemon balm, echinacea
Thirst	ginseng, cooked rehmannia	licorice, lycii	American ginseng, pueraria, raw rehmannia
Throat (inflammation)	ginger	licorice	echinacea, eyebright, raw rehmannia
Throat (sore)	ginger, bayberry, garlic, cayenne	licorice, slippery elm	echinacea, comfrey, peppermint, raw rehmannia, honeysuckle
Tinnitis	——————	ginkgo leaf	——————
Tiredness (see Energy)			
Tissue (tones, heals)	bayberry	——————	comfrey
Tongue Sores	——————	——————	raw rehmannia, gardenia, echinacea, marshmallow
Tonsillitis	——————	——————	comfrey, enchinacea
Toothache	cayenne, prickly ash, garlic, bayberry	yarrow	mullein, echinacea
Tuberculosis	fenugreek, ginseng, astragalus	licorice, lycii, slippery elm	marshmallow, American ginseng
Tumors	astragalus	slippery elm, reishi	chapparal, dandelion, red clover, oregon grape
Ulcers (intestinal)	wild cherry	calendula, licorice, slippery elm, lobelia	plantain, comfrey, marshmallow, St. John's wort, goldenseal
Ulcers (stomach)	cayenne, angelica, wild cherry, astragalus	calendula, licorice, slippery elm, lobelia	plantain, comfrey, gardenia, goldenseal, St. John's wort, marshmallow
Urination (frequent)	parsley, aconite, cornus	raspberry, yarrow, Chinese wild yam	——————

HOME REMEDIES

Symptom	Warm	Neutral	Cool
Urination (increases)	parsley, astragalus, Siberian ginseng	fu ling, shepherd's purse	dandelion, plantain, bur dock, nettle, uva ursi
Urinatiom (night time)	aconite, parsley, cinnamon	raspberry	———————
Uterus (tonic)	parsley	blackberry	aloe, black haw
Uterus (bleeding)— see bleeding			
Uterus (tumor)	bayberry, turmeric		
Vaccination (effects of and reactions)	———————	———————	echinacea
Vaginal Discharge	bayberry, garlic, schisandra	raspberry, yarrow	goldenseal, gentian, peony, squawvine
Vaginal Itch	———————	———————	gentian
Valvular Heart Disease	hawthorn	———————	———————
Varicose Veins	bayberry	calendula, yarrow	comfrey, St. John's wort
Viruses	———————	———————	chapparal, honeysuckle
Vitality and Low Energy (raises)	cinnamon, ginger, cayenne, codonopsis, ginseng, bayberry, astragalus	blackberries, licorice, reishi	bupleurum
Voice (hoarse)	cardamom	———————	———————
Vomiting	ginger, elecampane, fennel, cardamom, cinnamon, citrus, atractylodes, codonopsis	chamomile, slippery elm	peppermint, bupleurum
Warts	———————	———————	chapparal
Weakness	aconite, ginseng, jujube, atractylodes, codonopsis, astragalus	reishi	American ginseng
Weight (to gain)	ginseng, jujube	slippery elm	———————
Weight (to loose)	———————	seaweed	chickweed, barberry, dandelion

| \
HOME REMEDIES			
Symptom	**Warm**	**Neutral**	**Cool**
Wheezing	ginseng, ephedra, elecampane, schisandra	coltsfoot	_____
Whooping Cough	ginger, cinnamon, wild cherry	yarrow, licorice, coltsfoot, lobelia	lemon balm, comfrey, black cohosh, mullein
Wrinkles	ho shou wu		aloe
Worms	garlic, mugwort, parsley	_____	_____
Wounds	prickly ash, turmeric, tienchi	calendula, yarrow, slippery elm	comfrey, plantain, echinacea, aloe, marshmallow, mullein, yellow dock, St. John's wort, chapparal
Yeast	garlic, mugwort	_____	_____

A Few Tips for Mothers and Children

The many stages of carrying, birthing and raising a child entail different and varied health needs, both for the mother and the child. Several books are available focusing just on these issues and some are listed in the Bibliography. In addition, here are a few handy guidelines I'd like to pass along for treating babies and young children herbally.

Babies

The best way to treat nursing babies with herbs is to treat the mother. Any herbs you, the mother, take go directly into your milk and to the babe. Use the same herbs you would give for the baby's ailment and drink them in a tea. Start with teaspoon doses at first to make sure baby doesn't have a reaction. Increase to a cup, twice a day, if needed. Your baby will be able to accept and absorb the herbs through your milk. Mild herbs are quite safe to take during nursing. It is best to avoid laxative herbs, however, so that they don't cause diarrhea in the baby.

This same method is true of food. Whatever foods aggravate your baby's condition should be eliminated from your diet, while the foods that help should be eaten. Thus, if your nursing baby is sick it is important for you to examine your own diet and life habits. Because nursing babies are getting their sustenance from you, you may need to curtail certain foods, herbs or other substances which inevitably affect the baby.[1]

I have seen this occur many times. Once a mother was drinking 3 cups of peppermint tea a day, and her child began breaking out with red spots all over his body. As soon as the mother stopped drinking the tea, the spots went away. This is because peppermint is spicy and stimulates the pores to open. Another time, a mother was eating a lot of cheese, and her child continually had a stuffy nose. When the mother eliminated cheese from her diet, her child's nose cleared.

A third mom led a fairly chaotic life which, because she was immersed in it, didn't appear so to her. When she calmed her life, however, her "hyperactive" child calmed, too. It's important for nursing mothers to realize that what they are eating, drinking and doing has a dynamic impact on their babes, whether or not it is visually evident.[2]

Several herbs are excellent for increasing milk volume or for thickening your milk. These include *malva*, *marshmallow*, *blessed thistle*, *fennel*, *chaste berry*, *fenugreek*, *alfalfa* and *dandelion*. Drink 2-3 cups of tea a day of one or more of these herbs. For nourishing and enriching milk, *mochi* is an excellent food. This is a flattened "cake" of pounded sweet rice available in most natural foods stores. Heated goat's or raw milk with a little *ginger* added and followed by a taste of *honey* also enriches mother's milk.

For those who cannot nurse, there are several other effective ways to give babies herbs. A plastic eyedropper is useful for administering mild herbal teas. Squeeze a dropperful of the tea into the baby's mouth several times throughout the day. Keep the freshly made tea in the dropper bottle, and then it can conveniently travel with you and your babe throughout the day. This is a good method for treating colic. Try a combination of equal parts *chamomile*, *fennel* and *lemon balm* for this.

Herbal baths are also very effective and quite safe. The baby will absorb the healing properties of the herbs through the skin and into the blood stream. This can be done two to three times a day until the problem goes away. Fevers respond especially well to a bath of *poplar bark.*

Young Children

Teething can be a difficult time for mothers and babies. To help ease this process, both should drink *chamomile* tea in cup doses for the mother and teaspoon doses for the child. Mother can rub a little *birch, clove* or *St. John's wort* oils on baby's gums to help ease irritation. Chamomile homeopathic tablets can also be very effective.

Most children go through stages of intense activity and some are even hyperactive. Herbs very effectively ease any tension and calm the child. Try a combination of 2 parts each *chamomile, lemon balm, valerian* and *zizyphus seeds* and 1 part each *licorice root* and *hawthorn berries.* This is best made into a glycerine tincture. A little *cinnamon* and *anise oils* can be added for flavoring. Give 3-7 drops as needed throughout the day.

Hyperactivity is greatly affected, and caused, by diet. Excessive sugar, coke and other soft drinks, meat and treats all contribute to hyperactivity. The energy of foods affects children as it does adults. It is building their bodies and creating their future health. I have seen children with diarrhea, constant runny noses and/or frequent colds have these conditions quickly clear up just by eliminating their daily apple juice. A good diet supplemented with appropriate herbs helps a child grow strong and healthy.

---

[1] Those who are considering whether they should nurse or not definitely should. Formula is a very poor substitute for mother's milk. Nursing provides babies with a natural immunity, and the holding, caring and bonding that occurs helps create a more satisfied and fulfilled child.

[2] When we realize the direct and intimate connection created with our babes through nursing, it hopefully makes us nursing mothers think more than twice about what we put into our mouths. Alcohol, tobacco, caffeine, sugar, recreational drugs and poor food all go into your baby and create the same effects as you feel. The baby's body is then built from this. Any resulting sickness makes your life more difficult, not to mention the future it provides your child.

Macrobiotics and the System of Traditional Chinese Medicine

by Michael Tierra, L.Ac., O.M.D.

Perhaps one of the most unique contributions of this work is in the distinction between the predominant Yin-Yang classification of diseases, foods and herbs of the late George Ohsawa's macrobiotics and the Chinese energetic system. While basing it on the principles of traditional Chinese medicine, Ohsawa, when formulating and presenting his macrobiotic diet to the World, reversed some of the attributions and definitions of Yin and Yang. This has been the source of much confusion. With the rise of traditional Chinese medicine in the West, it would be regrettable indeed that the very worthwhile principles of the macrobiotic diet, based on traditional grain-based diets from around the world, may eventually be overlooked because of what may ultimately be considered as "Ohsawa's folly!"

The intent of Ohsawa's macrobiotics was to formulate a complete cosmological system which integrated diet and health with cosmic philosophy. To do this, Ohsawa reversed the traditional definitions of Yin and Yang in certain very important ways so that in contrast to the traditional approach of the Chinese, Yin is a rising energy and includes the sweet, sour and spicy flavors while Yang has a descending or dense energy and includes the salty and bitter taste.

The traditional Chinese designations used by thousands of trained Chinese herbalists and acupuncturists around the world is that Yin has a downward quality (earth) and includes the sour, bitter and salty flavors while Yang is upwards (heaven) and includes sweet and spicy as flavors. This unfortunate reversal of terms has been the source of annoying confusion among those who study and practice Traditional Chinese Medicine (TCM) and has resulted in the rejection of some otherwise very worthwhile macrobiotic principles, especially as they pertain to diet and nutrition.

Traditional Chinese medicine, while based upon Yin-Yang principles, generally tends to avoid making the classification of Yin and Yang to all foods, herbs and conditions. Instead it conjugates the qualities of Yin and Yang according to eight principles. Only if it becomes necessary to designate the Yinness or Yangness of an herb, food or condition would they be so regarded. Following the TCM definition of Yin and Yang as it pertains to health and healing, we have the following:

Yin—substantial, cold, deficient and moist;
Yang—ephemeral, hot, excessive and dry.

If anyone has had any experience attempting to define and utilize Yin-Yang theory with herbs and foods they would readily know how much confusion results. The same confusion occurs when attempting to classify foods according to acid-alkaline concepts. Basically, it centers around determining whether a given food or herb is Yin or Yang within itself or simply promotes those energies and qualities after being assimilated into the body.

Unlike macrobiotics, it seems that the Chinese wisely avoid making ultimate assignments of foods under the category of Yin or Yang. To them, assigning all foods and herbs as Yin and Yang, as is done in macrobiotics, is like resorting to the supreme court for all minor decisions. Instead, they seem to prefer to energetically classify foods and herbs primarily according to their hot or cold energies as represented by their flavors and actions (full or empty), allowing the classification of Yin and Yang to remain sometimes only vaguely implied. It is further interesting to note that by classifying herbs in terms of their hot or cold energies there is a pretty good equivalence in equating hot with acid-forming foods and cold with alkaline-forming foods.

I am happy to say that by consciously avoiding getting enmeshed in the Yin-Yang jungle, this book becomes important as the first to transmute the macrobiotics Yin-Yang classification of foods into the more traditional and less dogmatic, hot-cold, empty-full classification. By so doing, one preserves the tremendous value of macrobiotic philosophy (which, after all, has been one of the prime movers towards the wide acceptance of the value of high-fiber diets in the prevention of disease), offering a genuine potential to include a greater variety of foods according to more traditional energetic principles using the five flavors, the five energies of hot, warm, neutral, cool and cold together with empty and full to denote its nutritional content.

Bibliography

Western Herbals

Boericke, William, M.D., *Homeopathic Materia Medica*, New Delhi, India, Jain Publishers, 1976 (55/I, Arjun Narar, New Delhi 10016). Homeopathic medicine.

Christopher, Dr. John R., *School of Natural Healing*, Provo, UT, Biworld, 1976.

Courtenay and Aimmerman, *Wildflowers and Weeds*, Cincinnati, New York, Toronto, London, Melbourne, Van Nostrand Reinhold. A book useful for its many outstanding photographs of wildflowers and weeds, many of which are used medicinally.

Culpeper, Nicholas, *Culpeper's Complete Herbal* - 8th Edition, London, W. Foulsham and Co., LTD. A reprint of the original seventeenth century copy.

Clymer, R. Swinburne, M.D., *Nature's Healing Agents*, Quakertown, PA, The Humanitarian Society, 1973 (Box 77, Quakertown, PA 18951).

Ellingwood, Finley, *American Materia Medica Therapeutics and Pharmacognosy*, Portland, Oregon, 1983, Eclectic Medical Publications.

Felter, Harvey Wickes, M.D., *King's American Dispensatory*, Portland, OR, Eclectic Medical Publications, 1983 (11231 S.E. Market St.). This outstanding two-volume materia medica was first published during the latter part of the last century. A landmark work on Eclectic Medicine and the clinical use of North American herbs.

Foster, Steven, *East-West Botanicals*, Ozark Beneficial Plant Project (HCR Box 3, Brisey, MO, 65618). A cross-reference of medicinal herbs between North America and China.

Grieve, Mrs. M., *A Modern Herbal*, New York, Dover Pub., 1971. A two-volume reprint of the work originally published in 1931.

Hobbs, Christopher, *Chinese Herbs Growing in the Western U.S.*, Capitola, CA, Botanica Press (P.O. Box 742, Capitola, CA 95010). A cross-reference of a number of North American plants with similar species found growing in China.

Hoffmann, David, *The Herbal Handbook*, Rochester, Vermont, Healing Arts Press, 1987.

Hoffmann, David, *The Herb User's Guide*, Wellingborough, Northamptonshire and Rochester, Vermont, Thorsons Publishing Group, 1987.

Hoffmann, David, *The Holistic Herbal*, Scotland, Findhorn Press, 1983 (Findhorn Foundation, The Park, Forres IV36 OTZ, Scotland). Examines the systems of the body and gives herbal remedies.

Lust, John, *The Herb Book*, CA., Benedict Lust Pub., 1974. An introductory book on herbal medicine for the lay person.

Lust, John and Tierra, Michael, *The Natural Remedy Bible*, New York, Pocket Books, 1990. A compendium of ailments with their herbal and natural remedies.

Moore, Michael, *Medicinal Plants of the Mountain West*, Santa Fe, NM, Museum of New Mexico Press, 1979. An excellent book on Western medicinal herbs.

Nissim, Rina, *Natural Healing in Gynecolcogy*, New York, 1986, Pandora Publishers.

Parvati, Jeannine, *Hygieia, A Woman's Herbal*, Sevier, UT, Freestone Press, 1978 (960 South Ross Lane). Specific female conditions and their herbal allies.

Priest and Priest, *Herbal Medication*, Essex, England, L.N. Fowler & Co. LTD, 1982. An authoritative presentation of the clinical usage and principles of the British Institute of Medical Herbalists.

Rose, Jeanne, *Herbs and Things*, New York, NY, Grosset and Dunlap. An introduction to self-healing with herbs.

Schauenber, Paul and Paris, Ferdinand, *Guide to Medicinal Plants*, New Canaan, CT, Keats Publishing, 1977. A materia medica that organizes herbs according to their biochemical constituents.

Shook, Dr. Edward E., *Beginning and Advanced Treatise in Herbology*, Beaumont, CA, Trinity Center Press, 1978 (P.O Box 335).

Tierra, Michael, *The Way of Herbs*, New York, Pocket Books, 1983. An excellent beginning herbal introducing the energetics of herbs, Western and Chinese herbs and herbal therapy.

Tierra, Michael, *Planetary Herbology*, Santa Fe, Lotus Press, 1988. A precedent-setting and landmark publication applying the Chinese energetic system of classification to Western herbs. Ayurvedic principles are also included.

Tierra, Michael and Cantin, Candis, *The Herbal Tarot*, New York, U.S. Games, 1989. A unique and beautiful tarot deck and book with herbal assignments.

Weed, Susan, *Wise Woman Herbal for the Childbearing Year*, Woodstock, NY, Ash Tree Publishing, 1986.

Weiss, Rudolf Fritz, *Herbal Medicine*, 4830 N.E. 32nd Avenue, Portland, OR 97211, Medicina Biologica, U.S. Distributor, Pub. by AB Arcanum, Gothenburg, Sweden and Beaconsfield Publishers LTD, Beaconsfield, England. A modern text of medical herbalism with present-day research findings.

Willard, Terry, *Helping Yourself with Natural Remedies*, Reno, NV, CRCS Publications (P.O. Box 208950, Reno, NV 98515). An excellent practical book on herbal self-treatment.

Willard, Terry, *The Wild Rose Scientific Herbal*, Calgary, Alberta, Canada, Wild Rose College of Natural Healing Ltd., 1991.

Wren, *Potter's New Cyclopaedia of Botanical Drugs and Preparations*, Suffix, England, Health Science Press, 1907.

Green, James, The Male Herbal, Watsonville, CA., The Crossing Press, 1991.

Native American Herbals

Hutchens, Alma, *Indian Herbology of North America*, Canada, Merco, 1973. A study of Anglo-American, Russian and Oriental literature on Indian medical botanics of North America.

Moerman, Daniel E., *Medicinal Plants of Native America*, Ann Arbor, MI, University of Michigan Museum of Anthropology. A two-volume work on medicinal plants used by the Native Americans.

Mooney, James, *The Swimmer Manuscript of Cherokee Sacred Formulas and Medicinal Prescriptions*, first published by the U.S. government in 1932, reissued by Botanica Press, Capitola, CA. This is an important early document that is a first-hand account of the high art of Cherokee herbal medicine.

Vogel, Virgil H., *American Indian Medicine*, University of Oklahoma Press. A good historical presentation of the various herbal remedies used by tribes throughout the U.S.

Chinese Herbals

Beinfield, Harriet and Korngold, Efrem, *Between Heaven and Earth*, New York, N.Y., Ballantine Books, 1991. A fabulous introduction to Chinese medicine.

Bensky and Barolet, *Formulas and Strategies*, Seattle, Eastland Press, 1990. Chinese herbal formulas and their uses.

Bensky and Gamble, *Chinese Herbal Medicine Materia Medica*, Seattle, Eastland Press, 1986. A materia medica of Chinese medicinal herbs.

Chang, But, Yao, Wang and Yeung, *Pharmacology and Applications of Chinese Materia Medica*, Philadelphia, PA, World Scientific Publishing Company, 1986.

Cheung, C.S., *Treatment of Traditional Chinese Medicine*, San Francisco, Traditional Chinese Medical Publisher, 1980.

Connelly, Diane, *Traditional Acupuncture: The Law of the Five Elements*, Maryland, Center for Traditional Acupuncture, 1979. Presents an in-depth description of the fascinating system of Chinese five element theory.

Hong-Yen Hsu, *How to Treat Yourself With Chinese Herbs*, Los Angeles, Oriental Healing Arts Institute, 1980. A useful introductory book to the use of Chinese herbs.

Hong-Yen Hsu, Chau-Shin Hsu, *Commonly Used Chinese Herb Formulas With Illustrations*, Los Angeles, Oriental Healing Arts Institute, 1980.

Hong-Yen Hsu & Easer, Douglas, *Major Chinese Herbal Formulas*, Los Angeles, Oriental Healing Arts Institute, 1980.

Hsu, Dr. Hong-yen and Preacher, Dr. William G., *Chinese Herb Medicine and Therapy*, Los Angeles, CA, Oriental Healing Arts Institute. An introduction to the principles of Chinese herbology.

Hyatt, Richard, *Chinese Herbal Medicine*, New York, Schocken Books, 1978. An introduction to the principles of Chinese herbology and theory.

Kaptchuk, Ted, *The Web That Has No Weaver*, New York, N.Y., Congdon & Weded, 1983. A wonderful presentation of the fundamental principles of Chinese medicine.

Li Shih-Chen, *Chinese Medicinal Herbs*, San Francisco, Georgetown Press, 1973.

Ni, Maoshing, *Chinese Herbology Made Easy,* Los Angeles, The Shrine of the Eternal Breath of Tao and College of Tao and Traditional Chinese Healing, 1986 (117 Stonehaven Way, Los Angeles, CA).

Teeguarden, Ron, *Chinese Tonic Herbs*, New York, Japan Publications, 1984.

Tierra, Michael and Tierra, Lesley, *Chinese Planetary Herbal Diagnosis*, Santa Cruz, East West Publishing, 1989 (Box 712, Santa Cruz, CA 95061). A concise handbook for the clinical application of Chinese diagnostic principles.

The Revolutionary Health Committee of Hunan Province, *A Barefoot Doctor's Manual*, Seattle, Cloudburst Press, 1977. The manual used by the barefoot doctors of China. It lists over 520 herbs and mineral and animal derived substances used for medicine, many that are common with species and plants found in the West and other parts of the world.

Yeung, Him-che, *Handbook of Chinese Herbs and Formulas*, Vol. I and II, Los Angeles, Him-che Yeung, 1985. A two-volume materia medica and formulary on Chinese herbalism, highly practical and useable in clinical practice.

Zhen, Li Shi, *Pulse Diagnosis*, Brookline, MA, Paradigm Publications, 1981.

Bulletins of the Oriental Healing Arts Institute of U.S.A., Los Angeles, Oriental Healing Arts Institute. A quarterly journal on Chinese herbal medicine, including case studies, scientific investigations and clinical experiences of Chinese and occidental practitioners.

Ayurvedic Herbals and Philosophy

Frawley, Dr. David, *Ayurvedic Healing*, Salt Lake City, Passage Press, 1989.

Lad, Dr. Vasant, *Ayurveda, The Science of Self-Healing*, Santa Fe, Lotus Press, 1984. An excellent introduction to the principles of tridosha and ayurvedic medicine.

Lad, Dr. Vasant & Frawley, Dr. David, *The Yoga of Herbs*, Santa Fe, Lotus Press, 1986. Describes the use of Western herbs energetically, as they incorporate into the Ayurvedic system.

Natural Healing and Food Therapy

Ballentine, Rudolph, M.D., *Diet and Nutrition*, Honesdale, PA, the Himalayan International Institute, 1978. An important and comprehensive presentation on aspects of nutrition incorporating the traditional principles of Ayurveda with Western nutrition.

Colbin, Annemarie, *Food and Healing*, New York, Ballantine Books, 1980. An excellent presentation of the principles of macrobiotic food therapy and beyond by the author of the cookbook, *Book of Whole Meals*.

Flaws, Bob and Wolfe, Honora, *Prince Wen Hui's Cook*, Boulder, Blue Poppy Press (Chinese Dietary Therapy, 1810 Alpine Ave. #2, Boulder, CO 80302). A presentation of the priniciples of dietary therapy using foods and some herbs with many traditional herb-food recipes.

Kushi, Michio, *How to See Your Health: Book of Oriental Diagnosis*, Japan Rubl. Presents the principles of oriental diagnosis used with macrobiotics.

Kushi, Michio, *Book of Macrobiotics*, New York, Japan Publications, 1977. Presents the basic principles of macrobiotics.

Kushi, Michio, *Macrobiotic Home Remedies*, New York, Japan Publications, 1985. An excellent practical book on simple home remedies and treatments for a number of health problems.

Lu, Henry C., *Chinese System of Food Cures*, New York, Sterling Publishing Co., 1986. An outline of the principles of Chinese food therapy.

Muramoto, Naboro, *Healing Ourselves*, New York, Avon Press, 1973. Natural remedies and therapies, including food, for specific ailments.

Ni, Maoshing with McNease, Cathy, *The Tao of Nutrition* (Shrine of the Eternal Breath of Tao, 117 Stonehaven Way, Los Angeles, CA 90049.)

Satillaro, Anthony, *Recalled by Life*, New York, Avon, 1982.

Tara, William, *Macrobiotics and Human Behavior*, New York, Japan Publications, 1984.

Herbal Cultivation

Foster, Steven, *Herbal Bounty*, Salt Lake City, Peregrine Smith Books, 1984.

The History of Herbs and Foods

Griggs, Barbara, *Green Pharmacy*, New York, NY, Viking Press, 1981.

Griggs, Barbara, *The Food Factor*, New York, NY, Viking Press, 1986.

Robbins, John, *Diet for a New America*, Walpole, Stillpoint Publishing, 1987 (Box 640, Walpole, NH 03608).

The Relationship Between People and Plants

Tompkins, Peter and Bird, Christopher, *The Secret Life of Plants*, New York, N.Y., Harper Colophon Books, 1973.

Cookbooks

Colbin, Annemarie, *Book of Whole Meals*, New York, Ballentine Books, 1983.

Estella, Mary, *Natural Foods Cookbook*, New York, Japan Publications, 1985.

Kushi, Aveline, *Aveline Kushi's Complete Guide to Macrobiotic Cooking*, New York, Warner Books, 1985.

Kushi, Aveline, and Esko, Wendy, *The Changing Seasons Macrobiotic Cookbook*, Wayne, New Jersey, Avery Publishing Group Inc., 1985.

Turner, Kristina, *The Self-Healing Cookbook*, Grass Valley, CA, Earthtones Press, 1987.

Anatomy, Physiology, Pharmacognosy, Botany

Crittenden, Mabel and Telfer, Dorothy, *Wildflowers of the West*, Millbrae, CA, Celestial Arts, 1975.

Hickey, Michael and King, Clive, *100 Families of Flowering Plants*, New York, Cambridge University Press, 1981.

Tortora, Gerard J., *Principles of Human Anatomy,* New York, Harper and Row, 1980.

Tyler, Brady & Robbers, *Pharmacognosy*, Philadelphia, Lea & Febiger, 1981.

Vander, Sherman & Luciano, *Human Physiology*, New York, McGraw-Hill, 1980.

Library

The Lloyd's Library and Museum, 917 Plum Street, Cincinnati, OH 45202, 513-721-3707.

Some Places for Ordering These Books

East Wind Books
1435-A Stockton St., San Francisco, CA 94133, 415-781-3331.
Chinese herbals, Traditional Chinese Medicine theory, massage, acupuncture.

Lotus Press
Box 6265, Santa Fe, NM 87502, 505-982-5534.
Ayurvedic books, products, herb charts and information.

Oriental Healing Arts Institute
1945 Palo Verde Avenue, Suite 208, Long Beach, CA 90815.
Bulletins covering specific herbs, formulas and treatments of various disorders; also Chinese herbals and Traditional Chinese Medicine theory.

Redwing Book Company
44 Linden St., Brookline, MA 02146.
Books on acupuncture, Traditional Chinese Medicine theory, herbology, massage, natural medicine, homeopathy and more.

Herbal Resource Guide

The following is a list of resources for purchasing herbs and herbal products.

Western Herb Suppliers

Attar Herbs and Spices, Playground Rd., New Ipswich, NH 03071. They specialize in essential oils.

East-West Herb Products, Box 1210, New York, NY 10025, 1-800-542-6544. Retail mail orders of various Chinese, Ayurvedic and Western herbs and distributor of Planetary Formulas.

Frontier Co-op Herbs, Box 299 Norway, IA 52318.

Herbal Home Products, Bob Brucea, 3405 Angel Lane, Placerville, CA 95672.

Herbalist and Alchemist Inc., David Winston, P.O. Box 63, Franklin Park, NJ 08823.

Herb Pharm, P.O. Box 116, Williams, OR 97544.

Nature's Herb Company, Box 118, Dept. 34 Q, Norway, IA 52318, 1-800-365-4372. Wholesale or retail herbs and herb products.

Planetary Formulas, P.O. Box 533, Soquel, CA 95073, 1-800-776-7701. Manufactures and distributes Plantetary Formulas. (Ask for free catalogue.)

Reevis Mountain School, HC02 Box 1534, Roosevelt, AZ 85545

Trinity Herb Company, P.O. Box 199, Bodega, CA 94922.

Chinese Herb Suppliers

Great China Herb Company, 857 Washington St., San Francisco, CA 94108, 1-415-982-2195

East West Herb Products, 317 West 100th St., New York, NY 10025, in New York: 212-864-5508, outside New York: 1-800-542-6544

May Way Trading Corporation, 622 Broadway, San Francisco, CA 94133.

Tai Sang Trading Chinese Herb Company, 1018 Stockton, San Franscisco, CA 94108.

Chinese Medical Supplies

(moxibustion, cups, dermal hammers, magnets)

East West Herb Course, Box 712, Santa Cruz, CA 95061, 408-429-8066.

East West Herbs, Longston Priory Mews, Kingham, Oxforshire, OX7 6UP, England.

May Way Trading Company, 622 Broadway, San Francisco, CA 94133, 1-415-788-3646.

Oriental Medical Supplies, 1950 Washington St., Braintree, MA 02184, 1-800-323-1839.

Ayurvedic Herbs and Supplies

Lotus Express, 1505 42nd Ave., Suite 19, Capitola, CA 95010.

Lotus Light Distributing, Box 2, Wilmot, WE 53192, 1-800-548-3824 (out of state), 1-414-862-2395 (in state).

Organic Herb Farms

Pacific Botanicals, 360 Stephen Way Williams, Oregon 97544.

Trout Lake Herb Farm, Rt. 1 Box 355, Trout Lake, Washington 98650.

Wildcrafters

Blessed Herbs, Michael Volchok, Rt. 5, Box 191A, Ava, MO 85020.

Mike and Debby Minear, Rt. 1, Box 60, Little Hocking, OH 45742.

Reevis Mountain School of Survival, HCO2 Box 1534, Roosevelt, AZ 85545.

Ryan Drum, Waldron, WA 98297.

Herbal Teas

Frontier Herbs, Box 299 , Norway, IA 52318, Tao Teas.

Unitea Herbs, Box 8005, Suite 318, Boulder, CO 80306-8005, 1-800-864-8327 (out of state), 1-303-443-1248 (in state).

Live Herbs and Seeds

Shephards Garden Seeds, 6116 Highway 9, Felton, CA 95018.

Taylor's Garden, Inc., 1535 Lone Oak Road, Vista, CA 92083.

Herbal Resource Guide

Western Herb Suppliers

Attar Herbs and Spices, Playground Rd., New Ipswich, NH 03071. They specialize in essential oils.

East-West Herb Products, Box 1210, New York, NY 10025, 1-800-542-6544. Retail mail orders of various Chinese, Ayurvedic and Western herbs and distributor of Planetary Formulas.

Frontier Co-op Herbs, Box 299 Norway, IA 52318.

Herbal Home Products, Bob Brucea, 3405 Angel Lane, Placerville, CA 95672.

Herbalist and Alchemist Inc., David Winston, P.O. Box 63, Franklin Park, NJ 08823.

Herb Pharm, P.O. Box 116, Williams, OR 97544.

Nature's Herb Company, Box 118, Dept. 34 Q, Norway, IA 52318, 1-800-365-4372. Wholesale or retail herbs and herb products.

Planetary Formulas, P.O. Box 533, Soquel, CA 95073,1-800-776-7701. Manufactures and distributes Plantetary Formulas. (Ask for free catalogue.)

Planetary Herbal Products, P.O. Box 7145, Santa Cruz, CA 95061, 408-479-7074. Retail mail orders of various Chinese, Ayurvedic and Western herbs and distributor of Planetary Formulas.

Reevis Mountain School, HC02 Box 1534, Roosevelt, AZ 85545

Trinity Herb Company, P.O. Box 199, Bodega, CA 94922.

Chinese Herb Suppliers

Great China Herb Company, 857 Washington St., San Francisco, CA 94108, 1-415-982-2195

May Way Trading Corporation, 622 Broadway, San Francisco, CA 94133.

Tai Sang Trading Chinese Herb Company, 1018 Stockton, San Franscisco, CA 94108.

Chinese Medical Supplies

(moxibustion, cups, dermal hammers, magnets)

East West Herb Course, Box 712, Santa Cruz, CA 95061, 408-429-8066.

East West Herbs, Longston Priory Mews, Kingham, Oxforshire, OX7 6UP, England.

May Way Trading Company, 622 Broadway, San Francisco, CA 94133, 1-415-788-3646.

Oriental Medical Supplies, 1950 Washington St., Braintree, MA 02184, 1-800-323-1839.

Herbal Videos

Way of Herbs Video
by Michael Tierra
East West Herb School, P.O. Box 712, Santa Cruz, CA 95061

In his favorite element, the garden, Michael teaches the identification and detailed description and use of 12 medicinal herbs. From garden to kitchen, he covers folklore, growing and gathering herbs and simple herbal medicines and home remedies which can be easily made and used. Herbal rituals, dances and songs are also included.

A wealth of information, this 60-minute video celebrates herbal home medicine. The background music is Michael's own classical piano rendering of the American composer, Edward MacDowell's *Woodland Sketches*. The still photographs, cover photograph and narration are by Lesley Tierra. It is available in VHS and Beta.

Herbal Preparations and Natural Therapies
by Debra Nuzzi, MPH
Morningstar Publications, 997 Dixon Rd., Dept. H, Boulder, CO 80302.

Excellent presentation on making herbal preparations and therapies. Available with manual.

Edible Wild Plants
by Jim Meuninck and Dr. Jim Duke
Media Methods, 24097 North Shore Dr., Dept. W, Edwardsburg, MI 49112.

Excellent field guide to 100 useful wild herbs. Available with manual.

The Basics of Healthy Cooking
by Annemarie Colbin
Natural Gourmet Cookery School, 48 West 21 Street, New York, NY 10010.

Presents a complete course in the basics of cooking whole grains and beans and learning general guidelines of healthful cooking and menu planning.

Herb Seeker Press
Laura Clavio, P.O. Box 299W, Battle Ground, IN 57920, 1-317-567-2884.

Distributes herbal and garden videos.

Herbal Audio Cassettes

East West
by Lesley and Michael Tierra
East West Herb School, P.O. Box 712, Santa Cruz, CA 95061

A set of 24 one-hour audio cassettes comprising lectures on various topics relating to the study of herbal medicine, diagnosis and nutrition. These tapes are an edited version of an intensive weeklong seminar on Planetary Herbalism and Oriental diagnosis.

Herbal Magazines, Newsletters and Booklets

Planetary Formulas Newsletter
Author-Herbalist Roy Upton, P.O. Box 533, Soquel, CA 95073

Botanica Press
P. O. Box 7426, Capitola, CA 95010
Very informative booklets written on chaste berries, ginkgo, intestinal flora, immune system and many others by author, researcher and outstanding medical botanist, Christopher Hobbs.

American Herb Association Quarterly Newsletter
P.O. Box 353W, Rescue, CA 95672
This is the official newsletter of The American Herbalists Guild.

Business of Herbs
P.O. Box 559W, Madison, VA 22727
Reaches out to those involved with growing or marketing herbs.

Herbalgram
P.O. Box 12602W, Austin, TX 78711
An outstanding newsletter with up-to-date happenings and scientific studies on herbs and herbal medicine.

Herbal Perspectives
Planetary Formulas Quarterly Newsletter
P.O. Box 533W, Soquel, CA 95073
A free quarterly newsletter.

Medical Herbalism
P.O. Box 33080, Portland, OR 97233
An outstanding herbal journal.

Foster's Botanical and Herb Reviews
P.O. Box 106, Eureaka Springs, AR 72632

Journal of Ontario Herbalists' Association
7 Alpine Ave., Toronto, Ontario, Canada   M6P 3R6

Australian Journal of Medical Herbalism
P.O. Box 65, Kingsgrove, NSW, 2208, Australia

Business of Herbs
North Wind Farm, Rt. 2, Box 246C, Shevlin, MN 56676

Herbal Organizations

American Botanical Council
P.O. Box 201660W, Austin, TX 78720, 1-512-331-8868

American Herbalists Guild
Box 1683, Soquel, CA 95073
A professional body of herbalists dedicated to promoting and maintaining criteria for professional practice of herbalism in America.

American Herbal Products Association
P.O. Box 2410, Austin, TX, 512-320-8555
Devoted to herbal products, their manufacturing and quality.

Herb Research Foundation, 1007 Pearl St., Suite 200F, Boulder, CO 80302

American Herbalists Association
P.O. Box 1673, Nevada City, CA 95959

Rocky Mountain Herbalists Coalition
412 Boulder St., Boulder, CO 80302

Santa Cruz Herbalists Coalition
P.O. Box 1683, Santa Cruz, CA 95073

International Herb Growers and Marketers Association
Box 77123, Baton Rouge, CA 70879

Herbal Computer Programs

Falcor: Herbal Software
A New Era in Herbalism
by Steve Blake, N.D., D.Sc.
5831 Highway 9, Felton, CA 95018

All of the following programs are available for IBM and Mac computers:

Globalherb: The world's largest reference library for the computer, this program contains information from *all* of the other following programs and more. Over 700 herbs, formulas and other therapies at your fingertips! Information on each herb and the references which agree with that use of the herb are given. Comes with advanced research capabilities and features for exploring and adding knowledge.

Planetherb: This program unifies planetary approaches to herbal healing. Includes more than 490 herbs and formulas from the West, China and India covering over 1700 unique conditions. This program also includes the energy of each herb. It is easy to add new information or herbs and has automatic repeat entries and other advanced features. Based on Michael Tierra's book *Planetary Herbology*.

Proherb: An electronic library with the 15 most authoritative herbal references, you can choose an herb by the number of references which agree on that herb's use for a given condition. The herbs used in this program are the safest, easiest to find and most carefully studied. Not only are the number of references given, but the actual books and page numbers. It is truly "an herbal specialist in a box." Easy to use, it includes over 7200 book and page references, a revolution in comparative herbology. Proherb has a program to find formulas and a program to find the common herb name from any name listed. Perfect for the store, office or home.

Homeherb: This is a simple program to make finding herbs in the home easy. Information for each herb is listed with the number of references which agree with that use of the herb, including conditions, properties and dosage.

Food Therapy Studies

Creative Nutritional Cooking
Learn how to cook deliciously and nutritiously, including high-energy, low-fat menus, vegetarian dishes, healthy desserts and wheat, sugar, and yeast-free meals. Learn preventive nutrition, stress and weight management through diet, and methods to strengthen the immune system. Menu planning, cooking classes and individual consultations provided. For information contact:

> Creative Nutritional Cooking
> Joan Anderson
> c/o East West Herb Course
> 21 Hale Street
> Beverly, MA 01915

Weights and Measures

Weights and Measures

1 pound	=	453 grams
1 ounce	=	28.3 grams
16 ounces (dry)	=	1 pound
1 gallon	=	4 quarts
1 quart	=	2 pints
1 pint	=	2 cups
1 cup	=	8 fluid ounces
1 cup	=	16 tablespoons
1 teaspoon	=	60 drops
1 tablespoon	=	3 teaspoons
1 fluid ounce	=	2 tablespoons
1 fluid ounce	=	8 fluid drachms
1 fluid ounce	=	28.4 milliliters
1 fluid drachm	=	3.55 milliliters = 1 large teaspoon
1 kilogram	=	2 pounds, 3.27 ounces

Capsules and Powders

15.4 grains	=	1 gram		
1 gram	=	1000 milligrams		
contents 1 "00" capsule	=	about 650 milligrams	=	10 grains (well packed)
contents "0" capsule	=	about 500 milligrams	=	8 grains (well packed)
two gelatin capsules	=	1 teaspoon tincture		
two tablespoons tincture	=	1/2 cup tea		
1 ounce powdered herb	=	25-35 "00" well-filled capsules		
1 ounce powdered herb	=	35-45 "0" well-filled capsules		

LATIN INDEX

Latin Name	Common Name	Page
Achillea spp.	Yarrow	82
Aconitum carmichaeli	Aconite	84-85
Allium sativum	Garlic	63-64
Aloe barbadensis	Aloe	47
Althea officinalis	Marshmallow	70
Angelica archangelica	Angelica	48
Angelica sinensis	Dong Quai	88-89
Anthimis foles	Chamomile	55-56
Anthimis nobiles	Chamomile	55-56
Arctium lappa	Burdock	52
Arctostaphylos uva ursi	Uva ursi	80-81
Artemisia vulgaris	Mugwort	71
Astragalus membranaceus	Astragalus	85
Atracylodes alba	Atractylodes	85-86
Atractylodes macrocephalae	Atractylodes	85-86
Berberis aquifolium	Oregon Grape	73
Berberis vulgaris	Barberry	48-49
Borago officinalis	Borage	51-52
Bupleurum falcatum	Bupleurum	86
Calendula officinalis	Calendula	52
Capsella bursa-pastoris	Shepherd's Purse	77
Capsicum anuum	Cayenne	54
Cascara Sagrada	Cascara	54
Chyrsanthemum morifolium	Chrysanthemum	86
Chyrsanthemum parthenium	Feverfew	63
Cimicifuga racemosa	Black Cohosh	50
Cinnamomum verum	Cinnamom	57-58
Citrus reticulata	Citrus	87
Codonopsis pilosulae	Codonopsis	87
Cornus officinalis	Cornus	87
Crataegus oxyacantha	Hawthorn	67-68
Curcuma longa	Turmeric	80
Cyperus spp.	Cyperus	88
Dioscorea batata	Chinese Wild Yam	88
Dioscorea japonica	Chinese Wild Yam	88
Echinacea spp.	Echinacea	60-61
Elettaria cardamonmum	Cardamom	53
Eleutherococcus senticosus	Siberian Ginseng	78
Ephedra spp.	Ephedra	89
Euphrasia officinalis	Eyebright	61-62
Foeniculum vulgare	Fennel	62-63
Ganoderma spp.	Reishi	93-94
Gardenia jasminoides	Gardenia	90
Gentian spp.	Gentian	64-65

Ginkgo biloba	Ginkgo	66
Glycyrrhiza glabra	Licorice	68-69
Hydrastis canadensis	Goldenseal	66-67
Hypericum perforatum	St. John's Wort	79
Inula helinium	Elecampane	61
Lanoderma lucidum	Reishi	93-94
Larrea divaricata	Chaparral	56
Leonorus cardiaca	Motherwort	71-71
Lobelia inflata	Lobelia	69
Lonicera japonica	Honeysuckle	91
Lycium chinensis	Lycii	92
Mahonia repens	Oregon Grape	73
Matricaria chamomilla	Chamomile	55-56
Melissa officinalis	Lemon Balm	68
Mentha piperita	Peppermint	74
Mitchella repens	Squawvine	79
Myrica cerifera	Bayberry	49
Paeonia lactiflorae	Peony	92
Panax gineng	Ginseng	90
Panax pseudoginseng	Tienchi Ginseng	94-95
Panax Quinquefolium	American Ginseng	48
Petroselinum spp.	Parsley	73-74
Polygonum multiflorum	Ho Shou Wu	91
Poria cocos	Fu ling, Hoelen	89-90
Pipernigrum	Black Pepper	51
Plantago major	Plantain	74
Prunus serotina	Wild Cherry Bark	81-82
Prunus virginianna	Wild Cherry Bark	81-82
Puerariae lobata	Pueraria, Kuzu, Kudzu	92-93
Rehmannia glutinosa	Rehmannia	93
Rhamnus purshiana	Cascara	54
Rubus idaeus	Raspberry	75-76
Rubus villosus	Blackberry	50
Rumex crispus	Yellow Dock	82
Schisandra sinensis	Schisandra	94
Scutellaria lateriflora	Scullcap	77
Silybum marianum	Milk Thistle	70
Smilax officinalis	Sarsaparilla	76
Stellaria media	Chickweed	57
Symphytum officinale	Comfrey	59
Taraxacum officinale	Dandelion	59-60
Trifolium pratense	Red Clover	76
Trigonella foenum-graecum	Fenugreek	62-63
Tussilago farfara	Coltsfoot	58
Ulmus fulva	Slippery Elm	78-79
Urtica spp.	Nettle	72-73
Valeriana officinalis	Valerian	81
Verbascum thapsus	Mullein	72
Viburnum prunifolium	Black Haw	50
Vitex agnus-castus	Chaste Berry	56-57
Zanthoxylum americanum	Prickly Ash	75

CHINESE INDEX, MANDARIN

CHINESE INDEX, CANTONESE

chai wu	Bupleurum	86
chen pay	Citrus	87
da jo	Jujube Date	91-92
dong kway	Dong Quai	88-89
dong sum	Codonopsis	87
fuk ling	Fu Ling, Hoelen	89-90
fu jee	Aconite	84-85
gay jee	Lycii	92
gook fah	Chrysanthemum	86
gum nan fah	Honeysuckle	91
gwat gun	Pueraria	92-93
heung fu	Cyperus	88
ho sao wu	Ho Shou Wu	91
ma wong	Ephedra	89
ng way jee	Schisandra	94
san jee jee	Gardenia	90
san yu yok	Cornus	87
sang day	Raw Rehmannia	93
say yang sum	American Ginseng	48
shune cho yun	Zizyphus	95
som chuk	Tienchi Ginseng	94-95
so day huang	Cooked Rehmannia	93
yun sum	Ginseng	90
wai san	Chinese Wild Yam	88

GENERAL INDEX

aspirin, 43
assimilation, poor, 143,151,177
also see digestion, indigestion,
assisting herbs, in formulas, 40
Asteraceae Family, 41
asthma, 18,36,102,103,119,124,114,
128,133,137,138,149,156,159,
160,215
astragalus, 12,36,37,61,85,86,87,133,
143,178,181,187,193
astringent, 9,36,39,42,132,152,175,
180,190,199,204
athlete's foot, 210
atractylodes, 84,85-86,136,175,187,
193
autumn, 24, 170
avocado oil, 182
Ayurveda, iii,4,7,46,47,49,51,70,80,
87,135,152,159,163,166,181,182,
195,201,202

-B-

baby, babies 56,78,87,191,193,204,
234-235
bacon, 120
bacteria, 35
baking soda, 139
balm, 68
banana, 106
bancha tea, 136,141
barberry, 38,48,49,73,80,127,175
barley, 100,106
basil, 36,152
baths, 235
    preparation, 175
    remedies, 131-132,
bay, 134,181,192
bayberry, 13,36,37,49,75,132,139,
152,175,181
bearberry, 80
bed sores, 216
bedwetting, 216
beef, 106,134,200
bee stings, 216
beeswax, 187,199
beet, 107
belching, 216

benzoin tincture, 173,182,186,
187,199
Berberidaceae Family, 41
beriberi, 106,112
beta-carotine, 92
bile, 9,36,39,60,67,73,83,151,
152,175
    secretions, 38,60
binder, herbal, 175,183
biochemical components - *see*
    chemical constituents
birch, 181,235
birthing, 79,81
bites, 36,135,138,139,185,186,199,
210,216
bitters, 175
bitter, taste, 5,9,11,12,13,21,24,35,
36,38,39,43,46,86,99,127,128,
142,190,236
    principles, 39
    tonics, 49
black bean, 130,141
    tea, 141
blackberries, 9,39,50
blackberry, 39,40,50
    root, 35,40,50,75
black cohosh, 35,36,37,50,79,207
black haw, 38,39,50-51
black pepper, 37,51,107,129,135,
152,182
    corns, 141
black sesame seeds, 107
black soya bean, 107
black tea, 141,187
black walnut, 35
    hulls, 139
Bladder, 9,129
bladder, 10,43,46,73,133,134,152,
157,212
    infection, 14,15,16,36,70,74,77,
    80,85,132,133,156,157,210,
    215,223
    strain, 114
    stones, 37,114
    tract, 10,11,39
bland taste, 13,24
bleeding, 9,36,38,39,106,108,110,
112,113,114,142,156,181,
210,216
    uterine, 216
blemishes, 135

blepharitis, 216
blessed thistle, 234
bloatedness, 21,36,45,102,104,128,
133,142,143,153,203,211
bloating, 11,40,112,123
blood, 10,62,67,84,91,92,93,112,
113,124,128,133,134,142,145,
155,200,202
    building and strengthening, 216
    circulation, 9,36,37,107,108,111,
    175,178,192,202,216
    clots, 216
    poisoning, 216
    pressure high, 9,36,38,127,141
    pressure low, 225
    stimulation, 37
    sugar, 48, 106,216
    stagnation, 108,113
    tonics, 24
    toxicity, 35
bloodroot, 191
bloody stools, 114
blurred vision, 107,109,110,112,217
body ordor, 107
    hair, 9
boils, 107,108,110,138,184,217
bolus,
    preparations, 175-176
    remedies, 132
bones, 106,109,113,128,153,157
    aching, 10
    broken, 5,157,217
    marrow soup, 152
boneset, 35,36,106,193
borage, 51-52
botany, 39
bowels, 9,54,59,72,127,175,202
    elimination, 9,39
    inflammation, 224
    movements, 36,39,59,72,112,113
brain, 66,107,141,145
branch of disease, 15,22
brandy, 175,193
Brassicaceae Family, 41
bread, 101,144
breast, 57,60,73,91,137,184
    cancer, 137
    sores, cysts 216
breathing, difficult, 156,158
breathing exercises, ii,145-148
Brigham Tea, 89

miscarriage, 51,71,226
Missouri snakeroot, 195
mochi, 234
molasses, 83
monkshood, 84
moon, harvesting according to, 172
    for making tinctures, 190
Mormon Tea, 89
morning sickness,
51,106,112,136,226
morphine, 38
mosquito bites, 139,186,210
mothers and children, 234-235
mothers milk, increases, 36,70,106,
        108,110,111,226
    decreases, 226
motherwort, 10,35,36,37,71
motion sickness, 113,136,226
mouth, dry, 219
    sores, 226
    wash, 192-193
moxibustion, 129,142,155-157,209
    smoke, 143,156
mucilage, 39,78
mucous membranes, 39,181,226
    linings, damaged, 39
mucus, 9,16,18,21,36,40,42,102,
        103,106,108,109,110,111,114,
        136,137,,138,139,140,142,162,
        182,184,188,198,199,203,226
    also see phlegm
    congestion, 9
    linings, 202
    lungs, 128,156,182,188
mugwort, 36,71-72,134,140,143,155,
        160,161,167,196,200
mullein, 35,36,42,53,69,72,132,135,
        140,160,182,194,196,203,203
mumps, 106,112,114,226
mung bean, 110,133,141
    tea, 141
Muramoto, 138
muscle, 37,128,134,136,138,199,
        201,210
    pain, stiffness, 35,107,139
    produce, 112
    relax, 132,180
    sore, aching, 132,139-140,181
    spasms, 36,132,157,184
    strained, 133,180
    tones, 36

mushrooms, 24,94
    common button, 110
    reishi, 37,93-94
    shitaki, 113
mustard, 36,37,136,152,163,181,184
    greens, 111
    plaster, 137-138
myrrh, 39,134,139,152,179,181,190,
    193,199
Myricaceae Family, 41

-N-

Nadishodhana, 145-147
nails, finger, 9
    toe, 9
nasal, drip, 102,129
    congestion, 111
    wash, 157-158
nasturtium, 142
Native American, 4,71,75,81,82,123,
    160,161,163,166,192
nausea, 107,109,136,156,212,226
navel, 136
NDGA, 56
neck, 45,103,184
neibol, 123
nerve, 38,39,43,135,175,201
channels, 145
    energy, 9
    weak, 107
    pain, 227
nervine, 37,152,191
nervous, conditions, 37,92
    exhaustion, 91
    system, 37,38,77,133,145,147,
        152,160,191
    tension, 37,43,91
nervousness, 37,124,145, 151,
    152,226
neti, netibol, 123,158,167
nettle, 9,13,72-73,127,130,186
neuralgia, 113,227
neurasthenia, 109,141
neutral energy, 8
Newtonian physics, 3
nicotine, 38, 160
night blindness, 227
night sweats, 19,227
night time urination, 156,157
nocturnal emission, 227

nose, 40,62,74,77,102,103,105
    inflammation, 224
nosebleed, 112,113,227
Nosebleed, 82
nostrils, 157
numbness, 126,132,149,227
nursing, 36,44,52,234,235
    also see mother's milk
nutmeg, 181
nuts, 100,127

-O-

oak, 2,152,192
    bark, 35,39
obesity, 36
Ohsawa, George, 236
obstructions, removes, 10,37,114
oils, 127,134,135,173,180,199,201
    castor, 152
    comparison of oils, 186
    preparing, 181-182
    remedies, 134-135
    sesame, 152
    shopping for, 199
old age, 61,67
oliguria, 114
olive, 111
    oil, 64,135,137,144,182,186
onion, 111,138,142,152
    plaster, 138
    poultices, 122
    syrup, 140
opium poppy, 38
orange, peel, 9,64,141
    oil, 182
oregano, 152,181
Oregon grape, 35,36,37,38,49,73,
    80,152,196
organic, 103,105
organs, enlarged, 184
    prolapsed,151,152, 228
osha, 163
outward, 42
over, concentrating, 128
    eating, 36
    weight, 103,123,202
    work, 61
oyster, 111
oxalic acid, 38
ox bones, 130,200

The Herbs of Life Workbook

Lesley Tierra with **East West Herb Course** offers a companion workbook to *The Herbs of Life*. Includes worksheets, questions, projects, specific applications, activities, study guides, recommended reading, supplementary materials and more to help you fully learn and absorb the important elements of herbalism. For information write:

> East West Herb Course
> P.O. Box 712
> Santa Cruz, CA 95061

———————————————————

The Crossing Press
publishes a full selection of
New Age and Health titles.
To receive our current catalog,
please call —Toll Free—800/777-1048.